Maternal Hemodynamics

Maternal Hemodynamics

Edited by

Christoph Lees
Imperial College, London

Wilfried Gyselaers
Hasselt University, Diepenbeek, Belgium

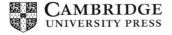

CAMBRIDGE
UNIVERSITY PRESS

University Printing House, Cambridge CB2 8BS, United Kingdom

One Liberty Plaza, 20th Floor, New York, NY 10006, USA

477 Williamstown Road, Port Melbourne, VIC 3207, Australia

4843/24, 2nd Floor, Ansari Road, Daryaganj, Delhi – 110002, India

79 Anson Road, #06–04/06, Singapore 079906

Cambridge University Press is part of the University of Cambridge.

It furthers the University's mission by disseminating knowledge in the pursuit of education, learning, and research at the highest international levels of excellence.

www.cambridge.org
Information on this title: www.cambridge.org/9781107157378
DOI: 10.1017/9781316661925

© Cambridge University Press 2018

First published 2018

Printed in the United Kingdom by TJ International Ltd. Padstow Cornwall

A catalogue record for this publication is available from the British Library.

Library of Congress Cataloging-in-Publication Data
Names: Lees, Christoph, editor. | Gyselaers, Wilfried, 1963– editor.
Title: Maternal hemodynamics / edited by Christoph Lees, Wilfried Gyselaers.
Description: Cambridge, United Kingdom ; New York, NY : Cambridge University Press, 2018. |
Includes bibliographical references.
Identifiers: LCCN 2017045274 | ISBN 9781107157378 (hardback)
Subjects: | MESH: Pregnancy Complications, Cardiovascular | Hemodynamics | Hypertension,
Pregnancy-Induced | Pre-Eclampsia | Plasma Volume | Fetal Growth Retardation – etiology
Classification: LCC RG580.H9 | NLM WQ 244 | DDC 618.3/6132–dc23
LC record available at https://lccn.loc.gov/2017045274

ISBN 978-1-107-15737-8 Hardback

....

Contents

Color plates are to be found between pp. 152 and 153

Contributors

Andreas Brückmann
Dept. of Obstetrics, University Hospital
Jena, Friedrich-Schiller University,
Germany

John R. Cockcroft
Dept. of Cardiology, University of Wales
College of Medicine, Cardiff, United
Kingdom

Jérôme Cornette
Dept. of Obstetrics, Erasmus Medical
Centre Rotterdam, the Netherlands

Anna David
Institute for Women's Health, University
College London, United Kingdom

Daniela Di Martino
Dept. of Obstetrics, Gynecology and
Neonatology, ICP – Buzzi Childrens'
Hospital, University of Milan, Italy

Johannes J. Duvekot
Dept. of Obstetrics, Erasmus Medical
Centre Rotterdam, the Netherlands

Thomas R. Everett
Dept. of Fetal Medicine, Leeds General
Infirmary, Leeds Teaching Hospitals NHS
Trust, United Kingdom

Daniele Farsetti
Department of Obstetrics and
Gynaecology, Policlinico Casilino, Tor
Vergata University, Rome, Italy

Enrico Ferrazzi
Dept. of Obstetrics, Gynecology and
Neonatolgy, ICP – Buzzi Childrens'
Hospital, University of Milan, Italy

Lin Fung Foo
Dept. of Cancer and Surgery, Imperial
College London, United Kingdom

Yuval Ginsberg
Institute for Women's Health, University
College London, United Kingdom

Wilfried Gyselaers
Dept. of Physiology, Hasselt University,
Diepenbeek, Belgium

Taminrit Johal
Dept. of Fetal Medicine, Rosie Hospital,
Addenbrooke's Hospital, Cambridge
University Hospitals, United Kingdom

Asma Khalil
Department of Fetal Medicine,
St George's University of London,
United Kingdom

Christoph Lees
Department of Surgery and Cancer,
Imperial College London,
United Kingdom

Carmel McEniery
Clinical Pharmacology Unit, University of
Cambridge, United Kingdom

Damiano Lo Presti
Department of Obstetrics and
Gynaecology, Policlinico Casilino, Tor
Vergata University, Rome, Italy

Victoria L. Meah
Centre for Exercise and Health, Cardiff
School of Sport and Health Sciences,
Cardiff Metropolitan University, Cardiff,
United Kingdom

Shireen Meher
Department of Obstetrics and
Gynaecology, Birmingham Women's and
Children's NHS Foundation Trust,
Birmingham, United Kingdom

Maria Muggiasca
Dept. of Obstetrics, Gynecology and
Neonatology, ICP – Buzzi Childrens'
Hospital, University of Milan, Italy

Gian Paolo Novelli
Department of Cardiology, San Sebastiano
Martire Hospital, Frascati, Rome, Italy

Louis L. Peeters
Dept. of Obstetrics, University Medical
Centre Utrecht, the Netherlands

Helen Perry
Department of Fetal Medicine, St George's
University of London, United Kingdom

Sylvia Salvi
Department of Fetal Medicine, St George's
University of London, United Kingdom

Marc Spaanderman
Dept. of Obstetrics, University Medical
Centre Maastricht, the Netherlands

Anneleen Staelens
Limburg Clinical Research Program,
Hasselt University, Diepenbeek, Belgium

Tamara Stampalija
Dept. of Obstetrics, Gynecology and
Neonatology, ICP – Buzzi Childrens'
Hospital, University of Milan, Italy

Eric J. Stöhr
Columbia University Irving Medical
Centre, Department of Medicine, Division
of Cardiology, Columbia University, New
York, USA

Jasmine Tay
Imperial College Healthcare
NHS Trust, Queen Charlotte's & Chelsea
Hospital, London, United Kingdom

Baskaran Thilaganathan
St George's University of London,
St George's University Hospitals NHS
Foundation Trust, London, United
Kingdom

Kathleen Tomsin
Limburg Clinical Research
Program, Hasselt University, Diepenbeek,
Belgium

Herbert Valensise
Department of Obstetrics and
Gynaecology, Policlinico Casilino, Tor
Vergata University, Rome, Italy

Barbara Vasapollo
Department of Obstetrics and
Gynaecology, Policlinico Casilino, Tor
Vergata University, Rome, Italy

Kristel Van Calsteren
Dept. of Obstetrics and Gynecology,
Catholic University Leuven, Belgium

Sharona Vonck
Limburg Clinical Research Program,
Hasselt University, Diepenbeek, Belgium

Ian Wilkinson
Div. Experimental Medicine
and Immunotherapeutics, University of
Cambridge, United Kingdom

Chapter

1

Maternal Hemodynamics in Health and Disease: A Paradigm Shift in the Causation of Placental Syndromes

Baskaran Thilaganathan

Summary

The belief that abnormal placentation causes preeclampsia (PE) and fetal growth restriction (FGR) has been championed for several decades – to the extent that they are collectively referred to as 'placental syndromes'. Although this may be true for the minority of early-onset disorders, consistent and emerging evidence suggests otherwise for the development of late-onset PE and FGR, which constitute the majority of cases. The inconsistencies with the placental origins hypothesis have been attributed to disease heterogeneity or explained as the maternal form of the disorders. These are neither adequate nor actual explanations of the causality of PE and FGR. It is increasingly clear that a stronger argument can be made for the role of the maternal cardiovascular system in the development of PE and FGR. While intrinsic placental dysfunction and the subsequent maladaptation of the maternal cardiovascular system is thought to lead to early-onset PE and FGR, late-onset disorders are more likely to be associated with acquired placental dysfunction as a result of the maternal cardiovascular system being unable to meet the excessive hemodynamic and metabolic demands of advancing pregnancy. Forming a better understanding of the precise etiology of so-called placental syndromes is critical for the development of accurate diagnostic aids, improved screening, better triage by disease severity and offering targeted preventative and therapeutic measures. This chapter, and other chapters in this volume, review the evidence that supports maternal cardiovascular involvement in the etiology of placental syndromes.

Conventional Beliefs Regarding the Causation of Placental Syndromes

Human placentation is uniquely associated with physiological remodeling of the spiral arteries, where deep placentation involves almost complete transformation of maternal spiral arteries to produce a low-resistance uterine circulation. Defective deep placentation has been associated with the persistence of a high-resistance uterine circulation, subsequent impaired placental perfusion and the development of PE and FGR [1]. Impaired trophoblast development and hypoperfusion is thought to result in the subsequent development of FGR, whereas a placental biochemical 'stress' response mainly composed of antiangiogenic factors is thought to lead to the endothelial cell dysfunction characteristic of PE (Figure 1.1). PE and FGR complicate some 10–15% of all pregnancies and are collectively termed placental syndromes. As the placenta is essential for these diseases to occur, defective placentation is believed to be central in the pathogenesis of PE and FGR. Furthermore, the cure for PE is delivery of the placenta, supporting the crucial etiological

1

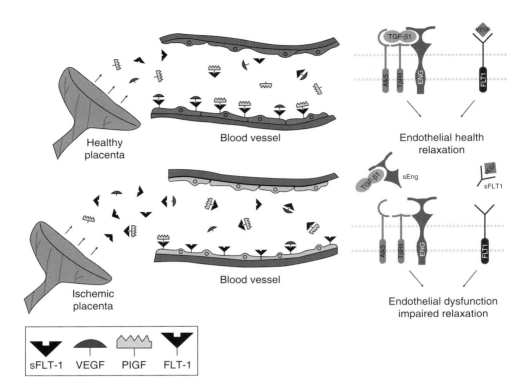

Figure 1.1 Healthy nonischemic placenta secretes normal (balanced) soluble fms-like tyrosine kinase (sFLT) leading to normal levels available for binding to fms-like tyrosine kinase 1 (FLT1) on endothelial cells systemically, leaving healthy and responsive endothelium. Ischemic placenta secretes increased sFLT, which binds circulating factors depleting their availability to FLT1 binding. The result is a dysfunctional endothelial cell leading to maternal systemic vasculopathy. (A black and white version of this figure will appear in some formats. For the color version, please refer to the plate section.)

role of the placenta in this disorder. The name 'placental syndrome' itself demonstrates the commonly accepted belief that the association between inadequate trophoblast invasion and the subsequent development of PE or FGR is causal in nature.

Placental Histology

A number of characteristic histological lesions of the placenta have been associated with the development of both PE and FGR – especially in early or preterm gestations [2]. A recent systematic review of large, well-conducted studies using objective diagnostic criteria demonstrated that preeclampsia was associated with a higher prevalence of both villous and vascular histological lesions of the placenta [3] (Figure 1.2). Importantly, the odds ratios for villous and vascular placental lesions in preeclampsia were consistently threefold lower in studies where the pathologist was blinded to the pregnancy diagnosis, demonstrating significant systematic operator bias in unblinded assessments. Furthermore, even though histological placental lesions are more prevalent in pathological pregnancies, the overall incidence is higher in normal pregnancies because the latter outnumber pathological pregnancies several-fold. This phenomenon is analogous to fetal aneuploidy, where the risk for trisomy may be higher in

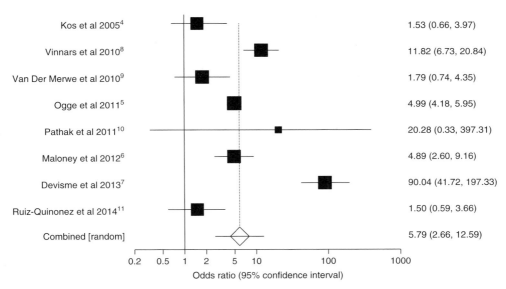

Figure 1.2 Forest plot, random-effects model of the odds ratio of villous lesions in the pregnancies complicated by preeclampsia and normotensive controls. The squares represent the studies included in the meta-analysis, arranged in time of publication order. In particular, the square boxes represent the effect estimates for each single study, and the horizontal line crossing the box shows the confidence interval, which is inversely proportionate to the reliability of the study. The diamante figure represents the summary effect and its width represents the degree of the heterogeneity. The vertical line intercepting 1 represents the line of no effect.

women ≥37yrs-old (point prevalence), but the majority of trisomic pregnancies occur in women <37yrs of age (population prevalence). Finally, the vast majority of FGR and PE pregnancies occur at term where these lesions occur far less frequently and are restricted to histology consistent with maternal under-perfusion of the placenta, such as perivillous fibrin deposition [4]. It therefore appears that the previously assumed characteristic placental lesions of PE and FGR are neither specific nor sensitive for the disorders – thereby questioning the validity of the histological basis for their placental etiology.

Birth Weight

An expected and anticipated consequence of poor placental development is impaired fetal growth, and, consistent with this, about 60% of early-onset PE cases before 34 weeks' gestation exhibit FGR. However, over 80% of PE cases occur at term and, using a large Scandinavian registry cohort, Rasmussen et al. demonstrated that there is a link between large for gestational age (LGA) birth and term preeclampsia, which is predominantly explained by maternal obesity [5]. The association of obesity and LGA birth with term preeclampsia is at odds with the universally accepted dictum that preeclampsia is a consequence of poor trophoblast development. The biochemical cascade responsible for preeclampsia is thought to occur as a consequence of a placental stress response – thought to be of placental origin in preterm preeclampsia. In the LGA form of term preeclampsia, maternal cardiac dysfunction and the inability to meet the metabolic demands of an enlarged fetoplacental unit may also result in placental stress. This hypothesis is supported by data showing that maternal cardiac dysfunction precedes preeclampsia, significant maternal cardiac maladaptation in term pregnancy and worsening hemodynamic function in obese women compared to those of normal weight [6–8].

Uterine Artery Doppler

The physiological remodeling of the spiral arteries by the invading trophoblast is thought to result in a low-resistance uterine circulation. Defective placentation is associated with the development of PE and FGR as well as a persistence of the high-resistance uterine circulation. Increased uterine artery Doppler resistance indices have long been presumed to be the consequence of incomplete trophoblast invasion of maternal spiral arteries resulting in a high-resistance placental circulation and under-perfusion of the fetoplacental unit [1]. The largest individual patient data meta-analysis of first trimester uterine artery Doppler assessment demonstrates a sensitivity of 48% and a specificity of 92% for the detection of early-onset PE [9] (Figure 1.3). The finding that maternal ophthalmic artery Doppler and other peripheral waveform measures are equally effective as uterine artery assessment in screening for FGR and/or PE suggests that maternal uterine artery Doppler assessments may be reflecting maternal cardiovascular performance rather than be specific to trophoblast development [10].

Uterine artery Doppler screening exhibits two characteristics – sensitivity for adverse outcome increases the later in pregnancy the test is performed, and the sensitivity for late-onset PE is poorer than for early-onset PE [9,11]. These features have conventionally been interpreted as lending support to the argument that early-onset PE is related to a dysfunctional placenta, while late-onset PE may have to be explained by a different etiology. An alternative explanation arises when one compares the similarities in test characteristics between uterine Doppler assessment and glucose tolerance tests in gestational diabetes – which is sensitive for early-onset gestational diabetes and shows improved performance the later in pregnancy it is performed [12]. Just as for pancreatic

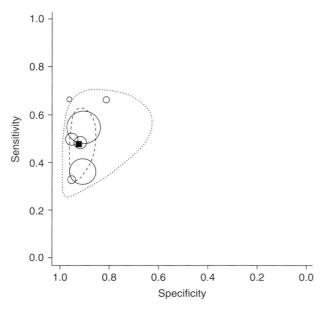

Figure 1.3 Summary estimates of accuracy of first-trimester uterine artery Doppler in the prediction of early-onset pre-eclampsia (a) and early fetal growth restriction (b) obtained with a bivariate model. Pooled sensitivity and specificity values were 0.48 (95% CI: 0.39–0.57) and 0.92 (95% CI: 0.89–0.95), respectively, for (a) and 0.39 (95% CI: 0.26–0.54) and 0.93 (95% CI: 0.91–0.95), respectively, for (b). Study estimate; summary point; 95% confidence region; 95% prediction region. Image reproduced by kind permission of Wiley.

function in gestational diabetes, early-onset PE may expose a pre-existing cardiovascular dysfunction, whereas late-onset PE may occur as a consequence of the maternal cardiovascular system's inability to deal with the excessive load of a term pregnancy. Corroborative evidence for this hypothesis is provided by MRI studies showing that early PE is associated with lower placental perfusion fractions compared to gestation-matched controls and late PE with larger placental perfusion fractions [13].

Placental Biomarkers

First trimester maternal serum levels of placental growth factor (PlGF) are reduced in pregnancies destined to develop preterm FGR and PE. In the studies with the best-reported screening performance, the sensitivity for early-onset PE using PlGF was around 60%, falling to approximately 15% for term PE for a fixed 5% false positive rate [14]. As with uterine artery Doppler assessment, these PlGF test performance characteristics were taken to support the placental origins hypothesis of early-onset PE, but allude to an alternative cause for late-onset PE. While PlGF is widely considered to be a pregnancy-specific hormone as it is produced by the trophoblast, it is also widely expressed in many extra-uterine tissues. PlGF has a significant role in cardiac adaptation to increased circulatory volume and resistance loads – where insufficient PlGF leads to impaired ventricular remodeling and cardiac maladaptation [15]. This is of particular relevance in PE, where low PlGF and high soluble fms-like tyrosine kinase-1 (sFlt-1) are characteristic of the PE phenotype. While low PlGF and high sFlt-1 have been considered to have an antiangiogenic adverse influence on the placenta, this combination of vascular factors also predisposes to increased systemic vascular resistance, abnormal ventricular remodeling and cardiac maladaptation – all hallmarks of PE. Just as for uterine artery Doppler and gestational diabetes, the pattern of PlGF screening performance for early and late PE may alternatively represent the difference between women with pre-existing cardiovascular dysfunction and those with acquired deficits due to the cardiovascular load of advanced pregnancy.

Environmental and Genetic Risk Factors for Preeclampsia

PE and FGR have predisposing similar clinical risk factors such as increased maternal age, ethnic origin, increased body mass index, diabetes and other maternal co-morbidities. PE is also believed to result from a complex interplay between genetic components and environmental factors. Familial clustering has been observed and reported in PE, which is relatively more common among daughters and sisters of preeclamptic women, suggesting that the condition may be partly attributable to genetic susceptibility [16]. Furthermore, the prevalence of PE also differs between various ethnic groups [17]. Numerous susceptibility genes for PE have been reported in the literature; however, reports have been inconsistent and the function of the majority of the identified genetic loci remains unknown. The most recent meta-analysis of genetic variants reproducibly associated seven genetic variants with PE [18]. Several of the variants that were associated with PE were also identified risk factors for developing cardiovascular disease. For example, carriers of select lipoprotein lipase (*LPL*) alleles as well as *SERPINE1* rs1799889, rs268, *FV* rs6025 and *F2* rs1799963 variants are all associated with adverse lipid profiles and coronary disease. It is therefore evident that the PE shares both genetic and environmental risk factors with cardiovascular disease, which may contribute both to the etiology of the disorder. The overlap in these predisposing environmental and genetic risk factors has been taken to imply that they have a deleterious impact on trophoblast development. However, it is important to acknowledge that these risk factors have long been associated with the development of cardiovascular disease in the nonpregnant population.

Maternal Cardiovascular Involvement in Preeclampsia

We have continued to observe that the placenta is a prerequisite and therefore crucial to the development of PE. There are inconsistencies in the placental origins hypothesis and the role of the maternal cardiovascular system deserves to be further evaluated to delineate whether cardiovascular derangement in PE is a secondary effect or the primary etiological factor. The concept that placental dysfunction is secondary to a maternal syndrome is not new when one considers the similarities between preeclampsia and gestational diabetes (Table 1.1). If we consider PE to be an analogous condition to gestational diabetes, where both conditions only develop in pregnancy and are cured by birth and passage of the placenta. In spite of these fundamental parallels between PE and gestational diabetes, the latter is not considered to be a placental disorder. In fact, it is well accepted that the glucose load and endocrine 'stress' of pregnancy results in the development of gestational diabetes when maternal pancreatic function is suboptimal. If similarities exist between so-called placental syndromes and gestational diabetes, then pregnancy will need to present a significant strain on the maternal cardiovascular system – as for pregnancy glucose levels and pancreatic function [19].

Maternal Cardiovascular Adaptation in Pregnancy

Maternal adaptation to pregnancy is expected to create optimal conditions for the growth and development of the unborn child without jeopardizing maternal health. Several studies have demonstrated progressive changes in cardiac geometry and ventricular function with advancing gestation. Pregnancy is associated with an increase in the intravascular compartment by about 1500ml, as well as an increase in the maternal heart rate. The combined effect of these two synergistic changes is to increase cardiac output – often misinterpreted as a maternal hyperdynamic state, but only because pregnancy metabolic demands are often significantly underestimated. In concert with the increase in cardiac output is a fall in systemic vascular resistance and redistribution of blood flow at a regional level [7]. By term, these profound changes in maternal hemodynamics result in an excessive increase in left ventricular mass by about 40%, adverse ventricular remodeling and even overt diastolic dysfunction in a small but significant proportion of apparently healthy women (Figure 1.4). To provide perspective, these cardiac changes are an order of magnitude greater than observed in elite athletes after several years of training and equate to changes seen in some pathological conditions in nonpregnant individuals.

Cardiovascular Maladaptation in Preeclampsia

At the time of PE diagnosis, there is evidence of abnormal ventricular geometry, impaired myocardial relaxation and diastolic dysfunction, and these findings are mirrored – to a slightly lesser extent – in FGR [20, 21]. Mild-moderate left ventricular diastolic

Table 1.1 Hypertension in pregnancy and gestational diabetes: disease similarities and apparent differences

	Gestational diabetes (GDM)	Pregnancy hypertension
Epidemiology		
Predisposing factors	Same as for type 2 diabetes	Same as for cardiac disease
Onset of disorder	Mid to late pregnancy	Mid to late pregnancy
Effect of parity	More common in primips	More common in primips
Recurrence risk	Increased risk if previously affected pregnancy	Increased risk if previously affected pregnancy
Fetal and placental effects		
Placental histology	Some histological lesions seen more often in GDM	Some histological lesions seen more often in pregnancy hypertension
Specificity of histology	None of the placental histological lesions are specific for the disorder	None of the placental histological lesions are specific for the disorder
Temporal nature of lesions	Seen more frequently in early-onset and/or severe disorder	Seen more frequently in early-onset and/or severe disorder
Placental function	Increased maternal-to-fetal transplacental glucose transfer	Impaired maternal perfusion of the uteroplacental bed
Fetus	Increased fetal glucose levels lead to macrosomia	Impaired placental function leads to impaired fetal growth
Screening/diagnostic tests		
Mechanism of screening	GTT gauges pancreatic reserve	Uterine Doppler, PlGF and BP are all measures of cardiac function
Performance of screening	Better for early-onset GDM	Better for early-onset PE
Timing of screening test	Improved sensitivity the later in pregnancy it is performed	Improved sensitivity the later in pregnancy it is performed
Diagnostic test	Supra-normal glucose levels in both pregnant and non-pregnant	High BP in both pregnant and nonpregnant population
Management		
Cure for disorder	Birth	Birth
Treatment/amelioration	Insulin – treats the biological deficit	Antihypertensive medications – treats a sign of the disorder
Long-term maternal health	50% develop type 2 diabetes by 10 years postpartum	20% develop chronic hypertension by 10 years postpartum

Table 1.1 (cont.)

	Gestational diabetes (GDM)	Pregnancy hypertension
Biology		
Maternal adaptation	Insulin requirements increase two- to three-fold in pregnancy	Cardiac output increases by about 50% in pregnancy
Early-onset phenotypes	Present with normal or lower insulin levels compared to non-pregnancy	Present with normal or higher cardiac outputs compared to non-pregnancy
Late-onset phenotypes	Present with supra-normal (high) insulin levels compared to non-pregnancy	Present with supra-normal (high) cardiac output compared to non-pregnancy
Aetiology	Inability of maternal pancreas to deal with the glucose load of pregnancy	Impaired trophoblast invasion or maternal cardiac maladaptation?

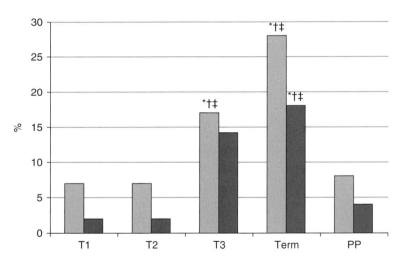

Figure 1.4 Summary of significant left-sided cardiac findings in pregnancy presented in a dichotomized analysis with indices rated as normal or dysfunctional. Myocardial diastolic dysfunction (white columns) was diagnosed with average early to late strain rate ratio of<1 and chamber diastolic dysfunction (black columns) according to the American Society of Echocardiography diagnostic algorithms. 1st indicates first trimester; 2nd, second trimester; 3rd, third trimester; NP, nonpregnant control; PP, 1-year postpartum; and Term, term of pregnancy. *$P<0.05$ v nonpregnant control; †$P<0.05$ v T1; ‡P0.05 v T2.

dysfunction is seen in approximately half of women with early-onset PE, with 20% of women having biventricular systolic dysfunction. This impairment in cardiac function is likely to be related to increase in cardiac afterload (high systemic vascular resistance) and abnormal left ventricular remodeling/hypertrophy. The abnormal pattern of remodeling observed in PE is similar to that observed in nonpregnant individuals with essential hypertension and is consistent with an impairment that is afterload-induced. The extent and severity of these findings explain the significant cardiovascular morbidity associated with PE and raise the possibility that these changes may be used for the early identification of abnormal maternal cardiovascular and volume adaptation leading to the development of PE. However, cardiovascular adaptations in pregnancy require both volume and resistance load to be raised significantly and for a prolonged period. Similarly to glucose tolerance testing, a conventional echo assessment prior to or in early pregnancy is unlikely to detect limited reserve capacity of the maternal cardiovascular system.

Postpartum Cardiovascular Legacy

The numerous parallels between placental syndromes and gestational diabetes also extend into the postpartum period. Women whose pregnancies were complicated by gestational diabetes have a 50% risk of developing diabetes in the subsequent decade. Similarly, women whose pregnancies were complicated with PE or FGR are predisposed to increased postpartum cardiovascular morbidity and mortality, including chronic hypertension, myocardial infarction, heart failure, stroke and death [22]. Detailed longitudinal follow-up with echocardiography in apparently healthy women after pregnancies complicated by placental syndromes has demonstrated persistent remodeling and left ventricular dys-function up to two years or more postpartum [23]. A more recent epidemiological study of hypertension rates demonstrated that the peak incidence of hypertension was in the first decade after birth and that the effect of pregnancy is to increase a woman's age-related hypertension risk as if she were two decades older [24] (Figure 1.5). Other population studies have suggested that the association of PE with adverse cardiovascular outcome postpartum may be due largely to shared prepregnancy risk factors rather than reflecting a direct influence of PE. Irrespective of whether the cardiovascular morbidity preceded the pregnancy or occurred as a consequence of the cardiovascular maladaptation in preg-nancy, these findings undermine the placental origins hypothesis for PE and stress the importance of continuing to monitor the cardiovascular health of these women.

Late-onset Uteroplacental Dysfunction and FGR

As with PE, late-onset FGR is considered to have a different etiological basis from the early-onset versions of the disorders. FGR near term is considered to have a different phenotype that suffers from absence of distinct placental pathology and lack of an effective screening test, as well as similar risk factors, cardiovascular disease changes and postnatal cardiovascular morbidity as PE [2,3,11,25]. These findings raise the possibility that late-onset FGR may not be a primary placental problem, but results from acquired uteropla-cental dysfunction as a consequence of maternal cardiovascular maladaptation near term. In support of this hypothesis, a recent population-based epidemiological study demon-strated a 2% increase in risk of term small-for-gestational-age (SGA) for every 1 mm Hg increase in maternal blood pressure within the normotensive range [26]. Although the authors suggested that maternal prehypertension may be a response to impaired placental function, consideration should be given to the possibility that the placenta is a perfusion-dependent organ and that impaired cardiovascular function may cause placental dysfunc-tion, rather than the other way round. Previous work has demonstrated maternal ven-tricular remodeling and diastolic function as well as significantly poorer placental perfusion in normotensive FGR pregnancies [21]. This evidence suggests that term FGR

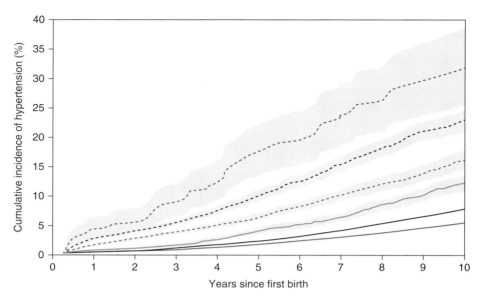

Figure 1.5 Ten-year cumulative incidences of hypertension by years since first pregnancy in women with and without a hypertensive disorder of pregnancy, by age at first delivery, Denmark, 1995-2012. Follow-up began in 1995 or 3 months postpartum, whichever came later; for women with a second pregnancy, follow-up ended at 20 weeks' gestation in the second pregnancy. Unbroken lines: women with no hypertensive disorder of pregnancy in their first pregnancy. Broken lines: women with a hypertensive disorder of pregnancy in their first pregnancy. Gray bands: 95% confidence intervals. Age at delivery: 20-29 years, blue; 30-39 years, green; 40-49 years, red. (A black and white version of this figure will appear in some formats. For the color version, please refer to the plate section.)

may well occur as a consequence of secondary placental dysfunction caused by impaired maternal cardiovascular function. This implies that both impaired maternal perfusion of the placenta (an extrinsic defect) and impaired placental development (an intrinsic defect) may lead to FGR.

Conclusions

A critical evaluation of maternal cardiovascular physiology reveals that there are profound changes in cardiac and hemodynamic performance in human pregnancy. The magnitude of these changes and maternal cardiovascular adaptation to pregnancy has previously been significantly underestimated. The consequences of these physiological findings only become apparent when considering the biological consequences of maternal cardiac maladaptation to increasing demands of advancing pregnancy. Placental dysfunction is fundamental to the pathophysiology of pregnancy complications such as PE and FGR, but, to date, the placenta has been considered in isolation without regard to the fact that its functioning is dependent on adequate maternal perfusion [27]. There is now incontrovertible evidence that failure of the maternal cardiovascular system to adapt to pregnancy is the primary mechanism leading to secondary placental dysfunction and so-called placental syndromes.

Key Points

- The placental origins theory seems aligned to the minority of cases of preeclampsia and/or FGR with early onset in pregnancy
- Placental dysfunction in late pregnancy may lead to the rapid development of preeclampsia and/or FGR without clear evidence of impaired or defective placentation
- The placental origins theory does not recognize that as an organ of perfusion, placental function may be dependent on maternal cardiovascular function (and related placental perfusion)
- Late-onset preeclampsia and/or FGR have epidemiological, biochemical, biophysical and clinical features which are in keeping maternal cardiovascular dysfunction leading to impaired placental function

References

1. Roberts JM, Redman CW. Pre-eclampsia: more than pregnancy-induced hypertension. *Lancet.* 1993;**341**:1447–51.

2. Ogge G, Chaiworapongsa T, Romero R, et al. Placental lesions associated with maternal underperfusion are more frequent in early-onset than in late-onset preeclampsia. *J Perinat Med.* 2011;**39**:641–52.

3. Falco ML, Sivanathan J, Laoreti A, Thilaganathan B, Khalil A. Placental histopathology associated with preeclampsia: a systematic review and meta-analysis. *Ultrasound Obstet Gynecol.* 2017;**50**(3):295–301.

4. Pathak S, Lees C, Hackett G, Jessop F, Sebire N. Frequency and clinical significance of placental histological lesions in an unselected population at or near term. *Virchows Arch.* 2011;**459**:565–72.

5. Rasmussen S, Irgens LM, Espinoza J. Maternal obesity and excess of fetal growth in pre-eclampsia. *BJOG.* 2014;**121**:1351–7.

6. Melchiorre K, Sharma S, Thilaganathan B. Cardiovascular Implications in preeclampsia: an overview. *Circulation.* 2014;**130**:701–14.

7. Melchiorre K, Sharma R, Khalil A, Thilaganathan B. Maternal cardiovascular function in normal pregnancy: evidence of maladaptation to chronic volume overload. *Hypertension.* 2016;**67**:754–62.

8. Kenchaiah S, Evans JC, Levy D, et al. Obesity and the risk of heart failure. *N Engl J Med.* 2002;**347**:305–13.

9. Velauthar L, Plana MN, Kalidindi M, et al. First-trimester uterine artery Doppler and adverse pregnancy outcome: a meta-analysis involving 55 974 women. *Ultrasound Obstet Gynecol.* 2014;**43**:500–7.

10. Kalafat E, Laoreti A, Khalil A, Da Silva Costa F, Thilaganathan B. Ophthalmic Artery Doppler Prediction of Preeclampsia: A Systematic Review and Meta-Analysis. *Ultrasound Obstet Gynecol.* 2018 Jan 12. doi:10.1002/uog.19002.

11. Allen RE, Morlando M, Thilaganathan B, et al. Predictive accuracy of second-trimester uterine artery Doppler indices for stillbirth: a systematic review and meta-analysis. *Ultrasound Obstet Gynecol.* 2016;**47**:22–7.

12. Andrietti S, Carlucci S, Wright A, Wright D, Nicolaides KH. Repeat measurements of uterine artery pulsatility index, mean arterial pressure and serum placental growth factor at 12, 22 and 32 weeks in prediction of pre-eclampsia. *Ultrasound Obstet Gynecol.* 2017;**50**:221–227.

13. Sohlberg S, Mulic-Lutvica A, Lindgren P, Ortiz-Nieto F, Wikstrom AK, Wikstrom J. Placental perfusion in normal pregnancy and early and late preeclampsia: a magnetic resonance imaging study. *Placenta.* 2014;**35**:202–6.

14. Poon LCY, Syngelaki A, Akolekar, Lai J, Nicolaides KH. Combined screening for preeclampsia and small for gestational age at 11–13 weeks. *Fetal Diagn Ther.* 2013;**33**:16–27.

15. Hochholzer W, Reichlin T, Stelzig C, et al. Impact of soluble fms-like tyrosine kinase-1 and placental growth factor serum levels for risk stratification and early diagnosis in patients with suspected acute myocardial infarction. *Eur Heart J.* 2011;**32**:326–35.

16. Nilsson E, Salonen Ros H, Cnattingius S, Lichtenstein P. The importance of genetic and environmental effects for pre-eclampsia and gestational hypertension: a family study. *BJOG.* 2004;**111**:200–6.

17. Steegers EA, von Dadelszen P, Duvekot JJ, Pijnenborg R. Pre-eclampsia. *Lancet.* 2010 21;**376**:631–44.

18. Buurma AJ, Turner RJ, Driessen JH, Mooyaart AL, Schoones JW, Bruijn JA, Bloemenkamp KW, Dekkers OM, Baelde HJ. Genetic variants in pre-eclampsia: a meta-analysis. *Hum Reprod Update.* 2013;**19**:289–303.

19. Thilaganathan B. Maternal death: a century of getting it wrong. TEDx talk on the origins of preeclampsia: www.youtube.com/watch?v=ELET24AHnEg

20. Melchiorre K, Sutherland GR, Baltabaeva A, Liberati M, Thilaganathan B. Maternal cardiac dysfunction and remodeling in women with preeclampsia at term. *Hypertension.* 2011;**57**:85–93.

21. Melchiorre K, Sutherland GS, Liberati M, Thilaganathan B. Maternal cardiovascular impairment in pregnancies complicated by severe fetal growth restriction. *Hypertension.* 2012;**60**:437–443.

22. Fraser A, Nelson SM, Macdonald-Wallis C, et al. Associations of pregnancy complications with calculated CVD risk and cardiovascular risk factors in middle age: the Avon Longitudinal Study of Parents and Children. *Circulation.* 2012;**125**:1367–1380.

23. Melchiorre K, Sutherland GR, Liberati M, Thilaganathan B. Preeclampsia is associated with persistent postpartum cardiovascular impairment. *Hypertension.* 2011;**58**:709–715.

24. Behrens I, Basit S, Melbye M, et al. Risk of post-pregnancy hypertension in women with a history of hypertensive disorders of pregnancy – a nationwide cohort study. *BMJ.* 2017. Jul 12;358:j3078. doi:10.1136/bmj.j3078.

25. Smith GC, Pell JP, Walsh D. Pregnancy complications and maternal risk of ischaemic heart disease: a retrospective cohort study of 129,290 births. *Lancet.* 2001;**357**:2002–6.

26. Wikstrom AK, Gunnarsdottir J, Nelander M, Simic M, Stephansson O, Cnattingius S. Prehypertension in pregnancy and risks of small for gestational age infant and stillbirth. *Hypertension.* 2016;**67**: 640–6.

27. Thilaganathan B. Placental syndromes: getting to the heart of the matter. *Ultrasound Obstet Gynecol.* 2017;**49**:7–9.

Cardiovascular and Volume Regulatory Functions in Pregnancy: An Overview

Louis Peeters

Summary

Pregnancy induces a high flow and low-resistance circulation accompanied by plasma volume expansion and renal hyperfiltration. These adaptive changes develop in response to an induced reset of various cardiovascular and volume regulatory receptors. Although neither the trigger for receptor resetting nor the purpose of the adaptive changes is clear, their importance for normal pregnancy is emphasized by their often defective development in pregnancies later on complicated by "placental syndromes." The common denominator of these syndromes is placental dysfunction presenting clinically as fetal growth restriction, gestational hypertension, preeclampsia, the HELLP syndrome and eclampsia in varying combinations. In this context it should be stressed that defective maternal cardiovascular adaptation to pregnancy may be the cause, but also an effect of these syndromes. This chapter provides an update of our current insights into how pregnancy resets cardiovascular and volume receptors and how these adjustments interact with one another. Finally, the current insights in the cardiovascular and volume adaptation to pregnancy will be used to speculate on how abnormal adaptation to pregnancy can be predicted prior to pregnancy to identify women at risk of having a pregnancy complicated by a placental syndrome.

Introduction

The maternal adaptation to pregnancy is expected to create optimal conditions for the growth and development of the unborn child without jeopardizing maternal health. Although most healthy women adapt normally to pregnancy, late-onset pregnancy complications are often preceded by initial abnormal adaptation. Pregnancy induces major structural and functional changes in the maternal cardiovascular and volume regulatory systems. This chapter focuses on these changes, how they are triggered, when they reach their maximum effect, how they interact with other changes and, last but not least, how women at risk for defective adaptation can be identified before pregnancy.

Mammalian pregnancy and parturition are natural processes that have been proven effective in the course of mammalian evolution. In natural conditions and without medical intervention, human pregnancy results in the birth of a healthy child in more than 80% of cases. Therefore, all maternal adaptive changes taking place in the course of pregnancy ought to be considered useful and necessary to achieve that one objective: healthy offspring without damaging maternal health. Nevertheless, it is a fact of life that the complex chain of events that begin at embryo implantation can be disturbed, eventually culminating in a pregnancy complication such as a placental syndrome or preterm birth. Obviously, our current insights into normal and defective adaptation to pregnancy are still incomplete.

Table 2.1 Hemodynamic and volume changes induced by pregnancy. The values presented have been derived from various reports specified elsewhere [2]. The pregnancy-induced changes in all variables are statistically significant except for the one in α-atrial natriuretic peptide (α-ANP).

	Nonpregnant	24–28 weeks amenorrhea
Cardiac output (L·min^{-1})	4.5	6.0
Heart rate (beats·min^{-1})	70	85
Stroke volume (mL)	65	72
Systolic blood pressure (mmHg)	110	105
Diastolic blood pressure (mmHg)	80	70
Total peripheral vascular resistance (dyne·cm^{-1}·sec^{-5})	1600	1000
Pulmonary vascular resistance (dyne·cm^{-1}·sec^{-5})	119	78
Colloid-osmotic pressure (mmHg)	21	18
Active plasma renin concentration (pg·mL^{-1})	16	41
α-ANP (pmol·L^{-1})	54	30
Osmolality (mOsm·L^{-1})	287	272
Plasma volume (mL)	2500	3800
Erythrocyte volume (mL)	1500	1800

Nevertheless, they do enable the differentiation between aberrant and normal maternal circulatory adaptation in the first trimester, thus paving the way for the development of early treatment and preventive strategies.

Pregnancy-specific Changes in Cardiovascular Function and Volume Homeostasis

1. *Global effects.* The first systemic effect of pregnancy on the cardiovascular system is generalized vascular relaxation, which induces the following set of compensations:
   1) baroreceptor activation to prevent a fall in blood pressure in response to the fall in cardiac afterload; 2) sodium and water retention to raise cardiac preload; 3) accelerated endothelial release of prostacyclin and nitric oxide to raise vascular compliance, so as to establish endothelial protection against the increased shear forces in the vascular bed; and 4) accelerated arteriovenous shunting to circumvent excessive influx of blood into the systemic capillary beds. These compensations enable the safe institution of a so-called "hyperdynamic circulation," defined as a raised cardiac output in the absence of a raised metabolic rate. This hyperdynamic circulation (individual changes detailed in Table 2.1) is maintained throughout pregnancy. Therefore, the associated extra cardiac work – defined as the triple product of heart rate, stroke volume and systolic blood pressure – induces cardiac remodeling to optimize cardiac efficiency for a prolonged period. The hyperdynamic circulation develops shortly after embryo implantation, most likely in concert with the sharp drop in plasma osmolality (Figure 2.1). Most of the changes reverse again within 6 months postpartum.

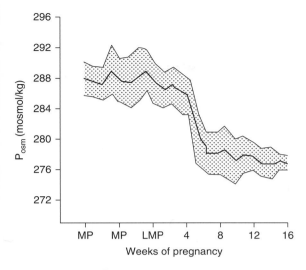

Figure 2.1 Mean osmolality (Posmol ± SD) measured at weekly intervals from before conception until 16 weeks pregnancy in nine healthy women with normal pregnancy outcomes. MP and LMP indicate menstrual and last menstrual periods, respectively. (Adapted and modified from [1]).

2. *Systemic vascular relaxation.* One of the most prominent pregnancy-induced circulatory changes is the fall in systemic vascular tone [3, 4]. The mechanism responsible for this effect is only partly elucidated because of its complexity requiring the presence of a pregnancy-specific steroid environment together with an orchestrated concomitant set-point resetting of various regulatory systems for vascular tone and intravascular volume [5, 6, 7]. An updated overview of the events involved in the primary systemic vasodilatation of pregnancy is presented in Table 2.2 and Figure 2.2.

3. *Effect of pregnancy on the arterial bed.* Indirect evidence suggests that the arterial baroreceptors located downstream in the arterial bed register "reduced transmural pressure" in response to the diminished effective arterial blood volume [4]. The acute response to the latter consists of vasoconstriction mediated by angiotensin-2, sympathetic mediators and vasopressin. Meanwhile, the slower response for the restoration of the effective arterial blood volume consists of combined vasopressin-mediated water retention and aldosterone-mediated sodium retention (Figure 2.3). In pregnancy the renal vasoconstriction in this mechanism is reversed to renal vasodilatation. The associated approximate 50% higher glomerular filtration rate maintains a relatively high distal tubular sodium and water delivery partly restricting their retention in favor of ≈ potassium conservation.

   The baroreceptors in the arterial bed and volume receptors in the atria and central veins reside in the vascular wall. This implies that their set-points are prone to change in conjunction with the overall pregnancy-induced rise in cardiovascular compliance. It is conceivable that the latter is responsible for the approximately 10 mmHg fall in diastolic blood pressure and approx. 5 mmHg fall in systolic blood pressure in early pregnancy, presumably developing in concert with the fall in plasma osmolality (Figure 2.1). To our knowledge, there are no reports in support of a concomitant change in the responsiveness of the carotid baroreceptors.

   Resting cardiac output and total blood volume increase gradually in the first trimester of pregnancy to a plateau of ≈ 40% above the prepregnant level in the second

Table 2.2 Contributors to the development of the primary systemic vascular relaxation in pregnancy involving concomitant changes at the endocrine, paracrine and reflex loop levels [3].

System involved	Target of changes	Altered 1) circulating levels, 2) postreceptor transduction, 3) renal hyperfiltration		Type of change
Endocrine system	Cardiovascular system	↑E2; ↑P; ↑relaxin	↓efficacy aldosterone and AVP, because of renal hyperfiltration	Systemic vasodilation; restricted K$^+$ loss
BP and volume regulatory systems	RAS system; vasopressine/ aNP kallikrein/ kinine	↑AT2 R; ↓ AT1 R ↑angiotensin- (1–7); ↓ACE; ↑bradykinin	↓aNP, due to raised set-point secondary to ↑ atrial compliance	Regional vasodilation
Paracrine regulation (local)	Endothelium; VSMC, sensorimotor nerves	↑CGRPs; ↑ADM; ↑Nitric oxide; ↑prostacyclin	↓ constrictive properties of endothelin	Local vasodilation

Abbreviations: E2: 17-ies of endothelin to ↑ atrial compliancenide.uctiRAS: renin–angiotensin-system; AT1 R: angiotensin-II-receptor-1 (signal transduction); AT2 R: angiotensin-II-receptor-2 (no signal transduction); ACE: angiotensin-converting enzyme; ANP: h an orchestrated concomiide; CGRP: calcitonin gene-related peptide.

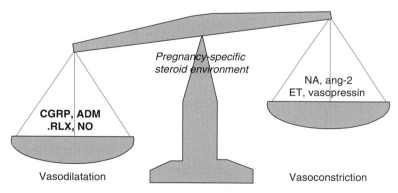

Figure 2.2 Simplified scheme summarizing the most important factors contributing to the development of systemic vasodilatation in early pregnancy as detailed previously [8]. NO: nitric oxide; ADM: adrenomedullin; RLX: relaxin; CGRP: calcitonin gene-related-peptide; ET: endothelin; NA: noradrenaline; ang-2: angiotensin-2.

trimester [9, 10]. Cardiac output is the product of heart rate and stroke volume. Until the 8th week of pregnancy cardiac output increases primarily by a rise in stroke volume. Additional rises in cardiac output afterwards are mostly achieved by a rise in heart rate. In the third trimester of pregnancy stroke volume decreases, most likely in conjunction with a rise in cardiovascular sympathetic tone. The latter is probably related to the increasing strain put upon the maternal metabolic and cardiovascular functions by the

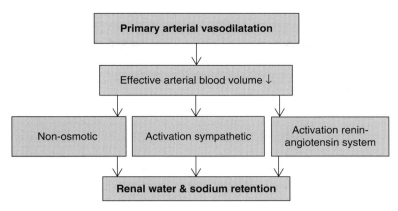

Figure 2.3 Response of the volume regulatory systems to the primary arterial underfill.

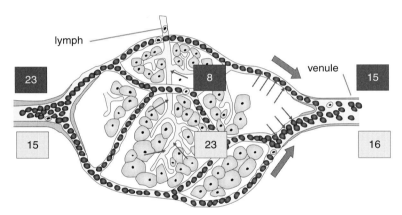

Figure 2.4 Driving forces for transcapillary fluid exchange based on the Starling principle. Hydrostatic and oncotic pressures (mmHg) at the precapillary sphincter, in the capillary bed and at the venular outflow site are listed in red and blue boxes, respectively. Pressure gradients enable serum to leave and re-enter the vascular bed during the passage of blood across the capillary bed. (A black and white version of this figure will appear in some formats. For the color version, please refer to the plate section.)

rapidly growing fetus and placenta. In this period heart rate increases to prevent the cardiac output from declining. Throughout pregnancy both heart rate and stroke volume increase by about 20% [9, 10].

4. *Effect of pregnancy on the systemic microcirculation.* The hemodilution together with the higher cardiovascular compliance can be expected to affect the transcapillary fluid balance in the systemic microcirculation (Figure 2.4). The hemodilution reduces the oncotic pressure of the circulating blood favoring fluid accumulation in the interstitial space. This effect explains the tendency of (orthostatic) edema formation. To our knowledge, it is still unclear whether the higher compliance in the arterial bed leads to a change in hydrostatic pressure at the level of the precapillary sphincters. In theory, a higher arterial compliance would enable the storage in the arterial wall of a larger fraction of the kinetic energy generated by the heart during systole to be released again

during diastole as extra volume flow. At the level of the precapillary sphincters this would translate into a larger volume flow at the expense of hydrostatic pressure. However, such an effect is highly unlikely as the microcirculation is tightly regulated by local mechanisms. Therefore, hydrostatic pressure is expected to remain unchanged during pregnancy with the generated excess flow being directed toward arteriovenous shunts.

5. *Effect of pregnancy on the venous bed.* About 70% of the total blood volume resides in the veins, which are 30 times more compliant than arteries, particularly in the splanchnic bed. Therefore, physiologic fluctuations in venous filling have a negligible effect on venous pressure. The venous system drains the blood from the peripheral tissues back to the heart, and – particularly the splanchnic bed – serves as a reservoir to maintain cardiac filling. The venous compartment consists of two imaginary components: the "unstressed" and "stressed volume". The unstressed volume represents two-thirds of the venous compartment and is defined as the volume that can be contained at zero transmural pressure. Meanwhile, the stressed volume refers to the one-third of the total venous blood volume that causes the transmural pressure to rise to the level of mean circulatory filling pressure, which is ≈ 7 mmHg [11]. The stressed volume determines cardiac preload and thus venous return [12]. A fall in cardiac output activates the baroreceptors in the carotid sinus triggering constriction of the most compliant part of the venous compartment: the splanchnic bed. This leads to an immediate shift of unstressed to stressed volume to preserve cardiac preload.

   Pregnancy induces venous relaxation and, with it, a condition of venous "underfill" activating the central volume receptors to accelerate volume retention by neuro-endocrine mechanisms. Indirect evidence supports the view that pregnancy also raises the set-point of the volume receptors for the release of atrial natriuretic hormone (α-ANP) by the atria [13]. Pregnancy also raises the responsiveness of the respiratory center to the CO_2 dissolved in the circulating blood, giving rise to a larger tidal volume. This effect creates a more negative intrathoracic pressure and, with it, a larger pressure gradient between central veins and the right atrium. The effect of the latter is a rise in cardiac preload and with it, venous return [14]. Figure 2.5 illustrates how the pregnancy-induced volume expansion accumulates in the venous compartment proportionally distributed between stressed and unstressed volume. The extra stressed volume enables the cardiac output to be maintained at approximately 40% above the prepregnant level for a prolonged period and with limited sympathetic drive.

   The venous pressure in the upper body changes little during pregnancy, in contrast to that in the lower body, which increases steadily from 10 to 25 mmH$_2$O after the 10th week of pregnancy [2]. This pressure rise in the lower body is mostly caused by a combination of stasis (gravity) and partial venous obstruction by the growing uterus. As a consequence, the venular pressure in the microcirculation of lower body tissues tends to rise with advancing pregnancy. Meanwhile, the colloid-osmotic pressure in the circulating blood is reduced in conjunction with the pregnancy-induced hemodilution and, with it, a 15% fall in serum albumin level. Both effects act in concert to hinder the reabsorption of interstitial fluid in the microcirculation. Therefore, orthostatic edema in advanced pregnancy is a normal physiologic phenomenon.

6. *Effect of pregnancy on blood pressure.* At 6-weeks amenorrhea the mean arterial pressure has already fallen by 3–5 mmHg relative to the prepregnant state with an additional

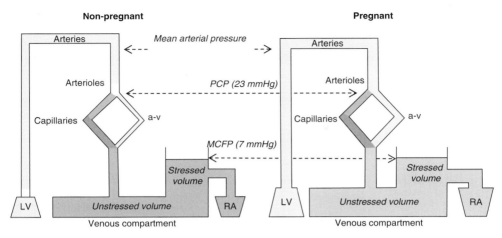

Figure 2.5 Diagram showing the pregnancy-induced change in cardiovascular function in general and the venous compartment in particular. Notice the larger venous compartment with preserved proportional distribution between stressed and unstressed volume. Excess cardiac output is directed toward arteriovenous shunts to protect the systemic microcirculation from excessive flow. Abbreviations: PCP = precapillary hydrostatic pressure; a-v shunts = arteriovenous shunts; MCFP = mean circulatory filling pressure; LV = left ventricle; RA = right atrium.

decline by 1 to 2 mmHg in the remainder of the first trimester [15]. The fall in diastolic pressure is slightly larger than that in systolic pressure, most likely in conjunction with the higher arterial compliance. After the 12th week the blood pressure begins to increase again, until 28 weeks and only by a modest ≈2 mmHg, but after the 28th week by ≈6 mmHg to reach almost prepregnancy levels near term. Therefore, the classical view of a blood pressure nadir in the second trimester ("midpregnancy dip") should be updated to 'first-trimester blood pressure dip.'

7. *Effect of pregnancy on volume homeostasis.* Volume homeostasis is determined by the balance between volume dissipation and retention. During pregnancy the intravascular compartment increases by about 1600 mL, comprising about 1300 mL extra plasma volume and 300 mL extra erythrocyte volume [2, 3, 10, 16]. Plasma volume expansion is the result of excess sodium and water retention in response to the initial fall in effective arterial blood volume (summarized in Figure 2.3). The plasma volume expansion along with more efficient cardiac filling (higher pressure gradient between central veins and right atrium) [14] increases venous return.

In the description of the volume homeostasis one should bear in mind possible concomitant changes in sodium and volume dissipation. During pregnancy, the most important causes of enhanced sodium and water dissipation are 1) the marked rise in renal blood flow giving rise to renal hyperfiltration [13, 16] and thus a higher distal tubular delivery of sodium and water [4]; 2) high circulating levels of progesterone competing with aldosterone for binding with its receptor in the distal tubules [17]; and 3) the rapidly growing fetus extracting sodium and water from the maternal compartment.

The balance between volume retention and dissipation in pregnancy is delicate. Disturbance of this balance will diminish the cardiovascular reserve capacity and thus the capacity to adapt to the primary fall in peripheral vascular resistance. If this happens, the

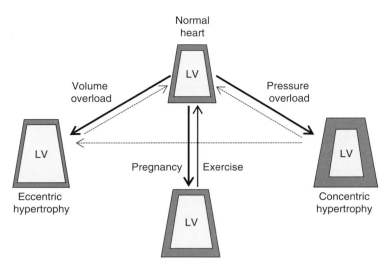

Figure 2.6 Physiologic remodeling of the heart in pregnancy as opposed to the pathologic forms of cardiac remodeling induced by volume or pressure overload. Note the proportional increase in left ventricular (LV) dimensions and wall thickness. The abnormal forms of cardiac remodeling are nonreversible[19].

so-called "fight or flight" back-up mechanism will be activated, which consists of an extra rise in the sympathetic contribution to the autonomic control of the cardiovascular system. This has adverse effects for pregnancy as it includes vasoconstriction at the implantation site. By 5 weeks pregnancy effective renal plasma flow (ERPF) and renal blood flow have already increased by one-third above the prepregnant level [13] and continue to rise to a plateau of ≈80% above the prepregnancy level by midpregnancy. The glomerular filtration rate (GFR) increases in concert with ERPF by only approximately 50%, resulting in a modest decline in filtration fraction (defined as the ratio of GFR and ERPF). The higher GFR is consistent with renal hyperfiltration, resulting in accelerated clearance of e.g. creatinine and urea. As the rise in renal hemodynamics does not raise intraglomerular pressure, the risk of renal damage is negligible. Nor does the renal hyperfiltration affect the maternal homeostasis of sodium and other electrolytes. The raised renal hemodynamics during pregnancy resolve within 2 weeks postpartum.

8. *Effect of pregnancy on the maternal heart.* Pregnancy induces *eccentric* myocardial hypertrophy resembling that in response to endurance sport [19, 22]. That is to say, both left ventricular end-diastolic diameter and left ventricular wall thickness increase by ≈15% (Figure 2.6). The increase in wall thickness is thought to minimize wall stress and maintain myocardial oxygenation in a state of increased cardiac pre- and afterload [22]. Cardiac remodeling in pregnancy develops in response to the following factors: 1) raised cardiac work; 2) higher cardiac preload; and, last but not least, 3) the endocrine environment of pregnancy. By midpregnancy cardiac work, defined as the triple product of heart rate (↑≈20%), stroke volume (↑≈20%) and systolic blood pressure (↓≈5%) [15, 19, 22] have increased by approximately one-third above prepregnancy levels. The cardiac remodeling involves a rise in left ventricular mass by as much as 50%, which regressed for over 90% in the first year postpartum without functional sequels [23].

During pregnancy, cardiac efficiency – defined as cardiac work per unit oxygen uptake – increases, mainly as a result of a rise in preload. Because of the latter cardiac filling is more efficient, enabling the Frank–Starling mechanism to generate a larger stroke volume. The high incidence of adverse pregnancy outcome in women who fail to raise their plasma volume adequately during pregnancy underlines the importance of volume expansion for normal pregnancy evolution [21]. To meet the higher demands for systemic blood flow, these women raise their heart rate and cardiac contractility by increasing the sympathetic tone in their cardiovascular system. This back-up mechanism has a high price as it includes redistribution of cardiac output at the expense of the uteroplacental blood flow (UBF).

With pregnancy advancing into the second half, the position of the heart adopts a more horizontal position within the thorax due to the upward movement of the diaphragm in conjunction with the rapidly growing uterus. As a consequence, the electrocardiogram (ECG) shows increasingly a leftward deviation of the QRS axis and flatter T-waves, often accompanied by abnormal T-waves [24]. Meanwhile, at cardiac auscultation the higher cardiac output without concomitant widening of the aortic annulus produces an ejection murmur.

9. *Effect of pregnancy on regional blood flows.* During pregnancy the cardiac output not only increases, but is also redistributed. Shortly after embryo implantation, the blood flow to the breasts, kidneys and skin increases. The rise in mammary flow is probably secondary to the growth and higher metabolic rate of the mammary glands most likely induced by endocrine stimuli, notably pregnancy steroids, placental lactogen and prolactin. Meanwhile, relaxin has been identified with strong vasodilator properties in the kidneys [7]. The elevated skin flow probably reflects enhanced arteriovenous shunting of excessive systemic flow generated by the hyperdynamic circulation [25]. With pregnancy advancing into the second trimester, UBF increases progressively, most likely at the expense of shunt flow, as suggested by the concomitant increase in maternal basal metabolic rate without additional rise in cardiac output [26].

10. *Early identification of abnormal maternal cardiovascular and volume adaptation.* Even though it is still unclear why pregnancy induces a primary fall in effective arterial volume, the maternal response to preserve the integrity of the cardiovascular function is pivotal for normal pregnancy course and outcome. This is emphasized by the shallow or even absent rise of ERPF and GFR in pregnancies later complicated by placental syndromes [27].

Pregnancy requires both cardiac work and the size of the intravascular compartment to be raised by $\approx30\%$ for a prolonged period. A conventional physical check-up in baseline conditions prior to pregnancy is not sensitive enough to identify limited reserve capacity of these organs. Therefore, a prepregnancy risk assessment in women at increased risk of developing a placental syndrome in their next pregnancy should focus on determining the prepregnant functional reserve capacity of the heart, the arterial and venous beds and the kidneys. This may consist of first evaluating by questionnaire her exercise habits, eating habits, stress management and medical and family history, and, second, a number of targeted tests, such as 1) an aerobic bicycle test [28] to determine her ability to raise stroke volume, 2) the assessment of the endothelium-derived vasodilator response of the forearm arterial bed [29] and 3) some blood/urine tests to determine endothelial and renal health, and to identify signs consistent with chronic inflammation.

Key Points

- A fall in systemic vascular tone at approximately 5 weeks pregnancy is probably the first measurable maternal systemic cardiovascular adaptive response to pregnancy.
- The pregnancy-induced fall in systemic vascular tone triggers a fall in systemic vascular resistance and arterial pressure, and a rise in cardiac output.
  - The pregnancy-induced fall in *systemic vascular tone* alters the set-points of the circulatory receptors residing in the wall of the arteries (baroreceptors) and veins/atria (stretch receptors), resulting in hemodilution and a lower mean arterial pressure.
  - The pregnancy-induced fall in *microcirculatory vascular tone* alters the Starling equilibrium in the microcirculation favoring (orthostatic) edema formation.
  - The pregnancy-induced fall in *venous tone* leads to expansion of the venous compartment, enabling a prolonged rise in venous return (and, with it, cardiac preload/cardiac efficiency) without concomitant rise in sympathetic tone.
- The maternal response to the pregnancy-induced fall in systemic vascular tone not only reflects the maternal adaptive potential to accommodate the extra demands of pregnancy, it also provides insight in the actual maternal cardiovascular reserves.

References

1. Davison JM, Vallotton MB, Lindheimer MD. Plasma osmolality and urinary concentration and dilution during and after pregnancy: evidence that lateral recumbency inhibits maximal urinary concentrating ability. *Brit J Obstet Gynaecol* 1981;**88**:472–9.

2. Peeters LLH, Lotgering FK. Chapter 11: De normale zwangerschap: de zwangere vrouw. In: Heineman MJ, Evers JLH, Massuger LFAG, Steegers EAP, eds. Obstetrie en Gynaecologie, De voortplanting van de mens. Reed Business, Amsterdam 2012: 257–75 (ISBN 978 90 352 3489 5).

3. Valdes G, Corthorn J. Challenges posed to the maternal circulation by pregnancy (review). *Integrated Blood Pressure Control* 2011;**4**:45–53.

4. Schrier RW, Niederberger M. Paradoxes of body fluid volume regulation in health and disease – a unifying hypothesis. *West J Med.* 1994;**161**:293–408.

5. Tkachenko O, Shchekochikhin D, Schrier RW. Hormones and hemodynamics in pregnancy. (review) *Int J Endocrinol Metab* 2014;**12**:e14098.

6. Irani R, Xia Y. The functional role of the Renin-Angiotensin-System in pregnancy and preeclampsia. *Placenta* 2008;**29**:763–71.

7. Conrad KP. Emerging role of relaxin in the maternal adaptations to normal pregnancy: Implications for preeclampsia. *Semin Nephrol* 2011;**31**:15–32.

8. Van Eijndhoven HWF. Mechanisms of vasodilatation in early pregnancy. PhD Thesis, Maastricht University, Medical Faculty. 2009. pp. 93–8.

9. Robson SC, Hunter S, Boys RJ. Serial study of factors influencing changes in cardiac output during human pregnancy. *Am J Physiol* 1989;**256**:H1060–5.

10. Tan EK, Tan EL, Med M. Alterations in physiology and anatomy during pregnancy. *Best Pract Res Clin Obstet Gynaecol* 2013;**27**:791–802.

11. Pang CC. Autonomic control of the venous system in health and disease; Effects of drugs. *Pharmacol Ther* 2001;**90**:179–230.

12. Berlin DA, Bakker J. Understanding venous return. *Intensive Care Med* 2014;**40**:1564–6.

13. Spaanderman M, Ekhart T, van Eyck J et al. Preeclampsia and maladaptation to pregnancy: A role for atrial natriuretic peptide? *Kidney Int* 2001;**60**:1397–1406.

14. Cong J, Yang X, Zhang Y et al. Quantitative analysis of left atrial volume and function during normotensive and preeclamptic pregnancy: a real-time three-dimensional echocardiography study. *Int J Cardiovasc Imaging* 2015;**31**:805–12.

15. Nama V, Antonios TF, Onwude J et al. Mid-pregnancy drop in normal pregnancy: myth or reality? *J Hypertens* 2011;**29**:763–8.

16. Cheung KL, Lafayette RA. Renal physiology of pregnancy. *Adv Chronic Kidney Dis* 2013;**20**:209–14.

17. Oelkers WK. Effects of estrogens and progestogens on the renin-aldosterone system and blood pressure. *Steroids* 1996;**61**:166–71.

18. Arbab-Zadeh A, Perhonen M, Howden E, et al. Cardiac remodeling in response to 1 year of intensive endurance training. *Circulation* 2014;**130**:2152–61.

19. Chung E, Leinwand LA. Pregnancy as a cardiac stress model. *Cardiovasc Res* 2014;**101**:561–70.

20. Thornburg KL, Jacobson SL, Giraud GD, et al. Hemodynamic changes in pregnancy. *Semin Perinatol* 2000;**24**:11–14.

21. Aardenburg R, Spaanderman MEA, Ekhart TH, et al. Low plasma volume following pregnancy complicated by pre-eclampsia predisposes to hypertensive disease in a next pregnancy. *Brit J Obstet Gynaecol* 2003;**110**:1001–6.

22. Melchiorre K, Sharma R, Thilaganathan B. Cardiac structure and function in normal pregnancy. *Curr Opin Obstet Gynaecol* 2012;**24**:413–21.

23. Melchiorre K, Sutherland GR, Liberati M, et al. Preeclampsia is associated with persistent postpartum cardiovascular impairment. *Hypertension* 2011;**58**:709–15.

24. Sunitha M, Chandrasekharappa S, Brid SV. Electrocardiographic QRS axis, Q-wave and T-wave changes in the 2nd and 3rd trimester of normal pregnancy. *J Clin Diagn Res* 2014;**8**:BC 17–21.

25. Spaanderman MEA, Meertens M, van Bussel M, et al. Cardiac output increases independently of basal metabolic rate in early human pregnancy. *Am J Physiol Heart Circ Physiol* 2000;**278**:H1585–8.

26. Forsum E, Löf M. Energy metabolism during human pregnancy. *Annu Rev Nutr* 2007;**27**:277–92.

27. Lopes van Balen VA, Spaan JJ, Ghossein C, et al. Early pregnancy circulatory adaptation and recurrent hypertensive disease: an explorative study. *Reprod Sci* 2013;**20**:1069–74.

28. Aardenburg R, Spaanderman MEA, Courtar DA, et al. Formerly preeclamptic women with a subnormal plasma volume are not able to maintain a rise in stroke volume during moderate exercise. *J Soc Gynecol Investig* 2005 **12**:599–603.

29. Lommerse T, Aardenburg R, Houben AJHM, et al. Endothelium-dependent vasodilation in formerly preeclamptic women correlates inversely with body mass index and varies independently of plasma volume. *Reprod Sci* 2007;**14**:765–70.

Chapter 3

Cardiac Function

Herbert Valensise, Gian Paolo Novelli, Daniele Farsetti
and Barbara Vasapollo

Summary

Maternal cardiac function is subject to structural and functional changes during the course of normal pregnancy. Inadequate cardiac adaptations relate to gestational complications such as nonproteinuric or proteinuric hypertension with or without fetal growth restriction. A full comprehension of the normal gestational cardiac physiology and its assessment methods is therefore mandatory for prenatal care providers, in particular those involved in follow-up of women at risk for gestational hypertensive disease.

Introduction

The study of cardiac function requires a comprehensive understanding of hemodynamics. The various modifications of hemodynamic parameters that occur during pregnancy are closely related to changes in cardiac function. Therefore, it is important to analyze the hemodynamic changes that occur during pregnancy.

Blood Pressure

Systolic blood pressure (SBP), diastolic blood pressure (DBP) and mean arterial pressure (MPA) all decrease during pregnancy, with DBP and MPA showing the greatest decreases. Numerous studies suggest that SBP does not change during pregnancy, whereas DBP and MPA decrease. The changes in blood pressure associated with pregnancy are as follows: Blood pressure decreases gradually from the start of pregnancy and drops sharply between the sixth and eighth weeks of gestation. The nadir of blood pressure values occurs during the second trimester and begins to increase again during the third trimester, progressively returning to preconception levels by term [1, 2 & 3].

There is a correlation between blood pressure levels and body mass index (BMI). Blood pressure is more elevated in pregnant women with high BMI than in those with low BMI values [1].

Studies have shown that there is a more marked reduction in central blood pressure than brachial blood pressure. This is related to the fact that the aortic wall and the peripheral artery walls undergo different modifications during pregnancy [4].

Heart Rate

Heart rate (HR) increases by 15%–25% during pregnancy. Unlike other hemodynamic parameters, the greatest changes in HR do not occur in the second trimester; rather, HR increases gradually and reaches peak values during the third trimester [1, 2 & 3]. HR values return to normal at approximately 10 days after delivery [3].

Cardiac Output

Cardiac output (CO) is defined as the product of stroke volume (SV) and HR. CO increases by the fifth week of gestation, with a considerable increase occurring during the first trimester. Peak values are reached at 25–35 weeks of gestation, when CO increases by 30–50% [1, 2 & 3].

There are conflicting results regarding CO evolution during the third trimester, with studies variously reporting an increase, decrease, or constant values [1].

The increase in CO during pregnancy is differentially mediated by the parameters of SV and HR:

- Changes in early pregnancy are mostly caused by SV.
- HR gradually increases and contributes to CO changes, especially after the end of the second trimester (when SV remains stable) [2].

In twin pregnancies, CO values can be 15% higher than those observed in single pregnancies.[1]

In the first 2 weeks after delivery, CO decreases rapidly and continues to drop until 24 weeks postpartum, eventually returning to prepregnancy values [3].

Furthermore, when a pregnant woman is in the supine position, the uterus compresses the inferior vena cava, resulting in a reduction of venous filling load and subsequent decrease in CO.

Systemic Vascular Resistance

During pregnancy, there is a substantial decrease (35–50%) in systemic vascular resistance (SVR), which begins at 5 weeks after conception [2]. However, the greatest decrease in blood pressure occurs during the 16th week of gestation.

Similar to the other parameters, SVR reaches a nadir in the second trimester (various studies have reported that it occurs by 20–28 weeks of gestation) [2, 3 & 5].

Thereafter, SVR remains constant until around 32 weeks, with a small increase occurring from week 32 to term [2].

At 2 weeks after delivery, SVR returns to preconception values.

The modifications of SVR during pregnancy (referred to as afterload changes) influence CO and ventricular performance.

The afterload is composed of two elements:

- Steady component
- Pulsatile component

SVR represents the steady component of the ventricular afterload, and it is essentially defined by the caliber of the blood vessels.

Mean SVR is approximately 1400 dyn·s·cm^{-5} before conception, decreases to 1000 dyn·s·cm^{-5} in the third trimester, and returns to 1200 dyn·s·cm^{-5} at 12 weeks postpartum [3].

Different mechanisms are related to the decrease of SVR during pregnancy. The role of vasodilator factors such as estrogen, progesterone, prostaglandin, nitric oxide (NO) and relaxin, and the contribution of the low resistance of the uteroplacental unit, have been studied extensively.

Estrogen, progesterone, prostaglandins and prolactin reduce SVR.

Recent evidence suggests an important role of NO in vasodilation during pregnancy. For this reason, the effect of NO donors on multiple obstetric conditions is a subject of research.

Finally, relaxin plays a crucial role in the SVR decrease, in addition to its known functions in connective tissue composition changes, myometrial activity and softening of the maternal pubic symphysis [2].

Global Arterial Compliance

The pulsatile component of the afterload is defined by global arterial compliance, aortic characteristic impedance, and measures of wave propagation and reflection.

Global arterial compliance increases by 30% during the first trimester and remains stable throughout the last two trimesters [3].

The augmentation index (AIx), a measure of wave reflection and arterial stiffness, is reduced in pregnancy. In particular, both unadjusted and adjusted AIx for HR decrease considerably during pregnancy, reach a nadir in the second trimester and increase in the third trimester [6].

Heart Remodeling

The heart adjusts in response to the hemodynamic changes, which can lead to pregnancy-induced eccentric cardiac hypertrophy [7].

This hypertrophy is described as physiological because it is reversible. In addition, fetal gene induction is not upregulated, there is no fibrosis, angiogenesis is normal and the *signaling pathway* is activated in a manner similar to that of exercise-induced hypertrophy.

Nevertheless, there are differences between pregnancy-induced and exercise-induced hypertrophy.

The mild eccentric hypertrophy induced during pregnancy is characterized by a proportional increase in chamber dimension and wall thickness. In this condition, the increase in myocyte length is slightly higher than the increase in myocyte width, and the length-to-width ratio is well preserved.

In conclusion, pregnancy-induced hypertrophy is different from pathological eccentric hypertrophy (caused by volume overload) and from pathological concentric hypertrophy (caused by pressure overload) [8].

The data that will be taken into consideration were obtained by ultrasound imaging and cardiovascular magnetic resonance imaging.

Left Ventricular End-Diastolic and End-Systolic Dimensions

Left ventricular end-diastolic (LVED) and end-systolic (LVES) diameters and volumes increase during pregnancy [9].

The increase in preload caused by the blood volume overload increases the LVED dimensions and the left atrial volume. LVED dimensions increase by approximately 10% starting at 12 gestational weeks, reach a plateau at 24–32 weeks and remain constant until term [3–10].

LVES dimensions increase by 20% in pregnancy, and this parameter is related to HR and afterload [3].

Left Ventricular Wall

Left ventricular wall thickness increases by 15–25%, beginning at 12 weeks of gestation [3].

The increase has the effect of minimizing wall stress and maintaining myocardial oxygenation.

Left Ventricular Mass

Left ventricular mass (LVM) increases by approximately 50%, principally in the third trimester [3–9].

The LVM corrected for *BSA* (left ventricular mass index, LVMI) also increases, confirming that hypertrophy is associated with pregnancy-induced heart remodeling, and *the increase in ventricular mass is greater than that of body size* [3].

The myocardial hypertrophy of pregnancy is mideccentric, as it is associated with a chronic increase in preload and a dilated left ventricle, without changes in the ratio of wall thickness to ventricular radius [3].

The LVM normalizes by 3–6 months after delivery.

Left Ventricular Outflow Tract and Aortic Root

The changes in the cross-sectional area of the left ventricular outflow during pregnancy remain controversial. A small but significant increase in the cross-sectional area of the left ventricular outflow during pregnancy has been reported [3].

The aortic root and ascending aortic dimensions do not change substantially during pregnancy [9].

Right Ventricular Dimensions and Mass

Right ventricular dilatation can be observed during pregnancy.

Several published studies analyzed the changes in right ventricle dimensions and mass using ultrasound technologies and magnetic resonance imaging and reported dilatation of the right ventricle of ~18% during the third trimester of pregnancy [9].

Atrial Geometry

The dimensions of both atria increase during pregnancy, which is caused by the increase in preload.

The left atrial volume increases by 30–50% [9–11], showing a gradual increase starting at 5 weeks of gestation and a plateau at 28–34 weeks of gestation [3].

The right atrial dimensions increase by 34–50% [9]; however, the morphological changes of this cardiac chamber have not been studied extensively.

Electrocardiographic Changes

The physiological adaptations of the heart to pregnancy can be assessed by electrocardiogram (ECG).

During pregnancy, there is a leftward deviation of the QRS axis compared with the pattern in nonpregnant women. This is particularly evident in the third trimester [12].

This phenomenon can be ascribed to elevation of the diaphragm caused by displacement of abdominal viscera by the enlarging uterus, which pushes the heart upward and causes its rotation.

Another possible reason for deviation of the QRS axis is the increase in the left ventricular dimensions and mass, which is described as an eccentric hypertrophy. The authors explain that the axis deviation in early pregnancy is due to the increased preload sustained by the heart.

Other common ECG findings in pregnant women are prominent Q waves in leads II, III, aVF, V4l, V5 and V6, and abnormalities in the T wave, which can be flat or inverted. In addition, innocent depression of the ST segment can be present. The cause of these changes is unknown [12].

These alterations need to be considered when interpreting ECGs of pregnant women.

Metabolism

Pregnancy causes substantial changes in maternal hemodynamics and metabolic requirements.

Adjustments in cardiac metabolism are necessary to support these modifications and to satisfy fetal needs and the increased cardiac work.

To meet the energy demand associated with a 50% increase in cardiac mass and 20–30% increase in cardiac work, cardiac metabolism needs to increase.

However, animal studies have shown that cardiac mean oxygen consumption only increases by 15%, indicating that the heart becomes more efficient.

The increase in oxygen consumption is due to increased coronary blood flow rather than increased extraction. Studies have shown an activation of cardiac endothelial nitric oxide synthase (eNOS) during pregnancy [10–13].

The source of fuel for the heart changes during pregnancy. Glucose utilization decreases considerably and fatty acid oxidation increases (in nonpregnant women, glucose provides 30% of the fuel used by the heart and fatty acid oxidation provides 70%). The ATP produced by the heart is derived almost entirely from the use of fatty acids [10]. The molecular mechanism underlying this fuel shift remains unknown.

Hormones in the bloodstream (estrogen, progesterone, prolactin and placental hormones) play an important role in these metabolic modifications. Many of these hormones cause insulin resistance, and estrogen promotes the use of fatty acids.

Notably, a pathological heart tends to use glucose over fatty acids, as it expresses fetal genes and acquires a metabolism similar to that of the fetus [8].

Molecular Mechanisms

Pregnancy-induced hypertrophy is mediated by Akt and its downstream molecules. In addition, this signaling pathway is an important mediator of exercise-induced hypertrophy.

The Gq signaling pathway is also involved in pregnancy-induced hypertrophy. Extracellular signal-regulated kinase (ERK1/2) phosphorylation increases in midpregnancy, which differs from the pattern in exercise-induced cardiac hypertrophy. The activation of ERKs is probably mediated by progesterone [8].

Calcineurin, a calcium and calmodulin dependent serine/threonine protein phosphatase upregulated in early pregnancy, is required for pregnancy-induced hypertrophy. Calcineurin is considerably downregulated in late pregnancy, reflecting the importance of the regulation of different signaling pathways during pregnancy. It is possible that the hormonal milieu activates calcineurin during early pregnancy, and this protein phosphatase triggers Akt and ERK1/2 signaling, leading to physiological hypertrophy [8].

Systolic Function

Left ventricular systolic function has been studied using classical and new parameters obtained through ultrasound technologies and magnetic resonance imaging. However, there is no consensus regarding the changes in systolic function during pregnancy. Studies report normal, increased or depressed systolic function. However, morphological and loading changes associated with pregnancy can alter the evaluation of cardiac function using classical and new parameters.

Although cardiac performance expressed as left ventricle stroke work increases during pregnancy, these data are not consistent with other systolic function indices [5].

The objective of this chapter is to summarize the main results of studies on myocardial function. Myofibrils are grouped into bundles and aligned longitudinally. Different bundles of myofibrils with the same longitudinal alignment are arranged in different orientations, resulting in a myocardial mesh.

For this particular myocardial architecture, left ventricular systolic contraction cannot be attributed to shortening in a single direction (unlike skeletal muscle, which has specific insertion points).

The left ventricle shows four different types of deformation: longitudinal shortening, circumferential shortening, torsion and thickening of the wall. The most important element for SV remains controversial. However, torsion is strictly related to longitudinal shortening because it is determined by the contraction of oblique longitudinal fibers.

Myocardial deformation is caused by various factors; in order of their effect, these are myofibril contractility, tissue elasticity and preload and afterload conditions.

The indices that describe systolic function can be grouped into the following three categories:

- Radial function
- Longitudinal function
- Systolic myocardial deformation

Radial Function

Radial function, which is determined by the contraction of circumferential fibers, is described by parameters such as ejection phase and wall stress.

There are conflicting results regarding the usefulness of ejection-phase indices such as ejection fraction, fractional shortening and velocity of circumferential fiber shortening [3, 5, 7 & 14]. Therefore, LV systolic function estimated by this index is increased or unchanged during pregnancy. This could be due to the dependence of ejection-phase indices on HR, preload, and afterload, which are modified in pregnancy.

Wall stress, defined as the tension within the wall of the ventricle, is determined by the pressure in the ventricle, the ventricular radius and the ventricular wall thickness. Studies that assessed the relation between end-systolic wall stress and the velocity of circumferential fiber shortening reported different values [3].

Longitudinal Function

The longitudinal function is examined by assessing the left ventricular systolic longitudinal axis displacement or velocity. The long-axis displacement is limited by the HR.

The use of these parameters in various studies revealed that longitudinal function can either improve (e.g., the maximum value at 23 weeks was 11% higher that of nonpregnant controls) or deteriorate during pregnancy [3].

Systolic Myocardial Deformation

The new echographic parameters of systolic myocardial deformation are strictly related to cardiac function, and are highly sensitive for revealing subtle modifications [5].

Indices of myocardial deformation show a reduction in global and segmental myocardial strain and strain rate in pregnancy, with a postpartum return to normal values [3, 5, 7 & 15]. However, various interpretations of these data are reported. Cardiac function is described as decreased in some studies [15] and increased in others (these last studies take into consideration hemodynamic changes and heart remodeling) [3–5].

Diastolic Function

Diastolic function is the capacity of the ventricle to fill to a normal end-diastolic volume without an abnormal increase in LVED pressure.

It is evaluated by the left atrial dimension, mitral inflow and pulmonary venous flow indices. A new parameter has been introduced: assessment by pulsed tissue Doppler ultrasound imaging at the level of the annulus of the mitral valve. This latter parameter is less load-dependent [9].

Mitral Inflow

An important modality for assessing diastolic function is the mitral inflow signal. It reflects the pressure difference between the atrium and the ventricle and analyzes the contribution of each individual phase to filling. The ratio between early (E) and late (A) filling wave velocity is an interesting parameter for evaluating diastolic function, and it decreases during pregnancy [3, 9, 11, 16 & 17].

Tissue Doppler Imaging

Tissue Doppler imaging (TDI) measures myocardial velocity directly, in real time.

Numerous studies have employed the E1/A1 ratio as an index. E1 is early diastolic myocardial velocity, and is defined by the velocity of ventricle lengthening in early diastole. A1 is late diastolic myocardial velocity, and it reflects the velocity of ventricular lengthening in late diastole (the period that follows atrial contraction).

Studies that used TDI reported a decreased E1/A1 ratio associated with pregnancy, and this was correlated with diastolic dysfunction.

The increase in A1, and therefore in the atrial contribution, may be a compensatory effect of the increased LVM or afterload [3].

Indirect Filling Pressure Indices

Left atrial and LVED pressures can be used to assess the chamber filling pressure. This was found to remain unchanged during pregnancy [3], thus eliminating the hypothesis of diastolic dysfunction.

Cardiac Function and Uteroplacental Flow

Studies that assessed cardiac function and uteroplacental Doppler flow reported a link between cardiac function and placentation. In particular, cardiac dysfunction is strictly related to poor placentation, as revealed by abnormalities in uteroplacental Doppler flow. Poor placentation is associated with poor perinatal outcomes.

Preexisting subclinical abnormal cardiac function causes an anomalous adaptation to pregnancy that results in high uterine arterial resistance.

Studies have examined the relation between left ventricular function and physiologic placentation. Cardiac dysfunction causes placental hypoperfusion and subsequently abnormal placental development and uteroplacental flow [18].

Several recent studies have focused on the role of right ventricular function in correct placentation. One study demonstrated that women with preeclampsia show systolic dysfunction and compromised contractility, but also diastolic dysfunction and impaired myocardial relaxation of the right ventricle [3–18].

Labor and Delivery

Labor and delivery place additional demands on the cardiovascular system. Increased CO and blood pressure cause a substantial increment in cardiac work, which can result in damage in women with heart disease, hypertensive disorders or severe anemia.

Pain, uterine contractions and blood loss are important factors that need to be taken into account when analyzing the hemodynamic changes that occur during this period.

During labor, CO increases by 30% in the first stage of labor and by over 50% in the second stage [2]. The highest CO values are detected during labor and immediately after delivery [1].

In the first stage of labor, CO increases because of the increase in SV, whereas in the second stage, the pushing efforts are primarily involved in the CO increment [2].

Approximately 300–500 mL of blood are transfused in the circulation during each uterine contraction,[2] which increases the venous return and subsequently the SV.

Pain increases catecholamine levels, and the increase in sympathetic tone increases blood pressure and HR values.

Both SBP and DBP increase with uterine contractions. This increment is related to the increased CO because the SVR does not change considerably during labor [2].

Key Points

- In pregnancy, CO is thought to increase by between 30–50%, the peak occurring in the late second or early third trimester.
- On ECG, the axis of the QRS complex deviates to the left with an increase in LVM.

- In normal pregnancy, there is mild eccentric remodeling of the heart. Volume overload and pressure overload contribute to pathological eccentric and concentric cardiac hypertrophy respectively.
- SVR reduces maximally in the midtrimester and then modestly rises afterwards. It returns to prepregnancy values two weeks after delivery.

References

1. Sanghavi M, Rutherford JD. Cardiovascular physiology of pregnancy. *Circulation* 2014;**130**(12):1003–8.

2. Ouzounian JG, Elkayam U. Physiologic changes during normal pregnancy and delivery. *Cardiol Clin* 2012;**30**(3):317–29.

3. Melchiorre K, Sharma R, Thilaganathan B. Cardiac structure and function in normal pregnancy. *Curr Opin Obstet Gynecol* 2012;**24**(6):413–21.

4. Mahendru AA, Everett TR, Wilkinson IB, Lees CC, McEniery CM. Maternal cardiovascular changes from pre-pregnancy to very early pregnancy. *J Hypertens* 2012;**30**(11):2168–72.

5. Savu O, Jurcuț R, Giușcă S, et al. Morphological and functional adaptation of the maternal heart during pregnancy. *Circ Cardiovasc Imaging* 2012;**5**(3):289–97.

6. Mahendru AA, Everett TR, Wilkinson IB, Lees CC, McEniery CM. A longitudinal study of maternal cardiovascular function from preconception to the postpartum period. *J Hypertens* 2014;**32**(4):849–56.

7. Cong J, Fan T, Yang X, et al. Structural and functional changes in maternal left ventricle during pregnancy: a three-dimensional speckle-tracking echocardiography study. *Cardiovasc Ultrasound* 2015;**13**:6.

8. Chung E, Leinwand LA. Pregnancy as a cardiac stress model. *Cardiovasc Res* 2014;**101**(4):561–70.

9. Ducas RA, Elliott JE, Melnyk SF, et al. Cardiovascular magnetic resonance in pregnancy: Insights from the cardiac hemodynamic imaging and remodeling in pregnancy (CHIRP) study. *J Cardiovasc Magn Reson* 2014;**16**(1):1.

10. Liu LX, Arany Z. Maternal cardiac metabolism in pregnancy. *Cardiovasc Res* 2014;**101**(4):545–53.

11. Yosefy C, Shenhav S, Feldman V, Sagi, Y, Katza A, Anteby E. Left atrial function during pregnancy: A three-dimensional ecocardiographic study. *Echocardiography* 2012;**29**(9):1096–101.

12. Sunitha M, Chandrasekharappa S, Brid SV. Electrocradiographic Qrs axis, Q wave and T-wave changes in 2nd and 3rd trimester of normal pregnancy. *J Clin Diagn Res* 2014;**8**(9):BC17–BC21.

13. Williams JG, Rincon-Skinner T, Sun D, Wang Z, Zhang S, Zhang X, Hintze TH. Role of nitric oxide in the coupling of myocardial oxygen consumption and coronary vascular dynamics during pregnancy in the dog. *Am J Physiol Heart Circ Physiol* 2007;**293**(4):H2479–86.

14. Ando T, Kaur R, Holmes AA, Brusati A, Fujikura K, Taub CC. Physiological adaptation of the left ventricle during the second and third trimesters of a healthy pregnancy: A speckle tracking echocardiography study. *Am J Cardiovasc Dis* 2015;**5**(2):119–26.

15. Zentner D, du Plessis M, Brennecke S, Wong J, Grigg L, Harrap S. Cardiac function at term in human pregnancy. *Pregnancy Hypertens* 2012;**2**(2):132–8.

16. Estensen ME, Beitnes JO, Grindheim G, Aaberge L, Smiseth OA, Henriksen T, Aakhus S. Altered maternal left ventricular contractility and function during normal pregnancy. *Ultrasound Obstet Gynecol* 2013;**41**(6):659–66.

17. Bamfo JE, Kametas NA, Nicolaides KH, Chambers JB. Maternal left ventricular diastolic and systolic

long-axis function during normal pregnancy. *Eur J Echocardiogr* 2007;**8**(5):360–8.

18. Kampman MA, Bilardo CM, Mulder BJ, Aarnoudse JG, Ris-Stalpers C, van Veldhuisen DJ, Pieper PG. Maternal cardiac function, uteroplacental Doppler flow parameters and pregnancy outcome: A systematic review. *Ultrasound Obstet Gynecol* 2015;**46**(1):21–8.

Chapter 4

The Venous Compartment in Normal Pregnancy

Kathleen Tomsin and Wilfried Gyselaers

Summary

Throughout normal pregnancy, both vascular tone and cardiac function are considered key players in maternal hemodynamics. A drop in peripheral vascular resistance in early pregnancy leads to a cascade of cardiovascular changes, of which the facilitation of plasma volume expansion is important to optimize blood flow to the fetoplacental unit. A crucial determinant of cardiac output is the functionality of the venous compartment.

The Venous System

The human cardiovascular system integrates several functions toward distribution of the blood via a complex circuit of blood vessels. Based on their histological constitution and anatomical location, these blood vessels are categorized into three main compartments: the arteries, the microcirculation and the veins. The inner layer of a vessel wall contains a heterogeneous set of endothelial cells, which can be considered a dynamic organ lining of the entire vascular system, with different functions depending on its location [1]. Elastin and collagen, located in the adventitia, are passive tension elements which contribute to the distensibility of a vessel. This compliance partly influences the response of the vascular wall to the active tension that is created by the activation of the vascular smooth muscle cells of the tunica media [2]. Veins are richly innervated by sympathetic nerves and have a 30 times greater compliance than arteries, i.e. a great change in volume causes only a small change in pressure. Consequently, the veins are able to significantly influence the distribution of large volumes of blood throughout the human body, and therefore determine most of the vascular capacitance [3]. As veins, heart and arteries together constitute a closed circuit, venous return determines cardiac output. Specifically, a reflex-induced venoconstriction can mobilize stored blood to preserve venous return to the heart, and, hence, cardiac output, in specific circumstances like hypovolemia [4].

The blood flow in the lumen of the vessels is mainly driven by pressure gradients between the different entities of the cardiovascular system. Contraction of the ventricles during systole creates a positive pressure gradient between heart and arteries. This gradient pushes the blood toward the systemic microcirculation at a certain velocity. The amount of blood distributed by this activity can be quantified as cardiac output in liters per minute. Equivalently, relaxation during diastole of the cardiac atria generates a negative pressure gradient between veins and heart, producing a suction force, which is one of the most important driving forces for venous return, shifting blood from the venous compartment into the heart [4]. As a result, specific pressure-flow relationships can be generated for each vessel depending on its structure and location in this closed circuit: the arteries act as resistors, the microcirculation as a diffusion and filtration system and the veins as capacitors [2].

Venous Physiology

Regulation of blood flow throughout the entire cardiovascular system is a complex interaction between different systemic and local subsystems [5]. The balance between vasodilation and -constriction of the vascular smooth muscle cells determines the state of vascular tone. A basal or intrinsic tone can be observed at the arterial side of the circulation, but this has not been illustrated for the veins. Modulation of smooth muscle tone or vascular tone can occur via *direct* stimulation or *indirect* endothelium-dependent stimulation [6]. The most important function of venous tone is the peripheral-central distribution of blood volume, as described above.

Important to note is that each organ has its own regulation mechanisms for blood flow distribution, which can be roughly categorized into *local control mechanisms*, depending on the metabolic needs of the surrounding tissue, e.g. at the level of the brain, and *systemic control mechanisms* resulting from neural activity, e.g. at the level of the kidneys and splanchnic organs. This allows the human body to preserve the functionality of important vital organs during cardiovascular distress.

Direct Stimulation

Direct stimulation occurs through the sympathetic nervous system, which plays a significant role in the reflex control of the overall vasculature, for instance, in the regulation of arterial blood pressure. Moreover, the sympathetic nervous system is the most important vasopressor system in the control of venous capacitance [7]. Sympathetic activity enables mobilization of stored blood to the circulation due to venoconstriction [8]. In the presence of minimal sympathetic tone, 60–70% of total blood volume is hemodynamically inactive and constitutes a blood volume reservoir (unstressed volume) [9]. This unstressed volume is located mainly in the splanchnic circulation and the liver, but also in the multiple venous vascular networks distributed throughout the body [7]. This capacitance bed serves as a site of adjustable resistance, containing blood that does not participate in the active circulation, serving as a reservoir from which volumes can be mobilized when an increase of cardiac output is needed.

The parasympathetic nervous system acts only on a small proportion of the resistance vessels, and therefore the effect on total vascular resistance is relatively small. It is, however, capable of depressing the ventricular performance, mainly by counteraction of its antagonist, i.e. the sympathetic nervous system. In this way, it plays a role in the baroreceptor reflex modulation by regulating myocardial performance, in order to maintain normal blood pressure and heart rate.

Indirect Stimulation

Endothelial cells respond to hormones, neurotransmitters and vasoactive factors, thereby indirectly influencing the underlying vascular smooth muscle cells through release of nitric oxide, prostacyclin, thromboxane and endothelin, and by means of hyperpolarization [1, 6]. On top of this, the endothelium can be activated by changes in flow-dependent shear stress. Shear stress is the force applied on a vessel due to flowing of the blood in that vessel, which depends on its diameter, its resistance and blood viscosity [10]. Endothelial cells activate several intracellular molecular pathways, such as the level of prostaglandins and bradykinin, in response to this mechanical shear stress, which in turn will influence the blood flow by changing vascular tone through changes in the level of cyclic adenosine and guanosine monophosphate [11]. The bioavailability of nitric oxide and the sensitivity to shear stress seem to be of importance in processes such as aging and cardiovascular disease [12].

On top of this, venous return can be influenced by many physiological variables. Respiratory movements, especially during inspiration when the diaphragm contracts, raise venous return by increasing abdominal pressure and reducing intrathoracic pressure [13]. Orthostasis and thus gravity tends to reduce venous return temporarily, but this is restored by both a reflex-induced venoconstriction and the muscle pump activity at the level of the veins surrounded by skeletal muscular tissue, mainly in the lower extremities [4]. Moreover, veins are susceptible to external compression caused by a tumor, gravid uterus or intraperitoneal pressure, and this passively influences the content and distribution of venous blood.

Control of Capillary Function

The function of the capillary network is discussed elsewhere (see Chapter 5: The Microcirculation). Because of the anatomical position between the arterial and venous compartments, capillary blood flow is influenced by both arterioles and venes, in anterograde or retrograde directions respectively [28]. An increase of intravenular pressure from any of the mechanisms discussed above will cause a deceleration of capillary blood flow, even stasis of blood. This can be responsible for increased transcapillary exsudation of water, electrolytes and proteins into the surrounding tissues, causing local edema or leakage of blood products. The opposite happens when there is a decrease of intravenular pressure.

The autonomic nervous system coordinates arterial and venular function in regulating capillary blood flow. Increased intravenular pressure induces a reflex arteriolar constriction, which is responsible for a reduction of capillary influx. This reflex prevents capillary dysfunction and the formation of edema or loss of metabolites and proteins, but at the cost of reduced capillary flow. Consequently, arteriolar pressure increases, inducing local or generalized arterial hypertension [28].

From the physiologic properties discussed above, one can conclude that the venous compartment fulfills three main functions: 1) control of cardiac output, 2) storage and mobilization of reserve blood volumes and 3) regulation of microcirculatory flow.

The Venous Doppler Flow Wave

The way in which the blood flow wave propagates within a vessel can be visualized using Doppler ultrasonography. Ultrasound waves are reflected by the flowing red blood cells, thereby changing the wavelengths of the sound, which is called the Doppler effect [17]. The venous Doppler waveform is well described at the level of the internal jugular vein. The characteristics of the venous pulse wave relate to the cyclic changes of right atrial pressure (Figure 4.1). The A-wave represents transient venous deceleration or even reversal of forward flow, caused by retrograde pressure from the contraction of the right atrium by lack of a valve mechanism between the right atrium and the vena cava.

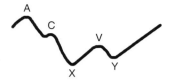

Figure 4.1 The venous Doppler waveform characteristics at the level of liver and kidneys resemble those of internal jugular veins.
The A-wave represents right atrial contraction. The X-wave relates to the fast filling phase of the right atrium, which can be interrupted by the closure of the tricuspid valve (c-wave). The V-wave represents the passive filling phase of the right atrium. The early ventricular diastole after opening of the tricuspid valve is reflected by the Y-wave.

The X-descent is a temporary acceleration of forward flow, which relates to the fast filling of the right atrium during atrial relaxation and the downward movement of the tricuspid valve during ventricular systole. The continuity of the X-wave may be interrupted by a small upward deflection (C-wave) at the time of tricuspid valve closure. The V-deflection is the deceleration of forward venous flow, at the moment of full passive filling of the right atrium when the tricuspid valve is still closed. Opening of the tricuspid valve in early ventricular diastole allows rapid emptying of the right atrium into the right ventricle. The fall in right atrial pressure induces a suction force with fast forward venous flow velocity, reflected in the Y-descent. When both ventricle and atrium are filled with blood, venous forward flow decelerates again, and this deceleration is reinforced by the new atrial contraction (18).

The typical venous waveform changes under physiological conditions, such as breathing, position and muscle activity, but is also different depending on the distance from the heart: central veins show a pattern similar to that of the internal jugular veins, whereas peripheral veins exhibit a flat pattern, representing more or less constant forward flow velocity. The changes in the venous Doppler waveform can be used to study venous physiology. Because of the multiple interfering variables, methodological standardization is needed, as is discussed in Chapter 12.

Similar to the calculation of the arterial resistivity index (RI), which is defined as (maximum velocity – minimum velocity)/maximum velocity, the maximum and minimum venous Doppler flow velocities can be used to calculate the venous impedance index. The venous impedance index is calculated as $(X - A)/X$ and offers some indirect information on the compliance of the vein [19]. As discussed above, the A-wave represents the retrograde jet of venous blood from the contracting atrium into the central veins and causes a) reversed venous flow at the level of hepatic and internal jugular veins, b) forward flow deceleration at the level of renal interlobar veins and c) no change at all in the peripheral veins.

In fact, the A-wave is the hemodynamic equivalent of the electrophysiologic P-wave of the electrocardiogram (ECG), which is known to induce the atrial contraction. The time interval between the corresponding physiologic signals A and P can be measured when a maternal ECG is simultaneously performed with the Doppler assessment (Figure 4.2). This PA time interval, corrected for the duration of the cardiac cycle or heart rate, represents the venous pulse transit time and is defined as PA/RR, where RR represents the time between two consecutive ECG R-waves [20]. More information on this procedure can be found in Chapter 12.

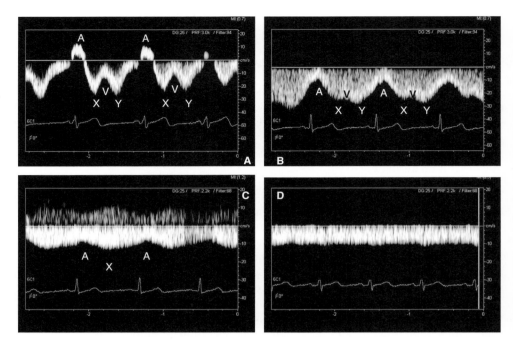

Figure 4.2 Different types of venous Doppler wave forms, as commonly seen in the hepatic and renal veins. (A black and white version of this figure will appear in some formats. For the color version, please refer to the plate section.)

Both the venous impedance index and pulse transit time at different locations of the human body are influenced by many physiologic variables, such as the intravascular volume (i.e. the filling status), the venous distensibility (i.e. venous tone), the pressure in the surrounding tissues (the intraabdominal pressure at the level of splanchnic organs or the muscle activity in the lower extremities) and pregnancy.

The Venous System in Pregnancy

The pattern of central venous blood flow and the venous Doppler waveform changes during the course of pregnancy [21]. These changes are reflected in the venous impedance indices and pulse transit times at the level of renal interlobar and hepatic veins.

Renal interlobar venous impedance index decreases throughout pregnancy, and this effect is more pronounced in the right than in the left kidney. Venous maximum Doppler flow velocities are consistently higher on the right than on the left side [22]. This difference can be explained by interrenal anatomical differences: the right renal vein is shorter than the left one, and the latter also drains blood from the left ovarian vein and is squeezed between the aorta and superior mesenteric artery. Next to this, the right renal vein has a larger diameter and contains more accessory branches than the left one [23]. According to the definition of venous impedance index as discussed above, higher maximum venous flow velocities are responsible for lower impedance indices. From the physiologic point of view, these Doppler flow characteristics illustrate that venous blood drains faster from the right than from the left kidney, and this effect becomes more pronounced during pregnancy.

At the level of the hepatic veins, a retrograde A-wave is present during the first trimester and converts to a continuous forward flow around 22–24 weeks of gestation: the early gestational triphasic pattern becomes flat in the third trimester [24]. This shift from triphasic to flat is also seen during valsalva maneuver or intraperitoneal gas insufflation at laparoscopy, which suggest a relation with intraperitoneal pressure. It has been demonstrated that intraperitoneal pressure is higher in third trimester pregnant women than in nonpregnant individuals, and that this pressure drops to normal values immediately after birth [27]. The link between flattening of the hepatic vein Doppler waveform and increasing intraperitoneal pressure during pregnancy offers a logic physiologic explanation for the reported increase of pressure in the femoral vein and the development of varicose veins in the lower limb during pregnancy.

Similarly, the evolution of venous pulse transit time shows a comparable evolution: the PA time interval increases during normal pregnancy and this change can be observed in both liver and kidneys [25].

The gestational changes of venous Doppler flow characteristics coexist with and may reflect some of the known physiological changes during pregnancy: a) the increased plasma volume and thus increased vascular filling, b) the decreased peripheral vascular resistance and thus increased vascular compliance [26] and c) external compression phenomena such as intraabdominal pressure and the gravid uterus [27].

Future Research of Venous Hemodynamics in Pregnancy

Regarding future research, several areas still need to be explored to further elucidate the role of maternal venous hemodynamics before, during and after pregnancy.

First, in early pregnancy, changes at the level of the uterine circulation are of great importance to ensure a high flow–low resistance bloodstream to the placenta. Here, the role of the uterine venous circulation is still unrevealed. More particularly, the presence of arteriovenous shunts is observed during early pregnancy, but their function is still unexplained [28].

As is explained above, hepatic venous hemodynamics is important for control of cardiac output via the storage of reserve blood in the capacitance reservoir or mobilization of volumes into the circulation. A correlation between hepatic vein Doppler indices and maternal cardiac output has been reported [29]. Next to this, neonatal birth weight is known to relate at least partly to maternal cardiac output, and a correlation between hepatic venous Doppler flow characteristics and birth weight has also been observed [29]. These observations invite further exploration of the role of hepatic hemodynamics in the control of maternal cardiac output and (indirectly) of fetal growth.

In the control of cardiac output, the heart and veins coordinate as one functional unit and venous return is influenced by cardiac diastolic function. Cardiac changes during pregnancy are discussed elsewhere (see Chapter 3: Cardiac Function). Cardiac diastolic dysfunction during gestational hypertensive disease has been reported, but its relation to venous hemodynamics is unknown.

Finally, studying the venous endothelium in relation with the function of endocardium and arterial endothelium may be helpful to better understand the changes of vascular tone during pregnancy.

Key Points

- The venous compartment serves three important physiologic functions: 1) cooperation with the heart in control and regulation of cardiac output, 2) blood volume capacitance and 3) contribution to the regulation of capillary function.
- Venous physiologic functions are altered by normal gestational adaptations.
- Venous flow can be assessed at the level of liver and kidneys using Doppler sonography.
- Hepatic and renal venous Doppler wave characteristics resemble those of internal jugular veins.

References

1. Sandoo A, van Zanten JJ, Metsios GS, Carroll D, Kitas GD. The endothelium and its role in regulating vascular tone. *Open Cardiovasc Med J.* 2010;**4**:302–12.

2. Boulpaep EL. Arteries and veins. In: Boron WF, Boulpaep EL, editors. *Medical physiology.* Philadelphia: Elsevier Inc.; 2003. pp. 447–62.

3. Gelman S. Venous function and central venous pressure: a physiologic story. *Anesthesiology.* 2008;**108**(4):735–48.

4. Berne R, Levy M. Control of cardiac output: coupling of heart and blood vessels. In: Berne R, Levy M, editors. *Cardiovascular physiology.* London: The C.V. Mosby Company; 2001. pp. 199–226.

5. Boulpaep EL. Integrated control of the cardiovascular system. In: Boron WF, Boulpaep EL, editors. *Medical physiology.* Philadelphia: Elsevier Inc.; 2003. pp. 574–90.

6. Dora KA. Coordination of vasomotor responses by the endothelium. *Circ J.* 2010;**74**(2):226–32.

7. Pang CC. Autonomic control of the venous system in health and disease: effects of drugs. *Pharmacol Ther.* 2001;**90**(2–3):179–230.

8. Segal SS. Special circulations. In: Boron WF, Boulpaep EL, editors. *Medical physiology.* Philadelphia: Elsevier Inc.; 2003. pp. 558–73.

9. Greenway CV, Lautt WW. Blood volume, the venous system, preload, and cardiac output. *Can J Physiol Pharmacol.* 1986;**64**(4):383–7.

10. Boulpaep EL. Organization of the cardiovascular system. In: Boron WF, Boulpaep EL, editors. *Medical physiology.* Philadelphia: Elsevier Inc.; 2003. pp. 423–46.

11. Lu D, Kassab GS. Role of shear stress and stretch in vascular mechanobiology. *J R Soc Interface.* 2011;**8**(63):1379–1385.

12. Collins C, Tzima E. Hemodynamic forces in endothelial dysfunction and vascular aging. *Exp Gerontol.* 2011;**46**(2–3):185–8.

13. Lewis B. The peripheral veins. In: Rumack CM, Wilson RD, Charboneau JW, Johnson JM, editors. *Diagnostic ultrasound.* Philadelphia: Elsevier Mosby; 2005. pp. 1019–35.

14. Khalil RA. *Regulation of Vascular Smooth Muscle Function.* San Rafael (CA): Morgan and Claypool Life Sciences; 2010.

15. Bank AJ, Kaiser DR. Smooth muscle relaxation: effects on arterial compliance, distensibility, elastic modulus, and pulse wave velocity. *Hypertension.* 1998;**32**(2):356–9.

16. Tomiyama H, Yamashina A. Non-invasive vascular function tests: their pathophysiological background and clinical application. *Circ J.* 2010;**74**(1):24–33.

17. Nelson TR, Pretorius DH. The Doppler signal: where does it come from and what does it mean? *AJR Am J Roentgenol.* 1988;**151**(3):439–47.

18. Martin N, Lilly LS. The cardiac cycle: Mechanisms of heart sounds and murmurs. In: Lilly LS, editor.

Pathophysiology of heart disease. Philadelphia: Lippincott Williams and Wilkins; 2007. pp. 29–44.

19. Bateman GA, Cuganesan R. Renal vein Doppler sonography of obstructive uropathy. *AJR Am J Roentgenol.* 2002;**178** (4):921–5.

20. Tomsin K, Mesens T, Molenberghs G, Peeters L, Gyselaers W. Time interval between maternal electrocardiogram and venous Doppler waves in normal pregnancy and preeclampsia: a pilot study. *Ultraschall Med.* 2012;**33**(7):E119–25.

21. Roobottom CA, Hunter JD, Weston MJ, Dubbins PA. Hepatic venous Doppler waveforms: changes in pregnancy. *J Clin Ultrasound.* 1995;**23**(8):477–82.

22. Gyselaers W, Mesens T, Tomsin K, Peeters L. Doppler assessment of maternal central venous hemodynamics in uncomplicated pregnancy: a comprehensive review. *Facts Views Vis Obgyn.* 2009;**1**(3):171–81.

23. Satyapal KS. Classification of the drainage patterns of the renal veins. *Journal of anatomy.* 1995;**186** (Pt 2):329–33.

24. Gyselaers W, Molenberghs G, Mesens T, Peeters L. Maternal hepatic vein Doppler velocimetry during uncomplicated

pregnancy and pre-eclampsia. *Ultrasound Med Biol.* 2009;**35**(8):1278–83.

25. Tomsin K, Mesens T, Molenberghs G, Gyselaers W. Venous pulse transit time in normal pregnancy and preeclampsia. *Reprod Sci.* 2012;**19**(4):431–6.

26. Sakai K, Imaizumi T, Maeda H, Nagata H, Tsukimori K, Takeshita A, et al. Venous distensibility during pregnancy. Comparisons between normal pregnancy and preeclampsia. *Hypertension.* 1994;**24** (4):461–6.

27. Staelens AS, Van Cauwelaert S, Tomsin K, Mesens T, Malbrain ML, Gyselaers W. Intra-abdominal pressure measurements in term pregnancy and postpartum: an observational study. *PLoS one.* 2014;**9**(8): e104782.

28. Gyselaers W, Peeters L. Physiological implications of arteriovenous anastomoses and venous hemodynamic dysfunction in early gestational uterine circulation: a review. *J Matern Fetal Neonatal Med.* 2013;**26**(9):841–6.

29. Vonck S, Staelens AS, Mesens T, Tomsin K, Gyselaers W. Hepatic hemodynamics and fetal growth: a relationship of interest for further research. *PLoS one.* 2014;**9**(12): e115594.

Chapter 5

The Microcirculation

Jérôme Cornette and Andreas Brückmann

Summary

The microcirculation and capillaries are important for normal blood supply to and drainage from tissues. This poorly understood part of the cardiovascular system is difficult to assess in clinical conditions. This chapter summarizes the most common technologies currently used to evaluate microcirculatory function, with respect to normal gestational adaptive changes.

Anatomy and Physiology

The circulatory system can be viewed as a closed circuit where the heart functions as central pump. With each beat, blood is driven through large elastic capacitance arteries and is then directed into more muscular arteries that distribute the flow to the organs according to their needs. In these tissues smaller arterioles further branch down into capillaries. Here, exchange of oxygen and nutrients for carbon dioxide and waste products takes place with tissue cells, which is in essence the primary function and ultimate goal of the circulation. Blood is then drained by venules into the venous system and returns to the heart.

The microcirculation includes vessels with a diameter (Ø) below 100 micrometer (µm) and mainly consist of the arterioles, capillaries and venules [1, 2]. It is by far the largest compartment of the circulatory system. Arterioles have a thin muscular layer and, along with precapillary sphincters, they regulate the blood flow toward the capillaries according to the tissues' needs on a microvascular level [2, 3]. Capillaries have a Ø below 20 µm, allowing erythrocytes to flow through them in a single column [4]. They consist of a layer of endothelial cells with a basal membrane. Three different types of capillaries can be distinguished based on the connection between the endothelial cells [2, 5, 6]. Continuous capillaries are the most commonly found type (e.g. nervous system, muscle, lung). They are characterized by narrow intercellular clefts where one cell directly connects to the next through tight junctions. Fenestrated capillaries have pores (transcellular cytoplasmatic holes) and are found in organs where more exchange between the intra- and extravascular compartment is required (e.g. endocrine glands, gastrointestinal tract and kidneys). Discontinuous capillaries are sometimes referred to as sinusoids and can be found in e.g. the liver, spleen and bone marrow. They have more significant gaps between adjacent cells and a discontinuous basal membrane. While exchange of gases and small molecules mainly occurs though diffusion and pinocytosis, gaps in or between the endothelial cells allow easier exchange of fluids and larger molecules. On the inside (lumen), the endothelial cells are covered with a gel-like structure called the glycocalyx [5–7]. It mainly consists of glycoproteins and soluble components and is sometimes referred to as the endothelial surface layer (ESL). It forms a film between the blood cells and the endothelium and improves rheology by preventing unnecessary interaction and adhesion of the erythrocytes, leucocytes and platelets with endothelial cells. The glycocalyx also plays an essential role in regulating the exchange of fluids and solutes (flux) between the intravascular compartment and the interstitium [8]. The classic Starling's principle, where exchange is driven by the opposing hydrostatic and oncotic forces, was revised as recent evidence suggest that the glycocalix reflects albumin into the intravascular compartments and creates a hypoalbuminamic space between the glycocalix and the endothelium [5, 6]. The inward flux created by the oncotic difference is not as large as previously assumed and most of the fluid returning from the interstitial space back into the circulatory system occurs through lymphatic drainage. Damage to the endothelial glycocalyx induces proteinuria in glomeruli and impaired permeability in systemic blood vessels [5].

Delivery of oxygen and nutrients to the tissues is essential to maintain cellular homeostasis and function but the required amounts are not constant. The circulatory system has several mechanisms to regulate the supply according to the specific needs and situations. Cardiac output can be adapted by modifying stroke volume and heart rate. Blood flow can be redirected to central organs or specific tissue areas and bypass others, by regulating the muscular tone of arteries and arterioles. In severe hemodynamic conditions such as septic shock, this redistribution might result in increased core organ perfusion on a macrovascular level but heterogeneous perfusion on a microvascular level, which can be detrimental for the tissues [1, 9, 10].

Delivering oxygen from the microvascular level to the cells occurs through two main mechanisms. The first is convective oxygen transport, which is dependent on the red blood cell velocity and the capacity of the red blood cell to carry oxygen. The second is diffusion, which is dependent on the pressure gradients between the red blood cell and the tissues and is inversely related to the distance between the capillary and the cell [11, 12]. With homogeneous capillary flow, tissues are steadily perfused in a continuous and equally distributed manner, allowing optimal exchange between the capillaries and the cells. During heterogeneous tissue perfusion the total amount of flow may be similar, but some parts closer to the capillaries are hyperperfused, while other cells further away receive less, resulting in suboptimal exchange and tissue dysfunction [1].

Methods of Assessing the Microcirculation

The study of the microcirculation has mainly been limited by technical difficulties. Major advances in the last two decades have permitted more rapid, easier and noninvasive assessment of microvascular beds of various organs with several different techniques. The microcirculation can be assessed morphologically by looking at the diameter or at the number of capillaries (capillary density (CD)), the appearance of capillaries or the integrity of the glycocalyx layer. Alternatively, one can assess microcirculatory perfusion by looking at red blood cell velocity in the microcirculation (microvascular flow index (MFI)) and/or heterogeneity of microvascular perfusion (heterogeneity index (HI)). Finally, the endothelial function in the microcirculation can be assessed by assessing the response to specific challenges such as drugs, flickering light, postischemic (occlusive) vasodilatation or thermal stimuli.

Which technique, site or parameter of microvascular assessment is most appropriate in a specific circumstance can be answered by addressing the four W questions.

Who: who is going to assess the microcirculation (e.g. a highly dedicated and skilled investigator for research purpose or a medical worker as part of routine clinical observations) and who is going to be assessed (e.g. a neonate or an adult, a patient with chronic rheumatologic disease or a patient with septic shock).

Why: why does one intend to assess morphology, perfusion or endothelial function (e.g. in order to understand pathophysiology or to monitor treatment).

Where: this refers to which microvascular bed is best assessed (e.g. sublingual, skin, nailfold, retina, gut, brain, vaginal mucosa) and in which setting (e.g. in a laboratory setting, outpatient clinic, at the bed side or during surgery).

When: when is one interested in single measurements, repeated intermitted or continuous measurements?

Video Capillaroscopy

Video capillaroscopy uses an intravital microscope coupled to a video camera to study the microcirculation in vivo [13–17]. The initial devices were quite bulky and cumbersome, limiting their use to research settings. Current video capillaroscopes are small hand-held devices that couple a microscope to a digital video camera [14, 16, 17]. They allow direct visualization of moving erythrocytes in the capillaries. The vessel wall is not visualized, and as such only perfused capillaries can be investigated. In the nailfold, capillaries run parallel to the skin and the technique can be used to assess the morphology of capillaries and estimate red cell velocities. It is used in rheumatic and skin conditions such as systemic sclerosis and Raynaud disease [15]. In the skin, the capillaries run perpendicular to the surface. They are observed as small red dots and the technique can merely be used to assess capillary density (basal capillary density (BCD)) and capillary recruitment (maximal capillary density (MCD)) after certain stimuli such as venous congestion, postocclusive reactive hyperemia and thermal challenges [17, 18]. Still, one has to bear in mind that skin perfusion is very heterogeneous and several sampling sites must be assessed and averaged in order to have reproducible measurements.

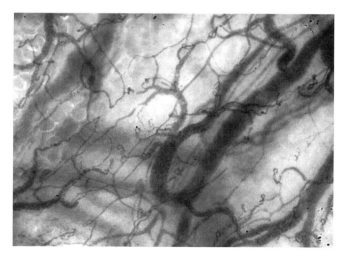

Figure 5.1 Snapshot image of IDF movie obtained from the sublingual microcirculation.

Orthogonal Polarization Spectral, Sidestream Dark Field Imaging and Incident Dark Field Imaging

These three types of hand-held videomicroscopes use green light (wave length of +- 530 nm),which penetrates the surfaces of organs to a depth of approximately 3 mm, to allow direct visualization of the superficial microcirculation. Green light of this wave length allows optimal absorption by hemoglobin in red blood cells. The surrounding tissues mostly reflect the light, which creates contrast. This is captured by a video camera, which allows visualization in high-contrast images of flowing red blood cells as little black moving targets in the superficial microcirculation (Figure 5.1). Here again the vessel walls are not visualized [19–22]. Depending on the size of the moving red blood cell column and the direction of flow, one can discern arterioles from capillaries and venules. Tissues with a thin epithelial layer are most easily studied. The sublingual mucosa is often used as it is easily accessible, located in close proximity to the brain and from the same embryologic origin as the gastrointestinal system, which is often substantially involved in the pathophysiology of conditions such as shock and sepsis [1, 10]. Nevertheless, other sites, such as the vaginal mucosa, cervix or skin, or the microcirculation of internal organs, such as bowel and brain during surgery, can be examined [23–27]. As such, these techniques allow immediate noninvasive visualization of the microcirculation at the bedside. They can be used in adults, children and even preterm neonates [28–30].

The recorded images need to be analyzed with specific software. These allow semiautomatic analysis and still require a substantial human input. Analysis is therefore often performed off-line and can be time consuming [31, 32]. Several aspects of the microvascular perfusion can be examined [4]. Vessels are divided according to their size into small (capillaries $\emptyset < 20\mu m$) and nonsmall vessels (arterioles and venules, $\emptyset$ 20–100 μm). For both groups vessel density (VD) and perfused vessel density (PVD) can be assessed. The MFI describes the predominant flow pattern with a semiquantitative score of 0–4 (0 =absent, 1 = intermittent, 2 = sluggish, 3 = normal, 4 = hyperdynamic flow) of both vessel types. The HI is an important parameter of microvascular tissue perfusion and is calculated from the MFI scores by subtracting the lowest score from the highest score divided by the mean score. The integrity of the glycocalyx can also be assessed with specific software by analyzing the dimensions of the red blood cell perfused boundary regions (PBR) [8, 33].

Usually 3–5 video clips are recorded and analyzed for the measurements. These are performed according to consensus recommendations of an international round table conference for standardization purposes, and the validation and reliability has been demonstrated in nonpregnant adults, pregnant women and neonates [29, 30, 34–37].

Orthogonal Polarization Spectral (OPS) (cytoscan cytometrics, Philadelphia, USA) was developed in the late 1990s and can be considered as the first generation of these hand-held video microscopes, which opened the field of bedside study of the superficial microcirculation [21, 22]. Further developments resulted in the second generation Sidestream Dark Field imaging technique (SDF) (MicroScan Video Microscope, MicroVision Medical, Amsterdam, the Netherlands), with improved image contrast and quality [20]. The mobility and ease of use at the bedside was improved by allowing battery depend operation. This device of approximatively 320 grams still contains an analogue video camera, necessitating conversion to digital images for time-consuming off-line analysis [29, 31, 32, 38].

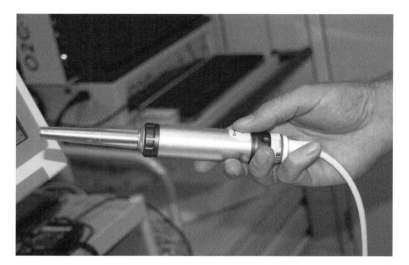

Figure 5.2 IDF probe. (A black and white version of this figure will appear in some formats. For the colour version, please refer to the plate section.)

Recently, a third-generation camera was developed using Incident Dark Field (IDF) illumination technique (cytocam Braedius medical, Huizen, the Netherlands) [19, 36] (Figure 5.2). It is the size of pen and weighs around 120 grams. Image quality was again substantially improved by the use of high-resolution optics, computer-controlled illumination units and a digital camera with computer-controlled high-resolution sensors. Image collection is further facilitated by a quantitative focus mechanism which determines and remembers an individual's characteristic focus depth for serial measurements.

The device also includes improved automatic-analysis software, which substantially quickens and facilitates analysis for several parameters and promises complete instant bedside analysis in the near future [19, 39]. This will permit the incorporation of microvascular as independent parameters for immediate clinical decision-making at the bedside.

Laser Doppler Imaging

With Laser Doppler Imaging, a beam of laser light is directed onto the skin with a wavelength that penetrates to a depth of approximatively 1 mm, and reflected light is measured. The principle is based on the wavelength change (Doppler shift) the light undergoes when hitting moving red blood cells in the superficial microcirculation of the dermis. This Doppler shift is related to the number and velocities of the blood cells. It provides an index of skin perfusion called flux, expressed in arbitrary units (AU), which is the product of average red blood cell velocity and concentration [13, 17, 40–43].

Initially, the technique was developed as laser Doppler flowmetry (LDF) or Laser Doppler perfusion monitoring (LDPM) assessing blood flow in a single area of less than 1 mm³. High sampling frequency allowed good temporal variability, making LDF interesting for the assessment of rapid changes in blood flow as a response to a stimulus [42]. Nevertheless, spatial variability and therefore reproducibility are limited due to the important heterogeneity in skin perfusion [44].

With Laser Doppler Imaging (LDI) or laser Doppler perfusion imaging (LDPI), all individuals' single measurement points are combined and a large area of interest is scanned by the laser beam (up to 50×50 cm^2) [13, 17, 44–47]. The backscattered light is analyzed and a 2-D color-coded image is created, with each pixel representing a perfusion value.

This overcomes the problem of spatial resolution and reproducibility encountered with LDF, but at the cost of reduced temporal resolution. As such, it cannot be used to assess rapid changes in microcirculatory perfusion. Nevertheless, recent developments in high-speed cameras, multichannel lasers and mapping algorithms permit much faster scanning [46, 47].

A recent technique is called laser speckle contrast imaging (LSCI) [48–50]. The laser light penetrates tissue to a depth of 300 μm and induces a phenomenon called laser speckle. This is the irregular backscattering pattern of the light created by irregularities in the tissue structure. This pattern is influenced by movements in the tissue, such as blood flow, creating a blurring of this pattern. Speckle contrast is a quantification of this blurring [45]. It allows instant scanning of larger areas, combining the advantages of LDF with LDPI, but measures a more superficial layer of the skin [51–53].

All these techniques are mostly used to assess microvascular skin reactivity to certain challenges, such as iontophoresis of vasoactive drugs, postocclusive reactive hyperemia and thermal challenges [17, 42–44, 54].

With iontophoresis a low-intensity current is used to deliver charged molecules into the dermis. Acetylcholine (Ach) and nitroprusside (SNP) are the most commonly used drugs, eliciting an endothelial-dependent and endothelial-independent vasodilatation respectively. In postocclusive reactive hyperemia, the increase in skin blood flow is analyzed after the relieve of a temporary arterial occlusion. Alternatively, the effect on skin perfusion of local heat or cold stimuli can also be analyzed. Nevertheless, the exact underlying biological mechanisms of all these reactions remain complex. As such, rather than specifically assessing distinct pathways, these tests merely reflect microvascular reactivity and function [17, 42–44]. Standardization remains essential in order to allow comparison between studies as many variables may influence the response and reproducibility of these tests.

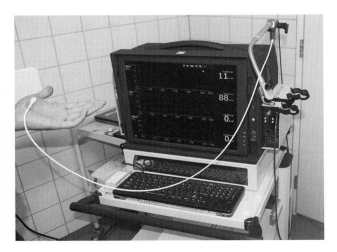

Figure 5.3 O2C monitoring device with glass fiber probe measuring microvascular perfusion on a hand palm. (A black and white version of this figure will appear in some formats. For the color version, please refer to the plate section.)

O2C

The O2C device (Lea Medizintechnik, Gießen, Germany) combines LDF with tissue spectrophotometry. It consists of a small glass fiber probe that can be attached to the skin, tongue or internal organs during surgery (Figure 5.3). The spectrophotometer transmits continuous wave laser light and white light into the tissue, and the reflected light is split into its spectral components by charge-coupled device array and converted into an electrical signal. It allows simultaneous, continuous (beat to beat) and operator-independent measurements of relative blood flow (in AU), blood flow velocity (in AU), capillary-venous oxygen saturation (in %, which reflects the oxygen reserve after extraction of oxygen by tissues) and relative amount of hemoglobin (in AU) in the microcirculation [55–60].

Retinal Vessel Analysis

With a nonmydriatic or mydriatic fundus camera retinal arterioles and venules can be noninvasively and directly visualized. Static imaging analysis of retinal vessels is the automatic measurement of the mean arteriolar and venular diameter, expressed as central retinal arteriolar equivalent (CRAE) and central retinal venular equivalent (CRVE) [61]. Therefore, the largest arterioles and venules within the superior temporal region are simply marked, using a Retinal Vessel Analyzer (e.g. RVA, Imedos, Jena, Germany; Figure 5.4). The superior temporal region represents a circular area of 0.5–2 disk diameters from the optic disc margin. As arteriolar constriction is often accompanied by venular dilatation, the arteriolar-to-venular ratio (AVR) is commonly used instead. Hence, a reduced AVR indicates arteriolar narrowing as a sign of hypertensive retinopathy, which is frequently seen in hypertension and even associated with 5-year incident-severe hypertension [62].

The dynamic behavior of retinal vessels can be solely assessed with a mydriatic fundus camera, which is part of the Dynamic Vessel Analyzer (e.g. DVA, Imedos, Jena, Germany; Figure 5.5)[63]. After 1% tropicamide administration to reach mydriasis, this device

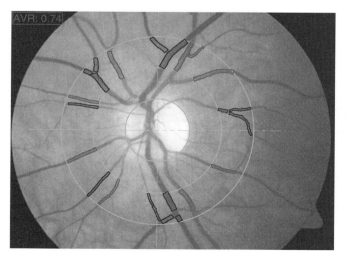

Figure 5.4 This retinal vessel imaging, recorded with a fundus camera (Retinal Vessel Analyzer, Imedos, Jena, Germany), demonstrates the direct measurement of retinal arterioles (red marks) and venules (blue marks) and the consequent automatic calculation of the mean arteriolar (CRAE) and venular (CRVE) diameter as well as the arteriolar-to-venular ratio (AVR). (A black and white version of this figure will appear in some formats. For the color version, please refer to the plate section.)

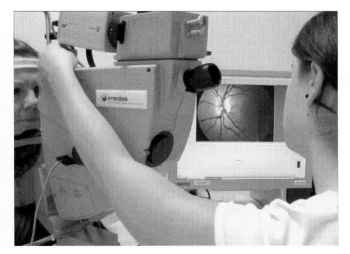

Figure 5.5 The static condition and dynamic behavior of the retinal microvasculature can be noninvasively visualized and analyzed with a fundus camera (Dynamic Retinal Vessel Analyzer, Imedos, Jena, Germany). (A black and white version of this figure will appear in some formats. For the color version, please refer to the plate section.)

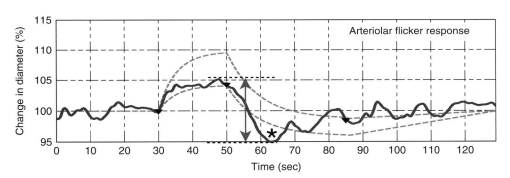

Figure 5.6 This sum curve of a dynamic retinal flicker analysis of a women with normal pregnancy outcome at 34 weeks gestation demonstrates the arteriolar flicker-induced dilatation (second black arrowhead), the physiologic maximum arteriolar constriction (asterisk) and the resulting arteriolar amplitude (blue double-headed arrow) along a normal distribution curve (dashed green lines). (A black and white version of this figure will appear in some formats. For the color version, please refer to the plate section.)

measures the arteriolar and venular diameter continuously, under the influence of flickering light stimulation. Retinal flicker response is a function of neurovascular coupling, caused by enhanced retinal ganglioneuronal activity, which primarily dilates capillaries. The secondary increase in blood flow thereby induces an NO-mediated dilatation of larger arterioles and venules, independently of perfusion pressure, with a physiological subsequent arteriolar constriction [64]. Therefore, the resulting sum curve of flicker analysis consists of a baseline diameter, flicker-induced dilatation (FID) and maximum arteriolar constriction component (MAC). The arteriolar amplitude is the percentage change from peak FID to MAC (Figure 5.6) [65]. Endothelium-dependent retinal flicker response, which includes FID and MAC, is impaired in chronic hypertension and aging, indicating pre-aged and stiffened retinal vessels with dysfunctional endothelium [66, 67].

Potential and Importance of Microvascular Measurements

With the recent developments of new techniques allowing direct visualization, the importance and potential of microvascular assessment for understanding the pathophysiology, predicting prognosis and directing therapy in conditions with hemodynamic imbalance is emerging. It is well known that macrocirculatory parameters such as cardiac output, blood pressure and filling pressures are poorly performing as predictors of outcome or endpoints for guiding therapy in conditions like sepsis and cardiac shock [68–71]. In pregnancy, discordance between macrovascular and microvascular parameters was demonstrated in women with severe preeclampsia, and changes in capillary perfusion were observed in women with HELLP syndrome [29, 72–74]. Parameters of microcirculatory perfusion are independently associated with outcome and can be better predictors of prognosis and response to treatment [10, 75–83]. Several experiments have shown that improving microcirculatory perfusion results in better outcome. If available at the bedside, microvascular assessment can become an important extension of conventional macrovascular hemodynamic monitoring in managing complex conditions with cardiovascular imbalance [11].

Even in normal pregnancy the cardiovascular system is severely challenged [84–86]. Most complications in pregnancy and causes of adverse maternal or fetal outcome, such as preeclampsia, growth restriction, cardiac disease, sepsis, diabetes, postpartum hemorrhage and thrombotic disease, result in or from substantial hemodynamic dysregulation and endothelial dysfunction, which suggests an involvement of the microcirculatory compartment [87–90]. Many of these complications are still poorly understood and major improvements are still to be achieved in their management. The advent of improved bedside techniques holds promise for research and clinical implication as it did in other conditions like sepsis and shock. Along with new noninvasive techniques for assessing macrocirculation and uteroplacental Dopplers, a concept of global fetomaternal hemodynamic monitoring or cardiovascular profiling can be developed to unravel many issues of these complex disease states [72].

As an example of the potential of microcirculatory assessment we will discuss fluid management, which is one of the most common therapeutic interventions performed in medicine for a variety of indications and disciplines, including obstetrics. In the literature, large scientific debates have been held on which type of fluid, either colloids or crystalloids, to use in case of shock [91–93]. However, on even more fundamental issues – such as when to start, how much to give and when to stop – for this common therapeutic act that is performed countless times on a daily base, one can hardly find any evidence or guidance. Clinical signs (e.g. hypotension, capillary refill test, decreased urinary production or consciousness), laboratory findings (lactate levels) and dynamic indices (CO, CVP, PCWP) are often arbitrary and do not offer information on how much to give and when to stop. The main goal of fluid management is to enhance oxygen delivery to the cells. As discussed previously, there are two main determinants of oxygen transport to the cells: convective transport and passive diffusion. The former is dependent on the red blood cell (RBC) velocity and oxygen-carrying capacity. Diffusion is dependent on the pressure gradient and inversely related to the distance between the RBC and the tissue. While colloids and crystalloids in themselves contain little components that might actually improve cellular function, they do so by increasing red cell velocity (thereby enhancing convective transport) and opening previously closed capillaries (thereby reducing diffusion distance between RBC and tissue). However, too much fluid will result in edema, which will increase diffusion distance. Despite increased perfusion this would lead to a reduction in cellular function. Finding the balance between knowing when to start and how much to give in order to improve tissue perfusion, but knowing when to stop before side effects prevail, can be helped by direct assessment of the microcirculation using OPS, SDF or IDF where convective transport is reflected by the MFI and the diffusion distance by functional capillary density (FCD). Fluid administration can be monitored and directed according to specific predefined MFI and FCD values. This concept is called functional microcirculatory hemodynamics [11, 12, 94].

The Microcirculation in Normal Pregnancy

Pregnancy is characterized by a major cardiovascular adaptation to meet the needs of growing a fetus. Early in pregnancy vascular resistance starts to fall and cardiac output rises. RBC mass is increased, but not as much as plasma volume, resulting in a physiologic hemodilution [84, 85]. In fact, perfusion of nearly all organs undergoes major changes. It is therefore likely that the microcirculatory compartment, which is the largest of the cardiovascular tree, is equally involved. Still, mainly due to technical limitations, very little is known about the microcirculation in normal pregnancy.

Using nailfold capillaroscopy two different groups showed a substantial increase in erythrocyte velocity during pregnancy and reduced vasodilatatory response after ischemia, which was attributed to the normal physiologic vasodilatation occurring in pregnancy [95, 96]. Recently, George et al. compared the sublingual microcirculatory perfusion between third-trimester healthy pregnant women and nonpregnant controls using SDF [97]. They found significant increase in MFI, reflecting increased RBC velocity. There were no changes in PVD. These values were similar to those of third-trimester healthy pregnant controls from another study assessing sublingual capillary perfusion in severe preeclamptic women, equally showing a PVD within normal nonpregnant reference ranges and a hyperdynamic capillary flow (MFI) [29]. Hasan et al. used intravital microscopy on the finger skin in 22 healthy pregnant women [98]. They initially showed an increase in BCD and MCD after venous congestion, reaching a peak at midgestation and mirroring a decrease in blood pressure. In a later study of 225 healthy primigravid Caucasian women, the same group using the same technique found opposite results with a reduction in BCD and MCD, but these changes also mirrored the rise in blood pressure with advancing gestation that was now observed in the population [99]. While these findings suggest that, as in other disease states, the microcirculation partly contributes to the regulation of blood pressure, it does not offer an explanation for the discrepancy in both microvascular and macrovascular findings between these two studies. Moreover, these findings of capillary rarefaction were not observed in the sublingual or nailfold microcirculation in other studies.

Knowledge about the effects of Ach and SNP challenges on microvascular forearm flow measured with laser Doppler during normal pregnancy is very limited, is mainly derived from small control groups and the results are not equivocal. Ramsay et al. found an increased dose-dependent vascular responsiveness to Ach and SNP during the third trimester as compared to several months postpartum [100]. Khan et al. observed a similar response for Ach but no difference for SNP [101]. In the same study there were no differences in vascular reactivity to Ach or SNP between 22–26 or 34 weeks of gestation, suggesting a steady increase in endothelium-dependent dilatation during normal pregnancy with return to normal values postpartum. The same group also showed an association between birth weight, augmentation index and endothelial function during pregnancy, suggesting microvascular involvement in the adaptation of the cardiovascular system to normal pregnancy [102]. Eneroth-Grimfors et al. could not find any difference between pregnant and nonpregnant woman, but they only used one charge stimulus and may not have reached a plateau level [103].

Physiological changes in the microcirculation can be visualized using static image analysis of retinal vessels, which provides insights into vascular tone and peripheral resistance. Similar to capillary density of the finger skin, the retinal arteriolar and venular diameter mirrored the fall and rise in blood pressure throughout pregnancy. The maximum retinal vascular diameter was reached at 19 weeks gestation, the nadir at delivery and baseline values at 6 months postpartum, which reflects a decreased vascular resistance at midgestation as one of the cardiovascular adaptations that occur during healthy pregnancy [104].

From this overview it is clear that knowledge about microvascular function in normal pregnancy is limited. There certainly is a necessity for further assessment in order to increase insights and to determine normal values as they are definitely different from the nonpregnant state. This would best be achieved longitudinally in a large population, preferably using the latest techniques and in conjunction with macrovascular hemodynamic parameters. We would suggest that this would be done using different techniques but in a standardized manner so as to allow comparison with other studies and/or with other health and disease states. We would also suggest assessing the microcirculation of several organ systems so as to discover which are most affected and which would best represent global microvascular function in pregnancy in future studies. Only when including the microcirculation within the concept of global fetomaternal hemodynamic profiling will we be able to better understand the complex cardiovascular adaptation to pregnancy and its disturbances that occur in many complications.

Key Points

- Capillary function is difficult to assess under in vivo conditions.
- Assessment of microvascular function is important to understand normal and abnormal blood supply to and drainage from tissues.
- Capillary and microvascular functions show important adaptations throughout normal pregnancy.

References

1. De Backer D, Ospina-Tascon G, Salgado D, Favory R, Creteur J, Vincent JL, Monitoring the microcirculation in the critically ill patient: current methods and future approaches. *Intensive Care Med*, 2010; **36** (11):1813–25.

2. Boron W, Boupaep E, *Medical Physiology, 2e Updated Edition.* 2012.

3. Sakai T, Hosoyamada Y, Are the precapillary sphincters and metarterioles universal components of the microcirculation? An historical review. *J Physiol Sci*, 2013; **63** (5):319–31.

4. De Backer D, Hollenberg S, Boerma C, et al. How to evaluate the microcirculation: report of a round table conference. *Crit Care*, 2007; **11**(5): R101.

5. Salmon, AH, Satchell SC, Endothelial glycocalyx dysfunction in disease: albuminuria and increased microvascular permeability. *J Pathol*, 2012;**226**(4): 562–74.

6. Woodcock, TE, Woodcock TM, Revised Starling equation and the glycocalyx model of transvascular fluid exchange: an improved paradigm for prescribing intravenous fluid therapy. *Br J Anaesth*, 2012;**108**(3):384–94.

7. Chappell, D, Jacob M, Role of the glycocalyx in fluid management: Small things matter. *Best Pract Res Clin Anaesthesiol*, 2014;**28**(3):227–34.

8. Donati, A, Damiani E, Domizi R, et al. Alteration of the sublingual microvascular glycocalyx in critically ill patients. *Microvasc Res*, 2013;**90**:86–9.

9. De Backer, D, Ortiz JA, Salgado D, Coupling microcirculation to systemic hemodynamics. *Curr Opin Crit Care*, 2010;**16**(3):250–4.

10. Trzeciak, S, Dellinger RP, Parrillo JE, et al. Early microcirculatory perfusion derangements in patients with severe sepsis and septic shock: relationship to hemodynamics, oxygen transport, and survival. *Ann Emerg Med*, 2007; **49**(1):88–98, 98 e1–2.

11. Ince, C, The rationale for microcirculatory guided fluid therapy. *Curr Opin Crit Care*, 2014; **20**(3):301–8.

12. Veenstra, G, Ince C, Boerma EC, Direct markers of organ perfusion to guide fluid therapy: when to start, when to stop. *Best Pract Res Clin Anaesthesiol*, 2014; **28**(3):217–26.

13. Allen, J, Howell K, Microvascular imaging: techniques and opportunities for clinical physiological measurements. *Physiol Meas*, 2014; **35**(7):R91–R141.

14. Grassi, W, De Angelis R, Capillaroscopy: questions and answers. *Clin Rheumatol*, 2007; **26**(12):2009–16.

15. Ingegnoli, F, Gualtierotti R, Lubatti C, et al. Nailfold capillary patterns in healthy subjects: a real issue in capillaroscopy. *Microvasc Res*, 2013;**90**:90–5.

16. Michoud, E, Poensin D, Carpentier PH, Digitized nailfold capillaroscopy. *Vasa*, 1994; **23**(1):35–42.

17. Roustit, M, Cracowski JL, Non-invasive assessment of skin microvascular function in humans: an insight into methods. *Microcirculation*, 2012;**19**(1):47–64.

18. Antonios, TF, Rattray FE, Singer DR, Markandu ND, Mortimer PS, MacGregor GA. Maximization of skin capillaries during intravital video-microscopy in essential hypertension: comparison between venous congestion, reactive hyperaemia and core heat load tests. *Clin Sci (Lond)*, 1999; **97**(4):523–8.

19. Aykut, G, Veenstra G, Scorcella C, Ince C, Boerma C. Cytocam-IDF (incident dark field illumination) imaging for bedside monitoring of the microcirculation. *Intensive Care Med Exp*, 2015; 3(1):40.

20. Goedhart, PT, Khalilzada M, Bezemer R, Merza J, Ince C. Sidestream Dark Field (SDF) imaging: a novel stroboscopic LED ring-based imaging modality for clinical assessment of the microcirculation. *Opt Express*, 2007;**15**(23):15101–14.

21. Groner, W, Winkelman JW, Harris AG, et al. Orthogonal polarization spectral imaging: a new method for study of the microcirculation. *Nat Med*, 1999;5(10):1209–12.

22. Mathura, KR, Vollebregt KC, Boer K, De Graaff JC, Ubbink DT, Ince C. Comparison of OPS imaging and conventional capillary microscopy to study the human microcirculation. *J Appl Physiol* (1985), 2001;**91**(1):74–8.

23. Lehmann, C, Abdo I, Kern H, et al. Clinical evaluation of the intestinal microcirculation using sidestream dark field imaging–recommendations of a round table meeting. *Clin Hemorheol Microcirc*, 2014;**57**(2):137–46.

24. Nilsson, J, Eriksson S, Blind PJ, Rissler P, Sturesson C. Microcirculation changes during liver resection–a clinical study. *Microvasc Res*, 2014;**94**:47–51.

25. Weber, MA, Milstein DM, Ince C, Oude Rengerink K, Roovers JP. Vaginal microcirculation: Non-invasive anatomical examination of the micro-vessel architecture, tortuosity and capillary density. *Neurourol Urodyn*, 2015;**34**(8), 723–9.

26. Weber, MA, Milstein DM, Ince C, Roovers JP. Is pelvic organ prolapse associated with altered microcirculation of the vaginal wall? *Neurourol Urodyn*, 2016; **35**(7):764–70.

27. Ijaz, S, Milstein DM, Ince C, Roovers JP. Impairment of hepatic microcirculation in fatty liver. *Microcirculation*, 2003; **10**(6): 447–56.

28. Abdo, I, Yang W, Winslet MC, Seifalian AM. Microcirculation in pregnancy. *Physiol Res*, 2014;**63** (4):395–408.

29. Cornette, J, Herzog E, Buijs EA, et al. Microcirculation in women with severe pre-eclampsia and HELLP syndrome: a case-control study. *BJOG*, 2014; **121**(3): 363–70.

30. Top, AP, Tasker RC, Ince C, The microcirculation of the critically ill pediatric patient. *Crit Care*, 2011; **15** (2):213.

31. Bezemer, R, Bartels SA, Bakker J, Ince C. Clinical review: Clinical imaging of the sublingual microcirculation in the critically ill–where do we stand? *Crit Care*, 2012; **16** (3):224.

32. Mik, EG, Johannes T, Fries M, Clinical microvascular monitoring: a bright future without a future? *Crit Care Med*, 2009;**37** (11):2980–1.

33. Lee, DH, Cornette J, Herzog E, Buijs EA. Deeper penetration of erythrocytes into the endothelial glycocalyx is associated with impaired microvascular perfusion. *PLoS One*, 2014. **9**(5): e96477.

34. Boerma, EC, Mathura KR, van der Voort PH, Spronk PE, Ince C. Quantifying bedside-derived imaging of microcirculatory abnormalities in septic patients: a prospective validation study. *Crit Care*, 2005;**9**(6):R601–6.

35. Hubble, SM, Kyte HL, Gooding K, Shore AC. Variability in sublingual microvessel density and flow measurements in healthy volunteers. *Microcirculation*, 2009;**16**(2):183–91.

36. van Elteren, HA, Ince C, Tibboel D, Reiss IK, de Jonge RC. Cutaneous microcirculation in preterm neonates: comparison between sidestream dark field (SDF) and incident dark field (IDF) imaging. *J Clin Monit Comput*, 2015; **16**(2): 183–91.

37. van den Berg, VJ, van Elteren HA, Buijs EA, et al. Reproducibility of microvascular vessel density analysis in Sidestream dark-field-derived images of healthy term newborns. *Microcirculation*, 2015;**22**(1):37–43.

38. Bezemer, R, Dobbe JG, Bartels SA, et al. Rapid automatic assessment of microvascular density in sidestream dark field images. *Med Biol Eng Comput*, 2011;**49**(11):1269–78.

39. Dobbe, JG, Streekstra GJ, Atasever B, van Zijlderveld R, Ince C. Measurement of functional microcirculatory geometry and velocity distributions using automated image analysis. *Med Biol Eng Comput*, 2008. **46**(7): 659–70.

40. Humeau, A, Steenbergen W, Nilsson H, Strömberg T.Laser Doppler perfusion monitoring and imaging: novel approaches. *Med Biol Eng Comput*, 2007;**45**(5):421–35.

41. Riva, C, Ross B, Benedek GB, Laser Doppler measurements of blood flow in capillary tubes and retinal arteries. *Invest Ophthalmol*, 1972;**11**(11):936–44.

42. Roustit, M, Blaise S, Millet C, Cracowski JL. Reproducibility and methodological issues of skin post-occlusive and thermal hyperemia assessed by single-point laser Doppler flowmetry. *Microvasc Res*, 2010;**79** (2):102–8.

43. Roustit, M, Cracowski JL, Assessment of endothelial and neurovascular function in human skin microcirculation. *Trends Pharmacol Sci*, 2013;**34**(7):373–84.

44. Cracowski, JL, Minson CT, Salvat-Melis M, Halliwill JR. Methodological issues in the assessment of skin microvascular endothelial function in humans. *Trends Pharmacol Sci*, 2006;**27** (9):503–8.

45. Eriksson, S, Nilsson J, Sturesson C, Non-invasive imaging of microcirculation: a technology review. *Med Devices (Auckl)*, 2014;**7**:445–52.

46. Leutenegger, M, Martin-Williams E, Harbi P, et al. Real-time full field laser Doppler imaging. *Biomed Opt Express*, 2011;**2**(6):1470–7.

47. Serov, A, Lasser T, High-speed laser Doppler perfusion imaging using an integrating CMOS image sensor. *Opt Express*, 2005;**13**(17):6416–28.

48. Briers, JD, Laser Doppler, speckle and related techniques for blood perfusion mapping and imaging. *Physiol Meas*, 2001;**22**(4):R35–66.

49. Forrester, KR, Tulip J, Leonard C, Stewart C, Bray RC. A laser speckle imaging technique for measuring tissue perfusion. *IEEE Trans Biomed Eng*, 2004;**51**(11):2074–84.

50. Mahe, G, Humeau-Heurtier A, Durand S, Leftheriotis G, Abraham P. Assessment of skin microvascular function and dysfunction with laser speckle contrast imaging. *Circ Cardiovasc Imaging*, 2012;**5**(1):155–63.

51. O'Doherty, J, McNamara P, Clancy NT, Enfield JG, Leahy MJ. Comparison of instruments for investigation of microcirculatory blood flow and red blood cell concentration. *J Biomed Opt*, 2009;**14**(3):034025.

52. Roustit, M, Millet C, Blaise S, Dufournet B, Cracowski JL. Excellent reproducibility of laser speckle contrast imaging to assess skin microvascular reactivity. *Microvasc Res*, 2010;**80**(3):505–11.

53. Tew, GA, Klonizakis M, Crank H, Briers JD, Hodges GJ. Comparison of laser speckle contrast imaging with laser Doppler for assessing microvascular function. *Microvasc Res*, 2011;**82**(3):326–32.

54. Cracowski, JL, Roustit M, Pharmacology of the human skin microcirculation. *Microvasc Res*, 2010;**80**(1):1.

55. Buise, MP, Ince C, Tilanus HW, Klein J, Gommers D, van Bommel J. The effect of nitroglycerin on microvascular perfusion and oxygenation during gastric tube reconstruction. *Anesth Analg*, 2005;**100**(4):1107–11.

56. Holzle, F, Loeffelbein DJ, Nolte D, Wolff KD. Free flap monitoring using simultaneous non-invasive laser Doppler flowmetry and tissue spectrophotometry. *J Craniomaxillofac Surg*, 2006;**34**(1):25–33.

57. Knobloch, K, Lichtenberg A, Pichlmaier M, et al. Microcirculation of the sternum following harvesting of the left internal mammary artery. *Thorac Cardiovasc Surg*, 2003;**51**(5):255–9.

58. Knobloch, K, Lichtenberg A, Pichlmaier M, Tomaszek S, Krug A, Haverich A. Palmar microcirculation after harvesting of the radial artery in coronary revascularization. *Ann Thorac Surg*, 2005;**79**(3):1026–30; discussion 1030.

59. Ladurner, R, Feilitzsch M, Steurer W, Coerper S, Königsrainer A, Beckert S. The impact of a micro-lightguide spectrophotometer on the intraoperative assessment of hepatic microcirculation: a pilot study. *Microvasc Res*, 2009;**77**(3):387–8.

60. Sommer, B, Berschin G, Sommer HM, Microcirculation Under an Elastic Bandage During Rest and Exercise – Preliminary Experience With the Laser-Doppler Spectrophotometry System O2C. *J Sports Sci Med*, 2013;**12**(3):414–21.

61. Nagel, E, Vilser W, Fink A, Riemer T. [Static vessel analysis in nonmydriatic and mydriatic images]. *Klin Monbl Augenheilkd*, 2007;**224**(5):411–6.

62. Smith, W, Wang JJ, Wong TY, et al. Retinal arteriolar narrowing is associated with 5-year incident severe hypertension: the Blue Mountains Eye Study. *Hypertension*, 2004;**44**(4):42–7.

63. Vilser, W, Nagel E, Lanzl I, Retinal Vessel Analysis–new possibilities. *Biomed Tech (Berl)*, 2002;**47** Suppl 1 Pt 2:682–5.

64. Lim, M, Sasongko MB, Ikram MK, et al. Systemic associations of dynamic retinal vessel analysis: a review of current literature. *Microcirculation*, 2013;**20**(3):257–68.

65. Brueckmann, A, Seeliger C, Lehmann T, Schleußner E, Schlembach D. Altered Retinal Flicker Response Indicates Microvascular Dysfunction in Women With Preeclampsia. *Hypertension*, 2015;**66**(4):900–5.

66. Kneser, M, Kohlmann T, Pokorny J, Tost F. Age related decline of microvascular regulation measured in healthy individuals by retinal dynamic vessel analysis. *Med Sci Monit*, 2009;**15**(8):CR436–41.

67. Pemp, B, Weigert G, Karl K, et al. Correlation of flicker-induced and flow-mediated vasodilatation in patients with endothelial dysfunction and healthy volunteers. *Diabetes Care*, 2009;**32**(8): 1536–41.

68. Cecconi, M, De Backer D, Antonelli M, et al. Consensus on circulatory shock and hemodynamic monitoring. Task force of the European Society of Intensive Care Medicine. *Intensive Care Med*, 2014;**40**(12):1795–815.

69. Hayes, MA,Timmins AC, Yau EH, Palazzo M, Hinds CJ, Watson D. Elevation of systemic oxygen delivery in the treatment of critically ill patients. *N Engl J Med*, 1994;**330**(24):1717–22.

70. ARISE Investigators; ANZICS Clinical Trials Group, Peake SL, et al. Goal-directed resuscitation for patients with early septic shock. *N Engl J Med*, 2014;**371**(16):1496–506.

71. ProCESS Investigators, Yealy DM, Kellum JA, et al. A randomized trial of protocol-based care for early septic shock. *N Engl J Med*, 2014;**370**(18):1683–93.

72. Cornette, J, Buijs EA, Duvekot JJ,et al. Haemodynamic effects of intravenous nicardipine in severe pre-eclamptic women with a hypertensive crisis. *Ultrasound Obstet Gynecol*, 2015;**47**(1): 89–95.

73. Perez-Barcena, J, Romay E, Llompart-Pou JA, et al. Direct observation during surgery shows preservation of cerebral microcirculation in patients with traumatic brain injury. *J Neurol Sci*, 2015;**353**(1–2):38–43.

74. Sarmento, SG, Santana EF, Campanharo FF, et al. Microcirculation Approach in HELLP Syndrome Complicated by Posterior Reversible Encephalopathy Syndrome and Massive Hepatic Infarction. *Case Rep Emerg Med*, 2014;**2014**:389680.

75. Ait-Oufella, H, Bourcier S, Lehoux S, Guidet B. Microcirculatory disorders during septic shock. *Curr Opin Crit Care*, 2015;**21**(4):271–5.

76. Ait-Oufella, H, Lemoinne S, Boelle PY, et al. Mottling score predicts survival in septic shock. *Intensive Care Med*, 2011;**37**(5):801–7.

77. Bateman, RM, Walley KR, Microvascular resuscitation as a therapeutic goal in severe sepsis. *Crit Care*, 2005;**9** Suppl 4:S27–32.

78. De Backer, D, Creteur J, Preiser JC, Dubois MJ, Vincent JL. Microvascular blood flow is altered in patients with sepsis. *Am J Respir Crit Care Med*, 2002;**166**(1):98–104.

79. De Backer, D, Donadello K, Sakr Y, et al. Microcirculatory alterations in patients with severe sepsis: impact of time of assessment and relationship with outcome. *Crit Care Med*, 2013;**41**(3):791–9.

80. Donati, A, Domizi R, Damiani E, Adrario E, Pelaia P, Ince C. From macrohemodynamic to the microcirculation. *Crit Care Res Pract*, 2013;**2013**:892710.

81. Donati, A, Tibboel D, Ince C. Towards integrative physiological monitoring of the critically ill: from cardiovascular to microcirculatory and cellular function monitoring at the bedside. *Crit Care*, 2013;**17** Suppl 1: S5.

82. Sakr, Y, Dubois MJ, De Backer D, Creteur J, Vincent JL. Persistent microcirculatory alterations are associated with organ failure and death in patients with septic shock. *Crit Care Med*, 2004;**32**(9):1825–31.

83. Top, AP, Ince C, de Meij N, van Dijk M, Tibboel D. Persistent low microcirculatory vessel density in nonsurvivors of sepsis in pediatric intensive care. *Crit Care Med*, 2011;**39**(1):8–13.

84. Cornette, J, Roos-Hesselink J. *Normal cardiovascular adaptation to pregnancy*, in *Evidence-Based Cardiology Consult*, K. Stergiopoulos, Editor. 2014, Springer: London. 423–32.

85. Duvekot, JJ, Peeters LL, Maternal cardiovascular hemodynamic adaptation to pregnancy. *Obstet Gynecol Surv*, 1994;**49**(12 Suppl):S1–14.

86. Melchiorre, K, Sharma R, Thilaganathan B, Cardiac structure and function in normal pregnancy. *Curr Opin Obstet Gynecol*, 2012;**24**(6):413–21.

87. Cantwell, R, Clutton-Brock T, Cooper G. Saving Mothers' Lives: Reviewing maternal deaths to make motherhood safer: 2006–2008. The Eighth Report of the Confidential Enquiries into Maternal Deaths in the United Kingdom. *BJOG*, 2011;**118** Suppl 1:1–203.

88. de Jonge, A, Mesman JA, Manniën J. Severe adverse maternal outcomes among women in midwife-led versus obstetrician-led care at the onset of labour in the Netherlands: A nationwide cohort study. *PLoS One*, 2015;**10**(5):e0126266.

89. Schutte, JM, Steegers EA, Schuitemaker NW. Rise in maternal mortality in the Netherlands. *BJOG*, 2010;**117**(4):399–406.

90. van Roosmalen, J, Zwart J, Severe acute maternal morbidity in high-income countries. *Best Pract Res Clin Obstet Gynaecol*, 2009;**23**(3):297–304.

91. Perel, P, Roberts I, Colloids versus crystalloids for fluid resuscitation in critically ill patients. *Cochrane Database Syst Rev*, 2012;**6**:CD000567.

92. Santry, HP, Alam HB, Fluid resuscitation: past, present, and the future. *Shock*, 2010;**33**(3):229–41.

93. Smorenberg, A, Ince C, Groeneveld AJ, Dose and type of crystalloid fluid therapy in adult hospitalized patients. *Perioper Med (Lond)*, 2013;**2**(1):17.

94. Pranskunas, A, Koopmans M, Koetsier PM, Pilvinis V, Boerma EC. Microcirculatory blood flow as a tool to select ICU patients eligible for fluid therapy. *Intensive Care Med*, 2013;**39**(4):612–9.

95. Linder, HR, Reinhart WH, Hänggi W, Katz M, Schneider H. Peripheral capillaroscopic findings and blood rheology during normal pregnancy. *Eur J Obstet Gynecol Reprod Biol*, 1995;**58**(2):141–5.

96. Ohlmann, P, Jung F, Mrowietz C, Alt T, Alt S, Schmidt W. Peripheral microcirculation during pregnancy and in women with pregnancy induced hypertension. *Clin Hemorheol Microcirc*, 2001;**24**(3):183–91.

97. George, RB, Munro A, Abdo I, McKeen DM, Lehmann C. An observational assessment of the sublingual microcirculation of pregnant and non-pregnant women. *Int J Obstet Anesth*, 2014;**23**(1):23–8.

98. Hasan, KM, Manyonda IT, Ng FS, Singer DR, Antonios TF. Skin capillary density changes in normal pregnancy and pre-eclampsia. *J Hypertens*, 2002;**20**(12):2439–43.

99. Nama, V, Antonios TF, Onwude J, Manyonda IT. Capillary remodeling in normal pregnancy: Can it mediate the progressive but reversible rise in blood pressure? Novel insights into cardiovascular adaptation in pregnancy. *Pregnancy Hypertens*, 2012;**2**(4): 380–6.

100. Ramsay, JE, Simms RJ, Ferrell WR, et al. Enhancement of endothelial function by pregnancy: inadequate response in women with type 1 diabetes. *Diabetes Care*, 2003;**26**(2):475–9.

101. Khan, F, Belch JJ, MacLeod M, Mires G. Changes in endothelial function precede the clinical disease in women in whom preeclampsia develops. *Hypertension*, 2005;**46**(5):1123–8.

102. Khan, F, Mires G, Macleod M, Belch JJ, et al. Relationship between maternal arterial wave reflection, microvascular function and fetal growth in normal pregnancy. *Microcirculation*, 2010;**17**(8):608–14.

103. Eneroth-Grimfors, E, Lindblad LE, Westgren M, Ihrman-Sandahl C, Bevegård S. Noninvasive test of microvascular endothelial function in normal and hypertensive pregnancies. *Br J Obstet Gynaecol*, 1993;**100**(5):469–71.

104. Lupton, SJ, Chiu CL, Hodgson LA, et al. Changes in retinal microvascular caliber precede the clinical onset of preeclampsia. *Hypertension*, 2013;**62**(5):899–904.

Plasma Volume Changes in Pregnancy

Marc E. A. Spaanderman and Anneleen S. Staelens

Summary

Under healthy conditions, only one-third of the plasma volume is located in the arterial compartment, whereas the remainder is located in the venous compartment to balance increased arterial demands. In normotensive formerly preeclamptic women, about half have low plasma volume, a condition paralleled by reduced venous compliance, blunted responsiveness to orthostatic stress and consistently higher sympathetic tone. Low plasma volume therefore seems to represent reduced venous reserve capacity. Functionally, prepregnancy low plasma volume predisposes to early-pregnancy circulatory maladaptation; clinically, it relates to increased risk on recurrent hypertensive disease, growth restriction and preterm birth. Modulation of the plasma volume compartment may therefore reduce the risk of recurrent gestational hypertensive sequellae in women with prepregnancy reduced plasma volume.

Introduction

The circulatory requirements rapidly increase early in pregnancy and onwards. Cardiac output rises, in absence of increased whole-body resting energy expenditure, as early as 5 weeks gestational age, most likely as the result of the opening of protective microcirculatory arteriovenous shunts and with it a tremendous drop in total peripheral vascular resistance [1]. Studies are mostly done in rodents and isolated vessels, who display comparable adaptation to pregnancy as humans, suggest that the most likely driver of this opening along with the later gestational hemodynamic adjustments seems to be endocrine, originating from the ovary, leading to vasodilation by upregulating endothelium-dependent NO pathway, decreasing responsiveness to vasoconstrictor stimuli, reducing myogenic reactivity and increasing arterial compliance [2–30] As observed in human early pregnancy, as a consequence of the early-pregnancy sudden drop in peripheral vascular resistance, arterial blood pressure drops, which, in turn, activates numerous compensatory mechanisms to balance the sudden reduction in cardiac afterload; sympathetic tone increases, heart rate and stroke volume rises, the volume-retaining renin–angiotensin–aldosterone system increases and venous tone increases to compensate for the reduced after load, until plasma volume has been restored and venous fullness, instead of tone, warrants preload [31, 32]. Mostly, the initial drop in peripheral vascular resistance can easily be balanced as unstressed venous circulatory volume, the virtual amount of blood not actively hemodynamically participating to meet the arterial demands, is large enough to compensate for the sudden loss of arterial filling, and, with it, pressure. It is generally thought that, in case of shallow venous reserves, problems in initial circulatory adaptation may arise, which, in turn, prelude to later clinical overt maternal hypertensive disease and fetal growth restriction (Figure 6.1).

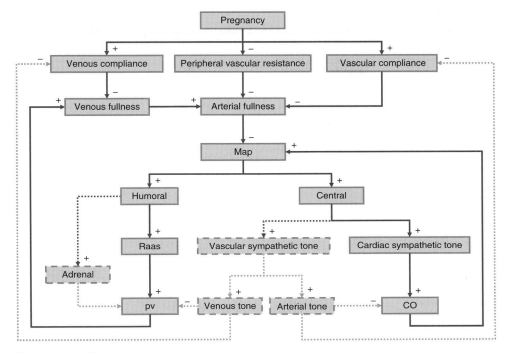

Figure 6.1 Initial first-trimester circulatory changes
Early pregnancy is characterized by a sudden drop in total peripheral vascular resistance, most likely as a consequence of hormonally driven opening of microcirculatory protective arteriovenous shunts, along with a rise in arterial and venous vascular compliance. As a consequence, cardiac afterload falls and blood pressure drops. The loss in arterial pressure initiates a cascade of compensating central autonomic and humoral changes, consisting of a rise in cardiac and vascular sympathetic tone, activation of the renin–angiotensin–aldosterone system (RAAS) and rise in adrenergic hormones (adrenal). The initial fall in afterload is balanced by turning unstressed venous volume into stressed arterial volume. The loss in venous reserve is counterbalanced by renin–angiotensin–aldosterone driven increase in plasma volume (PV), which in turn can be stored in the larger venous compartment, as venous compliance also increases (and atrial natriuretic peptide (ANP) indicating relative or absolute venous overfill does not rise). Moreover, the modest drop in mean arterial blood pressure (MAP) is compensated by baroreceptor-mediated rise in cardiac sympathetic tone raising cardiac output (CO) and restoring blood pressure at a lower set-point. If the gestational fall in afterload leads to substantial circulatory stress, when the hemodynamic system is more sensitive to vessel tone increasing stimuli or when the venous system is too shallow to accommodate the increased circulatory volume system, all of these relate to first-trimester circulatory maladaptation, affecting venous compliance and plasma volume expansion and with it restoration of adequate venous reserve capacity on the one hand, and arterial compliance and with it detrimental vascular shear stress as flow increases.
The dashed lines indicate circulatory responses associated with hemodynamic maladaptation when persistently present, whereas the solid lines represent normal gestational circulatory reactions.

Plasma Volume Largely Reflects Venous Reserves

Under healthy conditions, about two-thirds of the plasma volume is located in the venous compartment and functions as readily available buffer to compensate for continuous changes in arterial demands. In correspondence to early pregnancy, increased arterial needs are paralleled by arterial vasodilation and consequently venous unstressed stored blood will be directed toward the arterial system to compensate for the loss in arterial fullness. As all of our biological functions directly depend on the arterial perfusion capacity

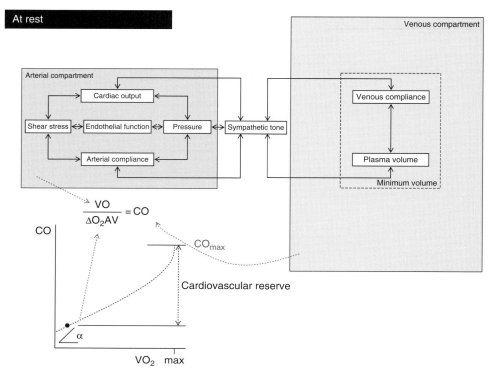

Figure 6.2 Plasma volume largely determines maximum oxygen uptake (VO$_2$ max)
At rest, about two-thirds of the plasma volume is localized at the venous compartment and serves as a readily available buffer to compensate for fluctuations in arterial demands. Both plasma volume and venous compliance determine the size of the venous compartment. As only part of the volume is needed as preload to deliver cardiac output (stressed volume), the remainder can be viewed as unstressed volume indicating the venous reserves. The autonomic system is able, by modulation of venous tone and plasma volume, to direct venous blood to the arterial compartment and vice versa. On the arterial side, the autonomic system exerts its regulation by modulation of flow (cardiac output), arterial compliance and blood pressure. These variables, in turn, affect endothelial shear stress and endothelial function. The arterial compartment requires flow-dependent deliverance of oxygen (VO2) to function, but microcirculatory oxygen extraction possibilities and efficiency do not, as indicated by the arteriovenous oxygen difference (ΔO2 AV). Oxygen uptake divided by effective oxygen extraction (ΔO2 AV) indicates cardiac output. During exercise the arterial needs increase, and while flow-dependent oxygen delivery rises to its maximum (VO2 max), heart rate (HR) and stroke volume increase until heart rate exceeds the threshold where ventricle filling time is too short to further increase stroke volume. VO2max is not affected by pregnancy [52]. During pregnancy, if the vital cardiovascular reserve capacity must be maintained throughout gestation, plasma volume must increase to allow maximum cardiac output to increase, compensating for the continuous increased resting cardiac output in order to remain maternal cardiovascular reserve.

in order to deliver oxygen and nutrients and to drain carbon dioxide and waste, at comparable arterial demands, shallow plasma volume most likely does not reflect arterial underfilling but reduced venous reserves (Figure 6.2).

In normotensive formerly preeclamptic women, under unstressed and unaffected conditions, in more than half of cases plasma volume is reduced [33]. Theoretically, reduced plasma volume could reflect arterial or venous underfilling. Based on numerous findings, reduced venous fullness instead of reduced arterial filling is most likely: on the one hand, during the early follicular phase, directly after the menstrual period, when

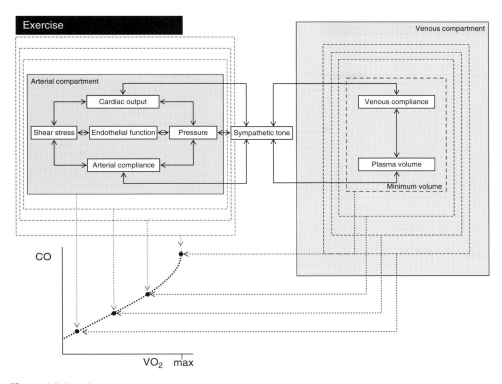

Figure 6.2 (cont.)

women can be considered at baseline hemodynamic condition since sex hormonal state affecting the circulation is comparable, women with low plasma volume do not display neuro-humoral alterations such as elevated renin, angiotensin and aldosterone levels or higher levels in epinephrine or norepinephrine [31, 32, 34, 35]. On the other hand, not only venous compliance is reduced in women with low plasma volume, but also the dynamic capacity to increase venous tone during orthostatic challenges and the static capacitance to hold extra-added venous fluid without increasing venous pressure and with it cardiac preload support the view of low plasma volume reflecting reduced venous reserve capacity [36, 37, 38].

What is the Origin of Low Plasma Volume?

But why is plasma volume low in these formerly preeclamptic women? On the one hand, in line with the Barker hypothesis, the venous compartment can be constitutionally smaller, affecting both capacity and capacitance. Recent observations detail the linear effect of birth weight on plasma volume in which multivariable analyses show that birth weight accounts for 14% of total adult plasma volume [39]. Human studies on venous functions related to the fetal origins of adult system biology are lacking. On the other hand, venous function can be reduced by functional changes through secondary increased sympathetic tone or increased autonomic sensitivity influencing capacity and, with it, increased smooth muscle contraction

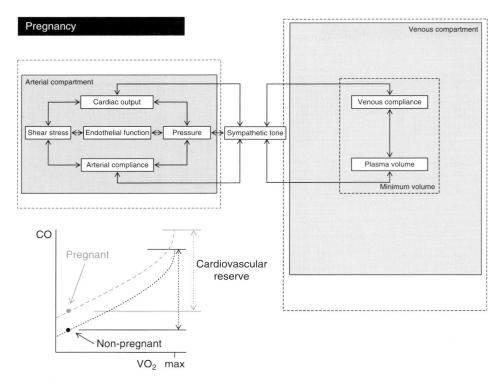

Figure 6.2 (cont.)

and later secondary increased muscle and collagen mass – the latter two primarily affecting capacitance. As stated, low plasma volume not only correlates with reduced venous compliance, it also relates to increased sympathetic tone and reduced venous capacitance. Moreover, the venous responsiveness to head up tilt is decreased in women with low plasma volume [37, 38, 40, 41]. These observations suggest at least an interrelated role for sympathetic dominance and low plasma volume. Whether or not the venous wall mass has gained increased stiffness through increased muscular or connective tissue remains to be elucidated. Finally, in theory, increased tone could also originate from reduced venous endothelial function. Recent observations not only indicate reduced arterial endothelial function in formerly preeclamptic women in the first year after birth, exercise proved capable of normalizing endothelial function toward that found in sedentary healthy parous women. Whether or not this observation can also extend to the venous endothelium is not known. The effects of modulation of the plasma volume compartment from healthy individuals, for instance by exercise known to affect hemodynamic as well as autonomic function, or more targeted interventions, such as central acting sympaticolytic agents, may shed light on the question of why the plasma volume is low [42, 43]. Although recent data support the view that exercise modulates sympathetic tone, arterial endothelial function and plasma volume, the clinical effects of these hemodynamic and autonomic improvements on the outcome of subsequent pregnancy must be awaited in women with chronically low plasma volume [40–43].

But Why Should We Bother About Plasma Volume?

Women with a history of preeclampsia are at increased risk for recurrent gestational hypertensive disease. More than half of these women have low plasma volume at follow-up in the first year after birth [33, 35]. Functionally, prepregnancy low plasma volume predisposes for subsequent early pregnancy circulatory maladaptation.[31] In this case, in response to the volume-retaining stimulus of early pregnancy, these women increase their plasma volume without increasing venous compliance. Meanwhile, atrial natriuretic peptide (ANP) rises – a rise, which in turn correlates with blunted plasma volume expansion. These data suggest venous overfill in early pregnancy. Apparently, the increased plasma volume cannot be accommodated in the venous compartment, leading to increased cardiac preload and with it the observed rise in ANP. Clinically, the lower the prepregnancy plasma volume, the higher the risk on recurrent gestational hypertensive disease, from about 1 in 20 in formerly preeclamptic women in the highest plasma volume quartile (corresponding normal plasma volume as observed in healthy parous controls) to 1 in 3 formerly preeclamptic women in the lowest plasma volume quartile [46]. Moreover, the size of the plasma volume is related to preterm birth and birth weight centile in these women. Therefore, even though the related recurrence rate varies between 1/20 and 1/3, knowing the plasma volume may be helpful in assessing personalized recurrence risks and severity of the situation when pursuing pregnancy. Lifestyle changes, such as exercise, have proven plasma-volume modulatory properties [40, 41, 42, 43]. Physical training before and during pregnancy may reduce the risk of preeclampsia [44, 45]. Since lifestyle changes lead to improved prepregnancy hemodynamic and autonomic function, it may be that in formerly preeclamptic women the resulting change in plasma volume relates to a corresponding change in recurrence risk. If so, knowing the person's plasma volume could also affect the type of advice given to these individuals.

Plasma Volume Changes Throughout Gestation

Plasma volume rapidly increases during human pregnancy (Figure 6.3). At the end of the third trimester, as compared to the nonpregnant condition, plasma volume has increased by about 14%, corresponding to a change from 2.45L to 2.63L, rising up to 20% (2.93L) at midgestation and 44% (3.51L) early in the third trimester, reaching its maximum expansion, over 50% (3.66L), after 36 weeks gestational age, irrespective of later maternal hypertensive complications or fetal growth restriction [48, 49, 50]. In the latter two subgroups, wherein the pregnancies are complicated by maternal or fetal placental syndrome, plasma volume is consistently lower throughout the course of gestation, long before these clinical problems manifest.[48] After pregnancy, plasma volume restores to normal in about 3 months.

In summary, under healthy conditions, about two-thirds of the plasma volume is located in the venous compartment. The venous compartment compensates for increased arterial demands. As such it represents the circulatory reserves. In formerly preeclamptic women, in absence of arterial signs of underfilling, about half have low plasma volume. Along with reduced venous compliance, responsiveness to orthostatic challenges, and increased sympathetic tone, low plasma volume seems to represent reduced venous reserve capacity. Functionally, prepregnancy low plasma volume relates to circulatory maladaptation; clinically, it relates to increased risk on recurrent hypertensive disease, growth restriction, and preterm birth. Modulation of the plasma volume compartment may therefore reduce the risk of recurrent gestational hypertensive sequellae.

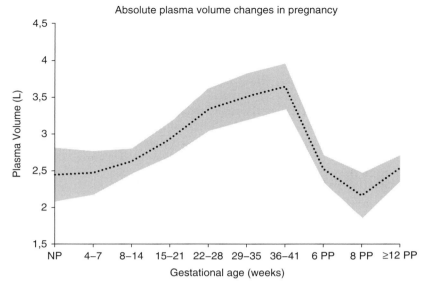

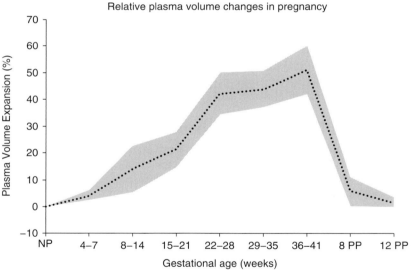

Figure 6.3 Absolute and relative changes in plasma volume throughout healthy gestation
Plasma volume increases steadily throughout gestation. When comparing changes, including studies which reported besides the observed plasma volume in pregnancy and also the prepregnancy, postpregnancy (≥6weeks), or nonpregnant companion, weighing sample size in the comparison, plasma volume reaches its maximum expansion late in the third trimester. Displayed relative changes slightly differ from absolute changes (weighted mean and SD), as for the latter only studies reporting nonindexed total plasma volumes could be included.
Pivarnik JM et al. Gynecol. 1994;83(2):265–9. Whittaker PG et al. Br J Obstet Gynaecol. 1993;100(6):587–92. Salas SP et al. Obstet Gynecol. 1993;81(6):1029–33. Brown MA et al. J Hypertens. 1992;10(1):61–8. Olufemi OS et al. Clin Sci (Lond). 1991;81(2):161–8. Abudu OO et al. Journal of the National Medical Association. 1988;80(8):906–12. Di Lieto A et al. Clinical and Experimental Hypertension – Part B Hypertension in Pregnancy. 1988;7(1–2):89–97. Abudu OO et al. Int J Gynaecol Obstet. 1985;23(2):137–42. Raman L et al. Indian J Med Res. 1985 Dec;82:528–33. Rajalakshmi K et al. Indian J Med Res. 1985;82:521–7. Hunyor SN et al. Hypertension. 1984;6(6 Pt 2):III129-32. Hunyor SN et al. Clin Exp Pharmacol Physiol. 1982;9(3):315–20. Gibson HM. J Obstet Gynaecol Br Commonw. 1973;80(12):1067–74. Pirani BB et al. J Obstet Gynaecol Br Commonw. 1973;80(10):884–7. Blekta M et al. Am J Obstet Gynecol. 1970;106(1):10–3. Honger PE. Scand J Clin Lab Invest. 1968;21(1):3–9. Retief FP et al. J Obstet Gynaecol Br Commonw. 1967;74(5): 683–93. Brody S et al. Acta Obstet Gynecol Scand. 1967;46(2):138–50. Bruinse HW et al. Eur J Obstet Gynecol Reprod Biol. 1985;20(4):215–9.

Key Points

- Plasma volume relates closely to function of the venous system.
- Normal plasma volume is important for cardiovascular functional integrity. Therefore, it is important to explore validated methods for plasma volume measurement.
- It is well known that plasma volume changes dramatically during pregnancy, and these changes are important if not mandatory for a normal gestational outcome.

References

1. Spaanderman ME, Meertens M, van Bussel M, Ekhart THA, Peeters LLH. The cardiac output increases independent of basal metabolic rate in early human pregnancy. *Am J Physiol* 2000;**278**:H1585–H1588.

2. Hermsteiner M, Zoltan DR, Doetsch J, Rascher W, Kuenzel W. Human chorionic gonadotropin dilates uterine and mesenteric resistance arteries in pregnant and nonpregnant rats. *Pflugers Arch* 1999;**439**(1–2):186–94.

3. Crandall ME, Keve TM, McLaughlin MK. Characterization of norepinephrine sensitivity in the maternal splanchnic circulation during pregnancy. *Am J Obstet Gynecol* 1990 May;**162**(5):1296–301.

4. Hermsteiner M, Zoltan DR, Doetsch J, Rascher W, Kuenzel W. Human chorionic gonadotropin dilates uterine and mesenteric resistance arteries in pregnant and nonpregnant rats. *Pflugers Arch* 1999;**439**(1–2):186–94.

5. Hermsteiner M, Zoltan DR, Kunzel W. The vasoconstrictor response of uterine and mesenteric resistance arteries is differentially altered in the course of pregnancy. *Eur J Obstet Gynecol Reprod Biol* 2001 Dec 10;**100**(1):29–35.

6. McLaughlin MK, Keve TM. Pregnancy-induced changes in resistance blood vessels. *Am J Obstet Gynecol* 1986 Dec;**155**(6):1296–9.

7. Parent A, St-Louis J, Schiffrin EL. Vascular effects of bradykinin and sodium nitroprusside during pregnancy in the rat. *Clin Exp Hypertens B* 1989;**8**(3):561–82.

8. Ren Y, Garvin JL, Liu R, Carretero OA. Cross-talk between arterioles and tubules in the kidney. *Pediatr Nephrol* 2009 Jan;**24**(1):31–5.

9. Baylis C, Davison JM. The Urinary System. In: Chamberlain G, Broughton Pipkin F, editors. *Clinical Physiology in Obstetrics*. Third edn. Oxford, UK: Blackwell Science; 1998. pp. 263–307.

10. Novak J, Danielson LA, Kerchner LJ, et al. Relaxin is essential for renal vasodilation during pregnancy in conscious rats. *J Clin Invest* 2001 Jun;**107**(11):1469–75.

11. Magness RR, Rosenfeld CR. Local and systemic estradiol-17 beta: effects on uterine and systemic vasodilation. *Am J Physiol* 1989 Apr;**256**(4 Pt 1):E536–E542.

12. Vacca G, Battaglia A, Grossini E, Mary DA, Molinari C, Surico N. The effect of 17beta-oestradiol on regional blood flow in anaesthetized pigs. *J Physiol* 1999 Feb 1;**514**(Pt 3):875–84.

13. Byers MJ, Zangl A, Phernetton TM, Lopez G, Chen DB, Magness RR. Endothelial vasodilator production by ovine uterine and systemic arteries: ovarian steroid and pregnancy control of ERalpha and ERbeta levels. *J Physiol* 2005;**565**(Pt 1).

14. Liao WX, Magness RR, Chen DB. Expression of estrogen receptors-alpha and -beta in the pregnant ovine uterine artery endothelial cells in vivo and in vitro. *Biol Reprod* 2005 Mar;**72**(3):530–7.

15. Rosenfeld CR, Cox BE, Roy T, Magness RR. Nitric oxide contributes to estrogen-induced vasodilation of the ovine uterine circulation. *J Clin Invest* 1996 Nov 1;**98**(9):2158–66.

16. Rosenfeld CR, Roy T, Cox BE. Mechanisms modulating estrogen-induced uterine vasodilation. *Vascul Pharmacol* 2002Feb;**38**(2):115–25.

17. Chang K, Lubo Z. Review article: steroid hormones and uterine vascular adaptation to pregnancy. *Reprod Sci* 2008 Apr;**15**(4):336–48.

18. Rupnow HL, Phernetton TM, Shaw CE, Modrick ML, Bird IM, Magness RR. Endothelial vasodilator production by uterine and systemic arteries. VII. Estrogen and progesterone effects on eNOS. *Am J Physiol Heart Circ Physiol* 2001 Apr;**280**(4):H1699–H1705.

19. Chen DB, Jia S, King AG, Barker A, Li SM, Mata-Greenwood E, et al. Global protein expression profiling underlines reciprocal regulation of caveolin 1 and endothelial nitric oxide synthase expression in ovariectomized sheep uterine artery by estrogen/progesterone replacement therapy. *Biol Reprod* 2006 May;**74**(5):832–8.

20. Ford SP. Control of blood flow to the gravid uterus of domestic livestock species. *J Anim Sci* 1995 Jun;**73**(6):1852–60.

21. Anderson SG, Hackshaw BT, Still JG, Greiss FC, Jr. Uterine blood flow and its distribution after chronic estrogen and progesterone administration. *Am J Obstet Gynecol* 1977 Jan 15;**127**(2):138–42.

22. Ezimokhai M, Osman N, Agarwal M. Human chorionic gonadotrophin is an endothelium-independent inhibitor of rat aortic smooth muscle contractility. *Am J Hypertens* 2000 Jan;13(**1** Pt 1):66–73.

23. Chesley LC, Talledo E, Bohler CS, Zuspan FP. Vascular Reactivity to Angiotensin II and Norepinephrine in Pregnant Woman. *Am J Obstet Gynecol* 1965 Mar 15;**91**:837–42.

24. Sladek SM, Magness RR, Conrad KP. Nitric oxide and pregnancy. *Am J Physiol* 1997 Feb;**272**(2 Pt 2):R441–R463.

25. Baylis C, Davison JM. The Urinary System. In: *Clinical Physiology in Obstetrics* (Third edn.), edited by Chamberlain G and Broughton Pipkin F. Oxford, UK: Blackwell Science, 1998, pp. 263–307.

26. Chesley LC, Talledo E, Bohler CS, Zuspan FP. Vascular Reactivity to Angiotensin II and Norepinephrine in Pregnant Woman. *Am J Obstet Gynecol* **91**:837–42, 1965.

27. McLaughlin MK, Keve TM. Pregnancy-induced changes in resistance blood vessels. *Am J Obstet Gynecol* **155**: 1986.

28. Sladek SM, Magness RR, Conrad KP. Nitric oxide and pregnancy. *Am J Physiol* **272**: R441–R463, 1997.

29. Slangen BF, Out IC, Verkeste CM, Peeters LL. Hemodynamic changes in early pregnancy in chronically instrumented, conscious rats. *Am J Physiol* **270**: H1779–H1784, 1996.

30. Van Eijndhoven HWF, Slangen BFM, van der Heijden OWH, Aardenburg R, Spaanderman ME, Peeters LLH. Hemodynamic changes in pseudopregnancy in chronically instrumented, conscious rats are preserved after hysterectomy. *Pflugers Arch.* 2002;**443**:427–31.

31. Spaanderman ME, Ekhart THA, van Eyck J, de Leeuw PW, Peeters LLH. Preeclampsia and maladaptation to pregnancy: a role for natriuretic peptide? *Kidney Int.* 2001;**60**:1397–406.

32. Spaanderman ME, Willekes C, Hoeks APG, Ekhart THA, Peeters LLH. The effect of pregnancy on the compliance of large arteries and veins in normal parous controls and formerly preeclamptic women. *Am J Obstet Gynecol* 2000:**183**;1278–86.

33. Scholten RR, Hopman MT, Sweep FC, et al. Co-occurrence of cardiovascular and prothrombotic risk factors in women with a history of preeclampsia. *Obstet Gynecol.* 2013 Jan;**121**(1):97–105.

34. Spaanderman ME, van Beek E, Ekhart THA, et al. Changes in hemodynamics and volume homeostasis with the menstrual cycle, in women with a history of preeclamsia. *Am J Obstet Gynecol* 2000;**182**:1127–34.

35. Spaanderman ME, Ekhart THA, van Eyck J, Cheriex EC, de Leeuw PW, Peeters LLH. Asymptomatic formerly preeclamptic women have latent

hemodynamic abnormalities. *Am J Obstet Gynecol* 2000:**182**;101–107.

36. Aardenburg R, Spaanderman ME, Courtar DA, van Eijndhoven HW, de Leeuw PW, Peeters LL. A subnormal plasma volume in formerly preeclamptic women is associated with a low venous capacitance. *J Soc Gynecol Investig.* 2005 Feb;**12**(2):107–11.

37. Krabbendam I, Janssen BJ, Van Dijk AP, et al. The relation between venous reserve capacity and low plasma volume. *Reprod Sci.* 2008;**15**(6):604–12.

38. Krabbendam I, Jacobs LC, Lotgering FK, Spaanderman ME. Venous response to orthostatic stress. *Am J Physiol Heart Circ Physiol.* 2008;**295**(4):H1587–93.

39. Scholten RR, Oyen WJ, Van der Vlugt MJ, et al. Impaired fetal growth and low plasma volume in adult life. *Obstet Gynecol.* 2011 Dec;**118**(6):1314–22.

40. Scholten RR, Thijssen DJ, Lotgering FK, Hopman MT, Spaanderman ME. Cardiovascular effects of aerobic exercise training in formerly preeclamptic women and healthy parous control subjects. *Am J Obstet Gynecol.* 2014 Apr 23. pii: S0002-9378(14)00385-8.

41. Scholten RR, Spaanderman ME, Green DJ, Hopman MT, Thijssen DH. Retrograde shear rate in formerly preeclamptic and healthy parous women before and after exercise training: relationship with endothelial function. *Am J Physiol Heart Circ Physiol.* 2014 Jun 6. pii: ajpheart.00128.2014.

42. Convertino VA. Blood volume: its adaptation to endurance training. *Med Sci Sports Exerc* 1991 December;**23**(12):1338–48.

43. Mueller PJ. Exercise training attenuates increases in lumbar sympathetic nerve activity produced by stimulation of the rostral ventrolateral medulla. *J Appl Physiol* 2007 February;**102**(2):803–13.

44. Rudra CB, Williams MA, Lee IM, Miller RS, Sorensen TK. Perceived exertion during prepregnancy physical activity and preeclampsia risk. *Med Sci Sports Exerc* 2005 November;**37**(11):1836–41.

45. Sorensen TK, Williams MA, Lee IM, Dashow EE, Thompson ML, Luthy DA. Recreational physical activity during pregnancy and risk of preeclampsia. *Hypertension* 2003 June;**41**(6):1273–80.

46. Scholten RR, Sep S, Peeters L, Hopman MT, Lotgering FK, Spaanderman ME. Prepregnancy low-plasma volume and predisposition to preeclampsia and fetal growth restriction. *Obstet Gynecol.* 2011 May;**117**(5):1085–93.

47. Bernstein IM, Ziegler W, Badger GJ. Plasma volume expansion in early pregnancy. *Obstet Gynecol.* 2001 May;**97**(5 Pt 1):669–72.

48. Salas SP, Marshall G, Gutierrez BL, Rosso P. Time course of maternal plasma volume and hormonal changes in women with preeclampsia or fetal growth restriction. *Hypertension.* 2006 Feb;**47**(2):203–8.

49. Hytten FE, Paintin DB. Increase in plasma volume during normal pregnancy. *J Obstet Gynaecol Br Emp.* 1963 Jun;**70**:402–7.

50. Pirani BB, Campbell DM, MacGillivray I. Plasma volume in normal first pregnancy. *J Obstet Gynaecol Br Commonw.* 1973 Oct;**80**(10):884–7.

51. Lopes van Balen VA, Spaan JJ, Ghossein C, van Kuijk SM, Spaanderman ME, Peeters LL. Early pregnancy circulatory adaptation and recurrent hypertensive disease: an explorative study. *Reprod Sci.* 2013 Sep;**20**(9):1069–74.

52. Lotgering FK, Struijk PC, van Doorn MB, Wallenburg HC. Errors in predicting maximal oxygen consumption in pregnant women. *J Appl Physiol* (1985). 1992 Feb;**72**(2):562–7.

Chapter 7

Arterial Function in Pathological Pregnancies

Asma Khalil and Silvia Salvi

Summary

Women undergo a variety of physiological cardiovascular adaptations in normal pregnancy, in order to support the development of the fetoplacental unit. Marked changes from the nonpregnant state can be seen from as early as 6 weeks of gestation. Women who develop pathological pregnancies, such as preeclampsia, fetal growth restriction, preterm birth and diabetes, have increased arterial stiffness in the form of elevated pulse wave velocity, augmentation index and central blood pressure. Some of these changes can be detected as early as 11 weeks' gestation, and some persist in the postpartum period. These women also have increased cardiovascular morbidity and mortality later in life. In fact, they might have cardiovascular predisposition even before the complicated pregnancy. The lack of the improved arterial compliance, which occurs in normal pregnancy, seems to play a critical role in the changes observed in these pathological pregnancies. Therefore, evaluating arterial function may play an important role not only in identifying women at higher risk of developing complications during pregnancy, but also those at highest risk of cardiovascular disorders later in life.

Arterial Function in Pathological Pregnancies

Arterial adaptation plays a critical role in the hemodynamic changes observed in normal pregnancy [1]. A compliant arterial system and normal arterial function are essential for optimization of the cardiovascular performance during pregnancy [2]. Moreover, the parameters reflecting arterial function have recently attracted attention since they have been shown to be independent predictors of cardiovascular morbidity. The pathologies of pregnancy which will be outlined in this chapter include hypertensive disorders in pregnancy, fetal growth restriction, diabetes and preterm birth.

Changes in Arterial Function in Hypertensive Disorders in Pregnancy

It is well established that women who develop hypertensive complications during pregnancy, such as preeclampsia, have a significantly greater risk of developing cardiovascular disease later in life, with a hazard ratio as high as 5.4 for women with severe preeclampsia/eclampsia [3]. Hypertensive disorders of pregnancy are not only significant causes of maternal and perinatal morbidity and mortality but are also risk factors for long-term cardiovascular mortality and morbidity. Women who develop hypertensive disorders during pregnancy are considered to have failed the cardiovascular "stress test" of pregnancy and therefore represent a cohort of women that deserve long-term cardiovascular monitoring and prevention. Because of this significant risk to the woman's health, the challenge for the

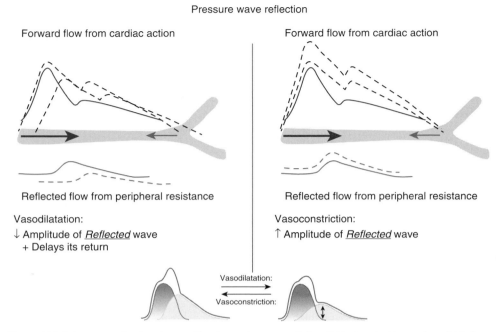

Pressure wave reflection

Forward flow from cardiac action

Forward flow from cardiac action

Reflected flow from peripheral resistance

Reflected flow from peripheral resistance

Vasodilatation:
↓ Amplitude of *Reflected* wave
+ Delays its return

Vasoconstriction:
↑ Amplitude of *Reflected* wave

Vasodilatation:

Vasoconstriction:

Figure 7.1 Pulse wave reflections in vasodilatation and vasoconstriction. (A black and white version of this figure will appear in some formats. For the color version, please refer to the plate section.)

near future is cardiovascular risk stratification, the aim of which is to identify the highest-risk women, for whom developing strategies for prevention and treatment is of utmost importance. Increased arterial stiffness is a recognized marker of future risk found in women who develop hypertensive disorders in pregnancy [4].

In pregnancies complicated by preeclampsia, there is an absence or loss of the normal adaptive mechanisms of pregnancy: increased arterial stiffness with reduced arterial compliance, with diffuse vasoconstriction and increased peripheral vascular resistance arising from the endothelial dysfunction [5]. The arteriolar tone (as measured by the total vascular resistance), which is the traditional measure of arterial load, is increased. Moreover, the large conduit arteries are globally affected. All the parameters describing the arterial stiffness and peripheral vasoconstriction in preeclamptic women have been found to differ significantly from normal pregnancies.

Women with preeclampsia had not only significantly higher total vascular resistance, but also reduced arterial compliance and elevated aortic impedance than the women with normal pregnancies. Total systemic vascular resistance incompletely characterizes arterial load because it does not take into account the pulsatile nature of aortic flow. Both the arterial compliance, as a measure of the vascular wall stiffness, and the aortic impedance, as an index of the elastic properties of the central arteries, are affected in preeclamptic patients (Figures 7.1 and 7.2) [6]. Hale et al. explored the relationship between arterial compliance before pregnancy and the risk of developing hypertensive disorders during pregnancy [7]. The Cardiac Output/Pulse Pressure (CO/PP) ratio has been used by these authors as an index of arterial compliance. A significant decrease in CO/PP ratio prior to pregnancy was

Pressure Wave Reflection

Forward flow from cardiac action

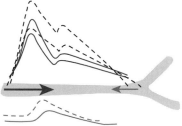

Stiff Aorta:
↑ Amplitude of _Incident_ wave
High amplitude _Reflected_
wave returns eariler

Reflected flow from peripheral resistance

Figure 7.2 Pulse wave reflections in pathological conditions with stiff aorta. (A black and white version of this figure will appear in some formats. For the color version, please refer to the plate section.)

found in women who subsequently developed hypertensive disorders, which suggests the existence of a predisposing phenotype. Using a different index (the ratio of stroke index to PP) as a measure of arterial compliance, women with preeclampsia demonstrated lower arterial compliance than those with uncomplicated pregnancies [1]. The reduced global arterial compliance is consistent with a generalized increase in vascular wall stiffness [8]. Moreover, the aortic impedance to pulsatile inflow from the contracting ventricle determines the aortic capacity to store a transient increase in blood volume. The higher value of aortic impedance observed in preeclamptic patients indicates that the elastic properties of the central arteries are impaired. It is also noteworthy that these parameters are virtually unchanged at 6 months postpartum [4].

In a systematic review which combined data from 23 studies evaluating the effect of preeclampsia on arterial stiffness, women with preeclampsia had elevated arterial stiffness both during and after pregnancy, and to a greater extent than in gestational hypertension (GH) [9]. Preeclampsia was associated with a 1 m/s increase in the carotid-femoral pulse wave velocity (cfPWV) and a 15% increase in augmentation index (AIx) [9]. This systematic review also demonstrated that more severe preeclampsia is associated with greater arterial stiffness. Robb et al. demonstrated that the cfPWV and AIx were raised in women with preeclampsia during and after pregnancy [10]. At 7 weeks postpartum, they both remained elevated, despite blood pressure returning to baseline. Estensen et al. showed that the systemic arteries of women with preeclampsia are significantly stiffer than those of healthy women at term; moreover, this phenomenon persisted at 6 months postpartum [4]. Mersich et al. found stiffness index to be significantly higher in preeclamptic women as compared to normotensive controls during the third trimester and up to 3 months postpartum [11]. Moreover, we have assessed the potential value of arterial stiffness at 11–13 weeks' gestation in predicting later preeclampsia and found that a screening test based on a combination of maternal variables, namely central aortic systolic blood pressure (SBP Ao), AIx and PWV, can identify women who subsequently develop preeclampsia with a detection rate of 57% at a false-positive rate of 10% [12]. Compared with women who remain normotensive, those who develop preeclampsia have greater arterial stiffness and higher SBP Ao, which are evident from the first trimester of pregnancy. Our findings have demonstrated that the mechanism of preeclampsia in these women was not mediated solely by impaired placental perfusion and function [12]. These findings support the concept that preeclampsia may be the common phenotypic expression of two distinct processes. One is based on a predisposition to cardiovascular disease that, under the physiological stress of pregnancy,

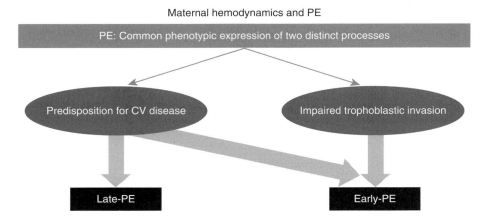

Figure 7.3 Proposed theory of the pathophysiology of preeclampsia

manifests as either early or late preeclampsia. The other results in early preeclampsia as a consequence of impaired trophoblastic invasion of the maternal spiral arteries (Figure 7.3). In a longitudinal study in women identified as being at high risk for pre-eclampsia following first-trimester screening, the maternal arterial function was assessed every 4 weeks. AIx, PWV and SBPAo were significantly higher from an early stage in pregnancy in women who developed preterm preeclampsia, compared to the normal group, with the difference from normal in AIx and PWV increasing, but that for SBPAo not changing with gestational age. In the term preeclampsia group, AIx, PWV and SBPAo did not differ significantly from those in the normotensive group. In GH, SBPAo was higher, but AIx and PWV did not significantly differ from those values in the normotensive group [13]. These results from longitudinal studies and the temporal relationship between the changes in arterial stiffness and the onset of preeclampsia suggest the possibility that arterial stiffness indices may have the potential to be used to predict the pregnancy outcome [12].

The finding of increased arterial stiffness in preeclampsia is in line with studies evaluating the PP and flow-mediated dilatation (FMD). Peripheral PP, a valuable surrogate measurement of arterial stiffness, is higher in women with preeclampsia [14]. An elevated PP during the first trimester is also associated with an increased risk of preeclampsia in nulliparous women [15]. Hale et al. found that PP was significantly higher in women who went on to develop preeclampsia [7]. This finding is of particular interest as PP has been used as an indicator of cardiovascular risk independent of pregnancy. PP has been commonly used as a measure of cardiovascular risk as it is often elevated prior to adverse cardiovascular events. PP is an indicator of blood vessel elasticity, where increased PP is a reflection of a stiffer vessel that exhibits reduced arterial compliance; so an increased PP is not only a marker of greater arterial stiffness but also an established cardiovascular risk marker. Studies examining FMD in preeclampsia have focused on three time periods, as follows: prior to disease (10–29 weeks), during preeclampsia and postpartum (2 weeks to 11 years) [16]. Interestingly, a lower FMD is demonstrated not only at the time of diagnosis but also in the first and second trimesters among high-risk women who subsequently developed preeclampsia [16–18]. Most studies suggest that FMD remains lower for up to 3 years postpartum in women who had preeclampsia [19, 20]. However, some researchers have reported that FMD increases by 4–6 weeks postpartum in women who had preeclampsia, suggesting a partial reversal of the endothelial dysfunction observed at diagnosis [21, 22]. The presence and magnitude of the effect may depend on the disease severity [16].

Among women who develop preeclampsia, arterial stiffness may also be used to stratify the severity of the disease: more severe preeclampsia seems to be associated with greater arterial stiffness [5, 9, 23, 24]. This is consistent with the findings in women with pre-eclampsia and GH. Two cross-sectional studies and one longitudinal study confirmed higher values of the arterial stiffness parameters (cfPWV, AIx) in preeclampsia patients when compared to pregnancies complicated by GH [23, 25]. However, FMD did not differ among women with mild and severe preeclampsia [21]. Evidence for differences in the vascular structures and functions between early and late-onset preeclampsia is highlighted by the study of Stergiotou et al.: late preeclampsia was characterized by a less pronounced increase in arterial stiffness as compared to early preeclampsia [26].

Arterial stiffness has been also investigated in women with a past history of preeclampsia. In formerly preeclamptic women, all of the indices of arterial elasticity and compliance are found to be reduced, indicating a longlasting vascular dysfunction. Hausvater et al. identified seven cross-sectional studies exploring whether a history of preeclampsia can cause lasting damage to the maternal vasculature; they showed increased arterial stiffness and decreased arterial compliance in women with a history of preeclampsia [9]. In their longitudinal study of pregnant women with a history of preeclampsia, Spaanderman et al. measured arterial compliance during weeks 5 and 7 of their second gestation. Their study demonstrated a failure of the normal increase in vascular compliance in women with a history of preeclampsia [27].

Several different mechanisms may contribute to the increased arterial stiffness found in preeclampsia: inflammation, oxidative stress and changes in the renin-angiotensin-aldosterone system are all contributors to the pathogenesis of preeclampsia and are all involved in determining arterial stiffness. What remains unclear is whether arterial stiffness is implicated in the pathogenesis of hypertensive complications of pregnancy or is simply a marker of an increased cardiovascular risk [2]. The increased arterial stiffness could simply be a marker of the pathological derangements that result in hypertensive complications of pregnancy or may promote the endothelial dysfunction and vascular damage, which in turn trigger the cascade that culminates in preeclampsia. Nevertheless, the increased arterial stiffness has multiple adverse circulatory effects based on an earlier return of the arterial pressure waveform. The arterial pressure waveform created by left ventricle ejection is known to be reflected back at branching or discontinuity of arteries and to combine with the forward arterial pressure waveform (Figures 7.1 and 7.2). As an artery stiffens, the PWV increases so that the returning (reflected) pulse wave meets the advancing wave during systole instead of during diastole. This increases the end-systolic stress on the left ventricle, amplifies systolic pressure and may impair coronary perfusion. Then, in preeclampsia, the elevated arterial stiffness may increase the load on the heart together with increased peripheral resistance and even predispose to structural changes, such as left ventricular hypertrophy. In a recent study, the heart of preeclamptic patients showed functional and structural changes as an adaptation to increased afterload, increased left ventricular mass, and left ventricular end-diastolic and end-systolic volumes [28]. Since increased arterial stiffness might also impair coronary perfusion, it further increases the deleterious impact of the hemodynamic changes in preeclampsia on the heart.

In summary, in preeclamptic patients, diffuse pathological arterial function is demonstrated by high PP and PWV, low arterial compliance and altered arterial stiffness. All of these features might be partly due to a physiological reaction to the high blood pressure [1]. However, in chronic hypertensive pregnancies, despite the significantly higher blood pressure values compared to uncomplicated pregnancies, the arterial stiffness is not as altered as in preeclampsia. The difference in arterial stiffness between preeclamptic and chronic hypertensive pregnancies could be explained by the exceptional properties of the arterial wall arising from the endothelial dysfunction in preeclampsia. In preeclampsia the endothelial dysfunction may impair vascular smooth muscle relaxation, enhancing arterial stiffness. On the other hand, endothelial dysfunction plays a role in the development of atherosclerosis and then in the development of the cardiovascular disease. Endothelial dysfunction may be the most plausible common link between the pathophysiology of preeclampsia and future cardiovascular disease in these women [16].

Changes in the Arterial Function in Pregnancies Complicated by Fetal Growth Restriction

The validity of any possible association between abnormal arterial function and fetal growth restriction is hampered firstly by the lack of distinction between fetal growth restriction with or without preeclampsia, and secondly by the lack of clarity around the difference between fetal growth restriction (FGR) and simply small for gestational age (SGA).

In pregnant women with chronic hypertension who subsequently develop both superimposed preeclampsia and fetal growth restriction, central systolic pressure (CSP), AIx, AIx-75, and the brachial systolic and PP measured at 26–32 weeks of gestation are all higher than those who did not develop superimposed preeclampsia or FGR [29]. In fact, AIx-75 was the only significant determinant of birth weight, even after adjusting for brachial systolic pressure, maternal height, smoking status, gestational age at testing and the presence of antihypertensive treatment at testing in a regression model [29]. The relation between arterial stiffness and FGR is further supported by the fact that AIx-75 was the only significantly elevated hemodynamic parameter in patients who developed fetal growth restriction but not superimposed preeclampsia. However, CSP was significantly elevated in the pregnancies complicated by superimposed preeclampsia but not fetal growth restriction.

One study compared women with SGA fetuses with and without preeclampsia [30]. Data gathered prospectively in the first trimester demonstrated high uterine artery pulsatility index (UAPI) and low-serum-pregnancy-associated plasma protein A (PAPP-A) in both groups in the first trimester. However, AIx, while normal in women with normotensive SGA pregnancies, was elevated in women who later presented with preeclampsia and SGA fetuses. Another study found no difference between the two groups in pulse wave velocity (PWV) [5]. Although this study did not discriminate between SGA and FGR fetuses, the difference suggests that the combination of impaired placentation (as evidenced by the high UAPI and low PAPP-A) and maternal vascular health (as evidenced by the high AIx) is what determines the phenotype of presentation in later pregnancy. In women with abnormal placentation, those with normal AIx may have sufficient cardiovascular reserve to avoid preeclampsia but women with raised AIx (indicating pre-existing endothelial dysfunction) are more likely to present with both preeclampsia and FGR. This model has previously been proposed, and a number of maternal factors have been identified that could cause endothelial dysfunction and interact with impaired placentation to produce preeclampsia [31]. These include insulin resistance, hyperlipidemia and disorders of coagulation. An alternative theory is that pre-existing maternal endothelial dysfunction may cause impaired placentation which then later presents with preeclampsia, whereas impaired placentation in otherwise healthy women produces only fetal effects.

A study using FMD to measure arterial stiffness in postnatal women demonstrated a persistent difference between women with pregnancies affected by FGR and those with appropriate-for-gestational-age (AGA) fetuses, whether hypertensive or not [32]. This difference was not seen when comparing glyceryl trinitrate (GTN) responsiveness between the two groups; this suggests that endothelial dysfunction (rather than vascular smooth muscle dysfunction) is the primary pathology. It is not possible to ascertain from this study whether the vascular dysfunction predated pregnancy in only the preeclamptic patients. Nor does it tell us how long these changes will persist in normotensive women affected by FGR, but the findings of Khalil et al. would suggest that this similarity in vascular resistance does not exist in the first trimester until the endothelial damage associated with FGR is triggered [30].

Changes in Arterial Function in Pregnancies Complicated by Preterm Birth

Preterm birth (PTB), which is the leading cause of perinatal mortality and morbidity, is also associated with an increased risk of maternal long-term cardiovascular disease and early death [33]. In a large screening study involving more than 7,000 singleton pregnancies where assessment of the arterial function was performed at 11–13 weeks' gestation, arterial stiffness and SBPAo were significantly increased if the PTB was iatrogenic but not if it was spontaneous. These findings were similar in women who experienced PTB at <37 weeks and at <34 weeks. Therefore, we hypothesized that the previously noted association between PTB and subsequent cardiovascular disorders is likely to be related to those who had iatrogenic delivery mainly for preeclampsia and FGR [34]. In this respect, the early delivery was a marker of the severity of this pre-existing pathology rather than a cause or co-pathology. This is further supported by the evidence that arterial stiffness correlates with the severity of preeclampsia, and is higher in early than late-onset preeclampsia. However, most studies reporting on the association between PTB and increased cardiovascular susceptibility failed to distinguish between iatrogenic and spontaneous delivery.

Changes in Arterial Function in Pregnancies Complicated by Gestational Diabetes

In nonpregnant individuals with impaired glucose tolerance and type 2 diabetes, SBPAo and arterial stiffness are raised [35]. Diabetes mellitus is associated with an increased risk of cardiovascular mortality and morbidity [36]. Elevated SBPAo and arterial stiffness in patients with diabetes mellitus is associated with this cardiovascular risk, suggesting its potential role as a predictive/prognostic marker in this population [37].

More than 60% of women with gestational diabetes mellitus (GDM) develop type 2 diabetes within the following 15 years. Both SBPAo and arterial stiffness are higher in women with established GDM and in those with pre-existing type 2, but not type 1, diabetes mellitus [38, 39]. The possible mechanisms for increased SBPAo and arterial stiffness in patients with established diabetes and those who develop GDM include alterations in the composition of the extracellular matrix and arterial remodeling due to hyperglycemia, advanced glycation end products, hyperinsulinemia, oxidative stress, chronic low-grade inflammation and endothelial dysfunction. Additionally, diabetes is associated with reduced nitric oxide production and increased homocysteine levels, which are strongly associated with increased arterial stiffness.

Furthermore, women who develop GDM have increased SBPAo and arterial stiffness, evident from the first trimester of pregnancy, suggesting its potential predictive value [40]. This observation provides further support for the proposal that pregnancy could be viewed as a stress test which unmasks diabetes and other medical conditions, such as hypertension, in women who are predisposed and have preclinical risk factors for these conditions. The mechanism linking abnormal vascular markers and GDM may be analogous to hypertensive disorders, in which women destined to develop cardiovascular disease in their 40s or 50s often present with preeclampsia in their 20s or 30s.

Conclusion

The lack of the expected arterial adaptation which occurs in normal pregnancy seems to play a critical role in the changes observed in pathological pregnancies. Therefore, evaluating arterial function may play an important role not only in identifying women at higher risk of developing complications during pregnancy, but also those at highest risk of cardiovascular disorders later in life.

Key Points

- Women who develop pathological pregnancies, such as preeclampsia, fetal growth restriction, preterm birth and diabetes, have increased arterial stiffness as compared to those who have uncomplicated pregnancies.
- Some of these maladaptive changes can be detected as early as 11 weeks' gestation.
- Women who show persistent arterial stiffness in postpartum have increased cardiovascular morbidity and mortality later in life.

References

1. Tihtonen KMH, Koobi T, Uotila JT. Arterial stiffness in preeclamptic and chronic hypertensive pregnancies. *Eur J Obstet Gynecol Reprod Biol.* 2006;**128**: 180–6.

2. Coutinho T. Arterial stiffness and its clinical implications in women. *Can J Cardiol* 2014; **30**:756–64.

3. McDonald SD, Malinowski A ZQ, Yusuf S, Dvereaux PJ. Cardiovascular sequelae of preeclampsia/eclampsia: a systematic review and meta-analyses. *Am Heart J* 2008,**156**:918–30.

4. Estensen ME, Remme EW, Grindheim G, Smiseth OA, Segers P, Henriksen T., Aakhus S. Increased arterial stiffness in pre-eclamptic pregnancy at term and early and late postpartum: a combined echocardiographic and tonometric study. *Am J Hypertens.* 2013;**26**:549–56.

5. Spasojevic M SS, Morris JM. Gallery ED: Peripheral arterial pulse wave analysis in women with pre-eclampsia and gestational hypertension. *BJOG* 2005;**112**: 1475–8.

6. Tomsin K, Mesens T, Molenberghs G, Peeters L, Gyselaers W. Characteristics of heart, arteries, and veins in low and high cardiac output preeclampsia. *Eur J Obstet Gynecol Reprod Biol.* 2013;**169**:218–22.

7. Hale S, Choate M, Schonberg A, Shapiro R, Badger G, Bernstein IM. Pulse pressure and arterial compliance prior to pregnancy and the development of complicated hypertension during pregnancy. *Reprod Sci.* 2010;**17**:871–7.

8. Hibbard JU, Korcarz CE, Nendaz GG, Lindheimer MD, Lang RM, Shroff SG. The arterial system in pre-eclampsia and chronic hypertension with superimposed pre. *BJOG* 2005;**112**:897–903.

9. Hausvater A GT, Sandoval Y-HG, Doonan RJ, et al. The association between preeclampsia and arterial stiffness. *J Hypertens* 2012;**30**: 17–33.

10. Robb AO, Mills NL, Din JN, Smith IB, Paterson F, Newby DE, Denison FC. Influence of the menstrual cycle, pregnancy, and preeclampsia on arterial stiffness. *Hypertension* 2009;**53**:952–8.

11. Mersich B, Rig OJ, Z LE, Studinger P, Visontai Z, Kollai M. Carotid artery stiffening does not explain baroreflex impairment in pre-eclampsia. *Clinical science* 2004;**107**: 407–13.

12. Khalil A, Akolekar R, Syngelaki A, Elkhouli M, Nicolaides KH. Maternal hemodynamics at 11–13 weeks' gestation and risk of pre-eclampsia. *Ultrasound Obstet Gynecol* 2012;**40**:28–34.

13. Khalil A, Garcia-Mandujano R, Maiz N, Elkhouli M, Nicolaides KH. Longitudinal changes in maternal hemodynamics in a population at risk for pre-eclampsia. *Ultrasound Obstet Gynecol* 2014;**44**:197–204.

14. Kaihura C, Savvidou MD, Anderson JM, McEniery CM, Nicolaides KH. Maternal arterial stiffness in pregnancies affected by preeclampsia. *Am J Physiol Heart Circ Physiol.* 2009;**297**:H759–64

15. Thadhani R EJ, Kettyle E, Sandler L, Frigoletto F. Pulse pressure and risk of preeclampsia: a prospective study. *Obstet Gynecol* 2001;**97**:515–20.

16. Weissgerber TL. Flow-mediated dilation: can new approaches provide greater mechanistic insight into vascular dysfunction in preeclampsia and other diseases? *Current hypertension reports* 2014;**16**: 487.

17. Noori M, Donald AE, Angelakopoulou A, Hingorani AD, Williams DJ. Prospective study of placental angiogenic factors and maternal vascular function before and after preeclampsia and gestational hypertension. *Circulation* 2010;**122**: 478–87.

18. Savvidou MD, Hingorani AD, Tsikas D, Frölich JC, Vallance P, Nicolaides KH. Endothelial dysfunction and raised plasma concentrations of asymmetric dimethylarginine in pregnant women who subsequently develop pre-eclampsia. *Lancet* 2003;**361**:1511–7.

19. Paez O, Alfie J, Gorosito M, Puleio P, de Maria M, Prieto N, Majul C. Parallel decrease in arterial distensibility and in endothelium-dependent dilatation in young women with a history of pre-eclampsia. *Clin Exp Hypertens.* 2009;**31**:544–52.

20. Chambers JC, Fusi L, Malik IS, Haskard DO, De Swiet M, Kooner JS. Association of maternal endothelial dysfunction with preeclampsia. *Jama* 2001;**285**:1607–12.

21. Mori T, Watanabe K, Iwasaki A, Kimura C, Matsushita H, Shinohara K, Wakatsuki A. Differences in vascular reactivity between pregnant women with chronic hypertension and preeclampsia. *Hypertens Res.* 2014;**37**:145–50.

22. Kuscu NK, Kurhan Z, Yildirim Y, Tavli T, Koyuncu F. Detection of endothelial dysfunction in preeclamptic patients by using color Doppler sonography. *Arch Gynecol Obstet.*2003; **268**:113–6.

23. Khalil A JE, Harrington K, Muttukrishna S, Jauniaux E. Antihypertensive therapy and central hemodynamics in women with hypertensive disorders in pregnancy. *Obstet Gynecol* 2009;**113**:646–54.

24. Avni B, Frenkel G, Shahar L, Golik A, Sherman D, Dishy V. Aortic stiffness in

normal and hypertensive pregnancy. *Blood pressure* 2010;**19**:11–5.

25. Elvan-Taspinar A FA, Bots ML, Bruinse HW, Koomans HA. Central hemodynamics of hypertensive disorder in pregnancy. *Am J Hypertens.* 2004;**17**:941–6.

26. Stergiotou I, Crispi F, Valenzuela-Alcaraz B, Bijnens B, Gratacós E. Patterns of maternal vascular remodeling and responsiveness in early- versus late-onset preeclampsia. *Am J Obstet Gynecol* 2013;**209**:558 e551-558 e514.

27. Spaanderman ME, Willekes C, Hoeks AP, Ekhart TH, Peeters LL. The effect of pregnancy on the compliance of large arteries and veins in healthy parous control subjects and women with a history of preeclampsia. *Am J Obstet Gynecol* 2000;**183**:1278–86.

28. Borghi C, Esposti DD, Immordino V, Cassani A, Boschi S, Bovicelli L, Ambrosioni E. Relationship of systemic hemodynamics, left ventricular structure and function, and plasma natriuretic peptide concentrations during pregnancy complicated by preeclampsia. *Am J Obstet Gynecol* 2000;**183**:140–7.

29. Tomimatsu T, Fujime M, Kanayama T, Mimura K, Koyama S, Kanagawa T, Endo M, Shimoya K, Kimura T. Abnormal pressure-wave reflection in pregnant women with chronic hypertension: association with maternal and fetal outcomes. *Hypertens Res* 2014;**37**:989–92.

30. Khalil A, Sodre D, Syngelaki A, Akolekar RNK. Maternal hemodynamics at 11–13 weeks of gestation in pregnancies delivering small for gestational age neonates. *Fetal Diagn Ther* 2012;**32**:231–8.

31. Ness RB, Sibai BM. Shared and disparate components of the pathophysiologies of fetal growth restriction and preeclampsia. *Am J Obstet and Gynecol* 2006;**195**:40–9.

32. Yinon Y, Kingdom JCP, Odutayo A, et al. Vascular dysfunction in women with a history of preeclampsia and intrauterine growth restriction: Insights into future vascular risk. *Circulation* 2010;**122**: 1846–53.

33. Catov JM, Newman AB, Roberts JM, et al. Health ABC Study. Preterm delivery and later maternal cardiovascular disease risk. *Epidemiology* 2007;**18**:733–9.

34. Khalil A, Elkhouli M, Garcia-Mandujano R, Chiriac R, Nicolaides KH. Maternal hemodynamics at 11–13 weeks of gestation and preterm birth. *Ultrasound Obstet Gynecol* 2012;**40**:35–9.

35. Schram MT, Henry RM, van Dijk RA, et al. Increased central artery stiffness in impaired glucose metabolism and type 2 diabetes: the Hoorn Study. *Hypertension* 2004;**43**:176–81.

36. Kannel WB, McGee DL. Diabetes and cardiovascular disease. The Framingham study. *JAMA* 1979;**241**:2035–8.

37. Cruickshank K, Riste L, Anderson SG, Wright JS, Dunn G, Gosling RG. Aortic pulse-wave velocity and its relationship to mortality in diabetes and glucose intolerance: an integrated index of vascular function? *Circulation* 2002;**106**: 2085–90.

38. Savvidou MD, Anderson JM, Kaihura C, Nicolaides KH. Maternal arterial stiffness in pregnancies complicated by gestational and type 2 diabetes mellitus. *Am J Obstet Gynecol* 2010;**203** 274.e1–274.e7.

39. Anderson JM, Savvidou MD, Kaihura C, McEniery CM, Nicolaides KH. Maternal arterial stiffness in pregnancies affected by Type 1 diabetes mellitus. *Diabet Med* 2009;**26**:1135–40.

40. Khalil A, Garcia-Mandujano R, Chiriac R, Akolekar R, Nicolaides KH. Maternal hemodynamics at 11–13 weeks' gestation in gestational diabetes mellitus. *Fetal Diagn Ther* 2012;**31**:216–20.

Chapter

8

Cardiac Dysfunction in Hypertensive Pregnancy

Herbert Valensise, Gian Paolo Novelli and Barbara Vasapollo

Summary

Multiple exceptional and exclusive changes in cardiac structure and function have been described in preeclampsia (PE), suggesting that these women display abnormal cardiac adaptation to pregnancy as compared to uncomplicated pregnancies. As such, preeclampsia is associated with altered cardiac geometry, impaired myocardial relaxation and biventricular diastolic dysfunction. Preterm, but not term, PE is also associated with severe left-ventricular hypertrophy and biventricular systolic dysfunction in a significant proportion of women. Many of these abnormal changes are already detectable in the latent phase of the disease. This chapter summarizes the most important pathophysiologic aspects of cardiac dysfunction in hypertensive pregnancy, with respect to their clinical diagnostic and therapeutic relevance.

Introduction

Pregnancy induces dramatic cardiovascular changes in order to ensure maternal and growing fetal metabolic needs are met. Along with progressive placental growth, blood volume increases and peripheral vascular resistance decreases. Cardiac output and heart rate also increase during pregnancy. Such changes result in compensatory cardiac remodeling. In pregnancy complicated by hypertension, abnormal pressure overloading would lead to different cardiac remodeling compared to normotensive pregnancies.

Preeclampsia (PE) is known to be associated with altered cardiac geometry, impaired myocardial relaxation and biventricular diastolic dysfunction [1]. Preterm, but not term, PE is also associated with severe left-ventricular hypertrophy and biventricular systolic dysfunction in a significant proportion of women.

More recent studies have better defined the cardiovascular profile in preeclampsia from the preclinical phase of the disease to the postpartum period and the long-term cardiovascular effect later in life. Multiple exceptional and exclusive changes in cardiac structure and function have been described in preeclampsia, suggesting that these women display abnormal cardiac adaptation to pregnancy [2].

Accurate knowledge of cardiovascular physiological adaptation to pregnancy is particularly important in elucidating the pathophysiology and management of hypertensive disorders of pregnancy. For this reason, in recent years several studies focused on the functional changes of the maternal heart during pregnancy: some authors demonstrated an enhancement of cardiac function in pregnancy, whereas others showed depressed cardiac function, and a few showed unchanged functional status [3].

These conflicting results are probably related to differences in clinical and pharmacological management already present before the hemodynamic evaluation. Other confounding variables are parity, maternal body fat mass distribution, the presence of other co-existing medical conditions and undiagnosed forms of chronic hypertension. Discrepant findings may also result from the complexity of the hemodynamic characteristics of hypertensive disorders in pregnancy, which can change and evolve during the pregnancy itself.

Classification of Hypertensive Disorders in Pregnancy

The International Society For The Study of Hypertension In Pregnancy's (ISSHP) classification of hypertensive disease in pregnancy includes preeclampsia, gestational hypertension, chronic hypertension (including essential or secondary) and preeclampsia superimposed on chronic hypertension.

Gestational hypertension is characterized by new onset of elevated blood pressure during the second half of pregnancy (after 20 weeks of gestation) without proteinuria that returns to normal by 12 weeks postpartum.

Preeclampsia is defined as blood pressure at least 140/90 mmHg (pre-existing or de novo) with significant proteinuria, and/or other signs of maternal-organ dysfunction and/or uteroplacental dysfunction with fetal growth restriction.

Chronic hypertension is defined as a blood pressure at least 140/90 mmHg predating pregnancy or less than 20 weeks of gestation, or diagnosed for the first time during pregnancy and does not resolve during postpartum.

Superimposed preeclampsia is defined as an exacerbation of hypertension that was previously well controlled requiring escalation of BP medications and/or new onset of proteinuria or sudden increase in pre-existing proteinuria that has to be substantial and/or sustained.

Preeclampsia affects 3–8% of pregnancies and represents a cause of increased maternal and perinatal morbidity and mortality [4, 5]. According to the onset time, the origin and hemodynamics, preeclampsia is classified as early (placental mediated, linked to defective trophoblast invasion with high incidence of altered uterine artery Doppler, and lower body mass index [BMI]) and late (related to higher BMI and no alteration of uterine artery Doppler), recurring in 15% of the subsequent pregnancies [6].

A New Point of View: Role of Maternal Heart

Preeclampsia is believed to result from abnormal trophoblasts or insufficient invasion into the myometrium and the spiral arteries, with subsequently shallow placentation and inadequate spiral artery transformation. In recent years, several studies focused on the pathogenetic role of the maternal cardiovascular system; in fact, women with both placental insufficiency and impaired left-ventricular (LV) function were more likely to develop preterm/early-onset preeclampsia. On the contrary, women with normal or enhanced LV function will be more likely to have an uncomplicated pregnancy. From these findings it can be assumed that maternal cardiovascular response to impaired placentation might be a key moment in the pathogenesis of preterm preeclampsia. This supports the theory of a more complex origin of preeclampsia, related not only to placental insufficiency but also to the ability of the maternal cardiovascular system to adapt to placental dysfunction, attributing a central role of the mother's heart [7].

Systolic Function

The hemodynamics of gestational hypertension and preeclampsia are a subject of controversy. Early studies indicated pregnancies complicated by both gestational hypertension and preeclampsia were characterized by normal or reduced cardiac output and elevated total vascular resistance values [8].

Model of Elevated Cardiac Output and Low Peripheral Resistance

Studies conducted by Easterling and Bosio [9, 10] found that cardiac output was consistently higher while total vascular resistance was not elevated during both the latent and the clinical stages of preeclampsia. During the evolution of the clinical phase of preeclampsia, they observed a marked reduction in cardiac output and an increase in peripheral resistance. On the contrary, women developing pregnancy-induced hypertension showed elevated cardiac output both before and during the clinical course of the disease. Thus, they proposed the existence of a hyperdynamic circulatory state during the latent or preclinical phase of preeclampsia and during gestational hypertension.

Elevated cardiac output and low peripheral resistance were found to be related to endothelial activation and inflammatory response.

The differences between these two "models" may be explained mainly by the fact that many of the women who developed preeclampsia in the studies from Easterling et al. and Bosio et al. had a high BMI, and obesity might in itself cause a hemodynamic state with high cardiac output and low total vascular resistance.

Model of Reduced Cardiac Output and Elevated Peripheral Resistance

Groenendijk and Wallenburg [11] found a pattern of high resistance and reduced cardiac output in untreated women with severe preeclampsia. Data from Nisell et al. [12] showed low cardiac output and elevated peripheral resistance in patients with pregnancy induced hypertension (PIH) complicated by fetal growth restriction (FGR). In our experience [13], PIH appears to be characterized by low cardiac output and elevated vascular resistance. Since the placental vascular bed contributes 20–26% of the reduction in total vascular resistance (TVR), high resistance at the level of the uteroplacental vascular bed in hypertensive patients may explain the higher TVR (compared to patients with normal uterine artery resistance). Moreover, the high TVR may be a possible cause of depressed systolic function. The elevated afterload found in PIH patients may therefore explain the lower cardiac output and ejection fraction compared to normotensive subjects [13].

The altered geometric pattern found in the same population appears to be generally associated with a depressed systolic function and high TVR.

More recently, our group had hypothesized two drastically different hemodynamic states at 24 weeks gestation preceding the appearance of early and late PE: early PE appears to be linked mainly to failed placental vascular remodeling and expresses through a high TVR–low CO response, whereas late PE might be more linked to maternal constitutional factors and is characterized by a low TVR–high CO [6].

Maternal echocardiography may be useful to evaluate maternal hemodynamics and LV geometry at 24 weeks of gestation and identifying women at increased risk of hypertensive complication. High maternal total vascular resistance, increased relative wall thickness of the left ventricle, small LV diameter and development of concentric LV hypertrophy have been related to early-onset preeclampsia, suggesting an involvement of the whole cardio-vascular system [13]. On the contrary, late-form preeclampsia showed low total vascular resistance, high cardiac output and increased diameter of the left ventricle with an inter-mediate relative wall thickness (eccentric geometry) as compared to controls and early preeclampsia.

Left Atrial Dimensions and Function

Women with PIH appear not to manifest the enhanced left atrial function typical of the second and third trimester of physiological pregnancy [13, 14]. These different adapta-tions of left atrial function are probably due to the different loading conditions of the left ventricle in normotensive and hypertensive pregnancies: during PIH, left atrial filling is reduced during the diastolic phase.

The modified intraventricular pressure present in PIH has an effect on the left atrial filling and emptying. Reduced left atrial filling during diastole has been demonstrated by low pulmonary vein flow. Left atrial fractional area-change, calculated either by automatic boundary detection methods or by planimetric tracing of the left atrial border, is lower in PIH compared to normotensive pregnancy. Hypertensive patients had a minimal area value that was higher than controls. This is probably secondary to the increased diastolic ven-tricular pressures affecting atrial voiding [13].

Left-Ventricular Dysfunction and Geometry

One of the most important findings in the literature is the physiological myocardial hypertrophy that characterizes normal pregnancy; it is the reversible increase in LV mass as a compensatory mechanism to a continuous physical effort that aims to maintain cardiac output despite the chronically increased load on the LV. Consequently, the heart needs to generate more energy and tension during systole, with an increase in myocardial work and oxygen consumption. This increase in energy demand is met initially by the increased utilization of fatty acids. In the long term the increased load on the LV increases further myocardial wall tension and stress. Subsequently, to reduce wall stress (and hence oxygen needs) the myocardium increases wall thickness and reduces the radius of the curvature. These mechanisms lead to an increase in LV myocardial rigidity and impaired diastolic function, which usually precedes systolic dysfunction. Progressively there is decreased LV compliance, increased end-diastolic pressure relative to diastolic volume, decreased rate of early diastolic filling and prolonged late filling phase and delayed relaxation [15].

LV global diastolic dysfunction was defined as the inability of the heart to fill to a normal volume without an increase in chamber filling pressures. One of the most important tools to estimate LV filling pressure in the general population and in patients with hypertension or preeclampsia is the ratio of transmitral flow E-wave velocity to myocardial e' velocity (E/e' ratio), which has been suggested to represent a more reliable index for evaluation of LV diastolic function than conventional indices based on transmitral flow E- and A-wave velocities (i.e. the E/A ratio).

LV remodeling is required during hypertensive disorders in pregnancy to minimize wall stress in the presence of increased afterload as a recognized mechanism for preserving the balance between myocardial oxygen demand and supply.

Our group evaluated if the presence of an altered LV geometric pattern in the early stages of untreated mild PIH might be predictive of future maternal and fetal complications.

We show that concentric geometry was an independent predictor of adverse events [16]. Of the 148 gestational hypertensive pregnancies reviewed, 68 (46%) showed a normal geometric pattern, of which 60 had an uneventful outcome and 8 developed complications. Eighty hypertensive women (54%) showed an abnormal geometric pattern (concentric remodeling and concentric hypertrophy), and abnormal geometry was more common in those who developed complications (37/47 (78%)) than in those with an uncomplicated course (31/101 (31%), < 0.0001).

In 2011 Melchiorre et al. [17] evaluated cardiac function and remodeling in preeclampsia occurring at term. This study shows that women with preeclampsia undergo significant heart remodeling, but approximately 20% of women demonstrate more evident myocardial damage and overt global diastolic dysfunction. Diastolic dysfunction usually precedes systolic dysfunction in the evolution of ischemic or hypertensive cardiac diseases and is of prognostic value in the prediction of long-term cardiovascular morbidity.

In another study, Melchiorre et al. [18] evaluated the maternal cardiovascular profile at midgestation in nulliparous normotensive women destined to develop preterm preeclampsia versus preeclampsia at term. In this study they demonstrated that the prevalence of LV remodeling/hypertrophy at midgestation was similar in both preterm preeclampsia and term preeclampsia women. This finding is likely to represent a compensatory response to the increased afterload that is evident from the higher midgestational mean arterial pressures seen in women with preeclampsia.

In patients who subsequently developed preterm preeclampsia, the authors demonstrated a very high prevalence (33%) of LV diastolic dysfunction at midgestation compared with women with term PE or uneventful pregnancy.

Long-term Outcome and Persistent Cardiac Dysfunction

There is growing evidence of an asymptomatic LV systolic and diastolic dysfunction, LV hypertrophy and prehypertension state one year postpartum in patients with previous early preeclampsia [19], and 40% of patients with persistent cardiac alterations develop essential hypertension within two years after early preeclampsia. Moreover, these patients are more likely to develop systemic hypertension and to die at an early age from cardiovascular disease [20]. In particular, postpartum follow-up of women with previous preeclampsia showed persistence of altered cardiac geometry and LV dysfunction.

A recent study showed impaired hemodynamic adaptation in a previous pregnancy, and the subsequent complications, such as preeclampsia, might imply an increased risk profile for both the woman and the fetus during a second pregnancy. In this study, patients with previous preeclampsia with persistent cardiac alterations one year after pregnancy are at risk for recurrent preeclampsia in subsequent pregnancies [21]. The main features of patients with recurrent preeclampsia were the low cardiac output, high total vascular resistance values (signs of an underfilled cardiovascular system) and the altered cardiac structure with a hypertrophied ventricle at 24 weeks of gestation.

The risk of developing cardiovascular disease (CVD) varies among studies. In small studies the risk of developing hypertension after having any kind of hypertensive disorder during pregnancy varied from 1.5 to 20 times. In more recent studies, after changes in the diagnostic criteria for hypertensive disorders of pregnancy and larger numbers of patients, the relative risk varied between 2.3 and 3.7, likely representing more accurate data [22].

For these reasons, the American Heart Association recommends to obtain a detailed history of pregnancy complications, including their severity, gestational age at onset, concomitance of FGR and need for iatrogenic preterm delivery as a consequence of disease severity. Early identification and intervention, such as lifestyle modifications, healthy diet, exercise, regular blood pressure and metabolic factors control, must be recommended after delivery during the asymptomatic phase of cardiac impairment and seems to reduce complications in subsequent pregnancies and long-term cardiovascular risk [23].

Acknowledgments

The authors thank all collaborating co-workers at Torr Vergata University, Rome, who contributed to this chapter: G. M. Tiralongo, G. Gagliardi, I. Pisani, D. Lo Presti, D. Farsetti and B. Vasapollo.

Key Points

- Concentric LV geometry in the early stages of untreated mild PIH is an independent predictor of future maternal and fetal complications.
- Early-onset preeclampsia presents with high maternal total vascular resistance, increased relative wall thickness of the left ventricle, small LV diameter and development of concentric LV hypertrophy, whereas late-onset preeclampsia is associated with low total vascular resistance, high cardiac output and increased diameter of the left ventricle with an intermediate relative wall thickness (eccentric geometry).
- There is growing evidence of an asymptomatic LV systolic and diastolic dysfunction, LV hypertrophy and prehypertension state one year postpartum in patients with previous early preeclampsia [19], and 40% of patients with persistent cardiac alterations develop essential hypertension within two years after early preeclampsia.

References

1. Melchiorre K, Sutherland GR, Liberati M, Thilaganathan B. Preeclampsia is associated with persistent postpartum cardiovascular impairment. *Hypertension* 2011;**58**:709–15.

2. Melchiorre K, Thilaganathan B. Maternal cardiac function in preeclampsia. *Curr Opin Obstet Gynecol* 2011;**23**:440–7.

3. Melchiorre K, Sharma R, Thilaganathan B. Cardiac structure and function in normal pregnancy. *Curr Opin Obstet Gynecol* 2012;**24**:413–21.

4. Rosser ML, Katz NT. Preeclampsia: an obstetrician's perspective. *Adv Chronic Kidney Dis* 2013;**20**:287–96.

5. Al-Jameil N, Aziz Khan F, Fareed Khan M, Tabassum H. A brief overview of preeclampsia. *J Clin Med Res* 2014;**6**:1–7.

6. Valensise H, Vasapollo B, Gagliardi G, Novelli GP. Early and late pre-eclampsia: two different maternal hemodynamic states in the latent phase of the disease. *Hypertension* 2008;**52**:873–80.

7. Melchiorre K, Sharma R, Thilaganathan B. Cardiovascular implications in preeclampsia: an overview. *Circulation* 2014;**130**:703–14.

8. Roberts J. *Pregnancy related hypertension.* In: Creasy R, Resnik R, eds. *Maternal fetal medicine: Principles and practice.* Philadelphia: WB Sounders, 1984:703–52.

9. Easterling TR, Benedetti TJ, Schmucker BC, Millard SP. Maternal hemodynamics in normal and preeclamptic pregnancies: a longitudinal study. *Obstet Gynecol* 1990;**76**:1061–9.

10. Bosio PM, McKenna PJ, Conroy R, O'Herlihy C. Maternal central hemodynamics in hypertensive disorders of pregnancy. *Obstet Gynecol* 1999;**94**: 978–84.

11. Groenendijk R, Trimbos JBMJ, Wallenburg HCS. Hemodynamic measurements in preeclampsia: preliminary observations. *Am J Obstet Gynecol* 1984;**150**:232–6

12. Nisell H, Lunell NO, Linde B. Maternal hemodynamics and impaired fetal growth in pregnancy induced hypertension. *Obstet Gynecol* 1988;**71**:163–6.

13. Valensise H, Novelli GP, Vasapollo B, DiRuzza G, Romanini ME, Marchei M et al. Maternal diastolic dysfunction and left ventricular geometry in gestational hypertension. *Hypertension* 2001;**37**: 1209–15.

14. Valensise H, Novelli GP, Vasapollo B, Borzi M, Arduini D, Galante A et al. Maternal cardiac systolic and diastolic function: relationship with uteroplacental resistances. A Doppler and echocardiographic longitudinal study. *Ultrasound Obst Gynecol* 2000;**15**:487–97.

15. Kametas NA, Mcauliffe F, Hancock J, Chambers J, Nicolaides KH. Maternal left ventricular mass and diastolic function during pregnancy. *Ultrasound Obstet Gynecol* 2001;**18**:460–6.

16. Novelli GP, Valensise H, Vasapollo B, Larciprete G, Di Pierro G, Altomare F, et al. Left ventricular concentric geometry as a risk factor in gestational hypertension. *Hypertension* 2003;**41**:469–75.

17. Gongora MC, Wenger NK. Cardiovascular complications of pregnancy. *Int J Mol Sci* 2015;**16**:23905–28

18. Valensise H, Vasapollo B, Gagliardi G, Novelli GP. Early and late pre-eclampsia: two different maternal hemodynamic states in the latent phase of the disease. *Hypertension* 2008;**52**:873–80.

19. Melchiorre K, Sharma R, Thilaganathan B. Cardiovascular implications in preeclampsia: an overview. *Circulation* 2014;**130**(8):703–14.

20. Goynumer G, Yucel N, Adali E, Tan T, Baskent E, Karadag C. Vascular risk in women with a history of severe preeclampsia. *J Clin Ultrasound* 2013;**41**:145–50.

21. Valensise H, Lo Presti D, Gagliardi G, et al. Persistent maternal cardiac dysfunction after preeclampsia identifies patients at risk for recurrent preeclampsia. *Hypertension* 2016;**67**:748–53.

22. Melchiorre K, Ross Sutherland G, Baltabaeva A, Liberati M, Thilaganathan B. Maternal cardiac dysfunction and remodeling in women with preeclampsia at term. *Hypertension* 2011;**57**:85–93

23. Mosca L, Benjamin EJ, Berra K, et al. Effectiveness-based guidelines for the prevention of cardio-vascular disease in women – 2011 update: a guideline from the American heart association. *Circulation* 2011;**123**:1243–62.

Chapter 9

Dysfunction of the Venous System Before and During Preeclampsia

Sharona Vonck and Wilfried Gyselaers

Summary

Dysfunction of the venous system, as observed by venous Doppler flow assessment, is present in preeclampsia but not in nonproteinuric gestational hypertension.

Early preeclampsia is characterized with triphasic venous flow patterns in the liver, where the wave characteristics A, X, V and Y are prominent and sharp. The Renal Interlobar Vein Impedance index (RIVI) in both the left and right kidney is high, due to the so-called venous pre-acceleration nadir (VPAN), which is more prominent in the left kidney than in the right kidney. The Venous Pulse Transit Time (VPTT) is shorter than in normal pregnancy. These abnormalities presents weeks before clinical onset of disease.

Compared to early preeclampsia, late preeclampsia has a more flattened hepatic wave pattern, but not as flat as in uncomplicated pregnancies. High RIVI values are found unilaterally and usually present at clinical onset of disease. VPTT is also short, although less pronounced than in early preeclampsia.

In gestational hypertension the venous flow patterns have the same properties as in normal pregnancy, which suggests that venous dysfunction is an important pathophysiologic feature in preeclampsia only.

Introduction

As explained in Chapter 4, the venous system is a very important but often underappreciated component of the cardiovascular circulation. It participates actively in maintenance of a hemodynamic steady state by its (a) capacitance function, which allows storage of blood, mainly in the liver and the splanchnic bed, (b) control of cardiac output in which it cooperates with the heart as one functional unit and (c) regulation of capillary function and interstitial fluid volume. It is well known that each of these functions may be troubled in gestational hypertensive diseases; e.g., in early-onset preeclampsia as compared to normal pregnancy, there is reduced plasma volume expansion, lower cardiac output and proteinuria with malleolar edema.

Venous Doppler Wave Changes in Preeclampsia

Venous Doppler wave patterns change dramatically during normal pregnancy: a) hepatic venous flow patterns shift from triphasic to flat, b) measured values and undulation of RIVI decrease [1] – this is more pronounced in the right than in the left kidney – and c) VPTT increases (Chapter 4). These changes are different in gestational hypertensive diseases than in normal pregnancy.

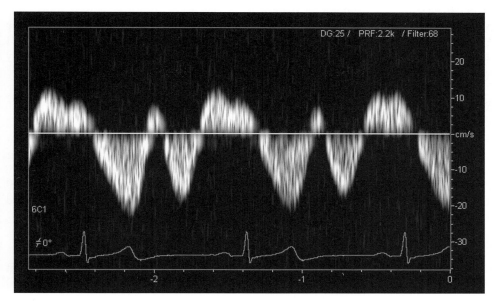

Figure 9.1 An example of tetraphasic hepatic venous Doppler waveforms. (A black and white version of this figure will appear in some formats. For the color version, please refer to the plate section.)

Hepatic Vein Waveforms

In preeclamptic patients, the normal transition from a triphasic to a flat pattern does not always occur in the hepatic veins (HV). During early-onset preeclampsia, triphasic HV patterns are observed instead of a flat pattern. This seemingly looks like the woman is either not pregnant at all or in the first part of pregnancy [2]. The wave characteristics A, X, V and Y are much more prominent and more sharply presented than in nonpregnant conditions, and sometimes even tetraphasic patterns are observed (Figure 9.1). In late-onset preeclampsia, however, flattening of the HV waveforms is mostly present, but to a lesser degree than in uncomplicated pregnancies [3]. It should be emphasized that the HV waveforms are not always identical at different locations of the hepatic venous tree: some parts of the liver may contain triphasic patterns whereas simultaneously other areas show flat types. This has been observed in normal pregnancy, preeclampsia and also during HELLP-crisis (unpublished data).

Renal Interlobar Vein Impedance Index

Renal Interlobar Vein Impedance Index (RIVI), defined as [(max flow – min flow)/max flow], is much higher in early-onset preeclampsia than in normal pregnancy [1,3]. In late-onset preeclampsia, however, these values are often within the normal range [4]. Increased RIVI values are mainly due to a sharp deceleration of forward venous flow, the so-called venous pre-acceleration nadir (VPAN), which is time-related to the P-wave of the maternal ECG. This represents backflow of venous blood during atrial contraction up to the level of the kidneys, which might be caused by a cardiac diastolic dysfunction or a reduced venous distensibility [2]. Increase of right renal RIVI values is found both in early- and late-onset preeclampsia, whereas increase of left renal RIVI values is observed mainly in early-onset preeclampsia [5]. The undulating pattern of weekly RIVI measurements is more pronounced in preeclampsia than in uncomplicated third trimester pregnancies, and, contrary to the nonpregnant conditions, presents simultaneous in both kidneys [1]. Abnormal RIVI values are observed weeks before clinical onset of preeclampsia, and, again, this is mainly true for early-onset preeclampsia [6].

Venous Pulse Transit Time

Venous pulse transit time (VPTT) is shorter in preeclampsia than in normal pregnancy, and this is more pronounced in early- than in late-onset preeclampsia [5, 7]. This indicates that during preeclampsia, the venous backflow of blood during atrial contraction travels faster and at a longer distance through the venous system than in uncomplicated pregnancy [5]. Preeclampsia-related shortening of pulse transit time occurs simultaneously at the arterial and venous sites [8], reflecting stiffening of the vascular wall, probably due to increased vascular tone.

Experimentally Induced Changes of Venous Wave Forms

Changes of hepatic venous waveforms have been studied in a group of healthy, nonpregnant individuals in order to better understand the background mechanisms behind normal and pathologic gestational HV Doppler flow changes [9].

Doppler sonography of HV was performed during an intravenous bolus of 500 ml normal saline: this volume load was responsible for increased and more pronounced deflections of the typical venous Doppler wave characteristics A, X and Y. This pattern is typically seen during early-onset preeclampsia. This suggests that the PE-related triphasic HV pattern seems to represent a state of intravascular overfilling and thus a reduced capacitance function of the venous system.

Valsalva maneuver, performed both before and after intravenous volume load, caused complete flattening of the HV Doppler wave form, which is the pattern seen during uncomplicated third trimester pregnancy. This flattening was also observed during intraperitoneal insufflation of CO_2-gas for operative laparoscopy. From this, it might be concluded that the normal gestational flattening of HV Doppler flow waves results from increased intraperitoneal pressure, due to the growing uterus in a poorly expanding abdominal cavity. A fall from increased intraperitoneal pressure to normal values has been measured by bladder catheterization before and after planned Cesarean section at term [10].

Venous Doppler Wave Changes in Nonproteinuric Gestational Hypertension

As explained above, PE-related venous Doppler wave changes are much more pronounced in early-onset than in late-onset preeclampsia. In nonproteinuric gestational hypertension, however, it has been observed that venous Doppler wave measurements have the same properties as a normal pregnancy [5, 8]. This suggests that venous hemodynamic dysfunction seems to be a pathophysiologic feature of preeclampsia but not gestational hypertension. In this perspective, the reported correlation between RIVI and degree of proteinuria in late-onset preeclampsia is very interesting [11].

The combination of these observations invites more research into the role of the venous compartment in the clinical presentation of gestational hypertensive disease, as two interesting hypotheses can be postulated. a) is it possible that the clinical symptoms of preeclampsia, apart from hypertension, may be evoked via the venous compartment? Or, to put it differently: is preeclampsia the gestational equivalent of the cardiorenal syndrome, [12]; and b) is it possible that there are two types of gestational hypertension: one presenting with venous hemodynamic dysfunction which is prone to soon develop proteinuria and become preeclampsia, and another with normal venous hemodynamics that will remain nonproteinuric?

Venous Doppler Measurements in Screening for Preeclampsia

As already discussed, abnormal RIVI values are observed weeks before clinical symptoms of (mainly early-onset) preeclampsia [6]. This opens perspectives to use venous Doppler measurements in screening for gestational hypertensive disease.

A preliminary study evaluated the cardiac, arterial and venous function according to standardized protocols in 242 pregnant women around 12 weeks of gestation, using impedance cardiography and combined ECG-Doppler ultrasonography [13]. This study showed a different cardiovascular physiology between uncomplicated pregnancies and those destined to develop gestational hypertension, preeclampsia or intrauterine growth retardation (IUGR). Mainly blood pressures and aorta flow velocity parameters were already abnormal at 12 weeks in the pathologic pregnancies. Venous Doppler parameters, however, were normal at 12 weeks in all pregnancies. Case observations in early- and late-onset preeclampsia showed an abnormal evolution of venous Doppler measurements between 12 and 20 weeks of gestation, as compared to the normal reference range [14]. Therefore, it seems that longitudinal assessments of venous hemodynamic function are necessary when venous Doppler parameters are used for prediction of preeclampsia. In this perspective, it might be interesting to evaluate the value of noninvasive measurements of the maternal cardiovascular system at 12 and 20 weeks in the prediction of and discrimination between types of gestational hypertensive disease, based on venous Doppler waves changes, potentially in combination with other techniques.

Conclusion

Venous Doppler flow abnormalities are an intrinsic feature of preeclampsia and present more prominently in early than in late-onset preeclampsia. They seem not to be present in nonproteinuric gestational hypertension. These observations invite exploration of the role of venous hemodynamic dysfunction in the clinical presentation of different types of gestational hypertensive diseases.

Key Points

- Abnormal venous Doppler wave patterns are a common feature in preeclampsia but not in gestational hypertension.
- In early-onset preeclampsia, abnormal venous Doppler measurements are very prominent due to the presence of a venous pre-acceleration nadir, presenting bilaterally and weeks before onset of clinical disease.
- In late-onset preeclampsia, abnormal venous Doppler measurements are less prominent than in early-onset preeclampsia, and usually present unilaterally from onset of clinical disease.

References

1. Gyselaers W, Mullens W, Tomsin K, Mesens T, Peeters L. Role of dysfunctional maternal venous hemodynamics in the pathophysiology of pre-eclampsia: a review. *Ultrasound Obstet Gynecol.* 2011;**38**(2): 123–9.

2. Gyselaers W. Hemodynamics of the maternal venous compartment: a new area to explore in obstetric ultrasound imaging. *Ultrasound Obstet Gynecol.* 2008;**32**(5):716–7.

3. Gyselaers W, Mesens T, Tomsin K, Molenberghs G, Peeters L. Maternal renal interlobar vein impedance index is higher in early- than in late-onset pre-eclampsia. *Ultrasound Obstet Gynecol.* 2010;**36**(1):69–75.

4. Gyselaers W, Molenberghs G, Van Mieghem W, Ombelet W. Doppler measurement of renal interlobar vein impedance index in uncomplicated and preeclamptic pregnancies. *Hypertens Pregnancy.* 2009;**28**(1):23–33.

5. Gyselaers W, Tomsin K, Staelens A, Mesens T, Oben J, Molenberghs G. Maternal venous hemodynamics in gestational hypertension and preeclampsia. *BMC Pregnancy Childbirth.* 2014;**14**:212.

6. Gyselaers W, Mesens T. Renal interlobar vein impedance index: a potential new Doppler parameter in the prediction of preeclampsia? *J Matern Fetal Neonatal Med.* 2009;**22**(12):1219–21.

7. Tomsin K, Mesens T, Molenberghs G, Gyselaers W. Venous pulse transit time in normal pregnancy and preeclampsia. *Reprod Sci.* 2012;**19**(4):431–6.

8. Gyselaers W, Staelens A, Mesens T, et al. Maternal venous Doppler characteristics are abnormal in pre-eclampsia but not in gestational hypertension. *Ultrasound Obstet Gynecol.* 2015;**45**(4):421–6.

9. Tomsin K, Vriens A, Mesens T, Gyselaers W. Non-invasive cardiovascular profiling using combined electrocardiogram-Doppler ultrasonography and impedance cardiography: An experimental approach. *Clin Exp Pharmacol Physiol.* 2013;**40**(7): 438–42.

10. Staelens AS, Van Cauwelaert S, Tomsin K, Mesens T, Malbrain ML, Gyselaers W. Intra-abdominal pressure measurements in term pregnancy and postpartum: an observational study. *PLoS One.* 2014;**9**(8): e104782.

11. Mesens T, Tomsin K, Staelens AS, Oben J, Molenberghs G, Gyselaers W. Is there a correlation between maternal venous hemodynamic dysfunction and proteinuria of preeclampsia? Eur J Obstet Gynecol Reprod Biol. 2014;**181**:246–50.

12. Pollock E, Nowak A. The cardiorenal problem. *Swiss Med Wkly.* 2014;**144**: w14051.

13. Oben J, Tomsin K, Mesens T, Staelens A, Molenberghs G, Gyselaers W. Maternal cardiovascular profiling in the first trimester of pregnancies complicated with gestation-induced hypertension or fetal growth retardation: a pilot study. *J Matern Fetal Neonatal Med.* 2014;**27**(16):1646–51.

14. Mesens T1, Tomsin K, Oben J, Staelens A, Gyselaers W. Maternal venous hemodynamics assessment for prediction of preeclampsia should be longitudinal. *J Matern Fetal Neonatal Med.* 2015;**28**(3): 311–15.

Chapter 10

Microvascular Findings in Pathological Pregnancy

Andreas Brückmann and Jérôme Cornette

Summary

Preeclampsia is considered as a disease of the maternal endothelium, and the proper function of the microvascular endothelium includes maintenance of a barrier and regulation of vascular tone. However, the extent to which microvascular dysfunction results from endothelial dysfunction, sympathetic influence, neuronal or myogenic disturbance, increased permeability or microangiopathy, at different levels of risk for preeclampsia and in different vascular beds, remains uncertain. Summarizing, it is hypothesized that in preeclampsia a pre-existing endothelial dysfunction and a consequently increased permeability results in a disturbed microvascular reactivity and autoregulation that also affects the placenta. Beyond the persistent peripheral vasoconstriction, due to sympathetic overactivity, the microcirculation exhibits blood flow regulative competence to counteract the impaired macrovascular endothelial function. The disruption of this microvascular autoregulatory competence, with further disease progression and the resulting atherosclerotic changes, which are partially genetically determined, indicate an increased risk for future cardiovascular disease. The analysis of the microcirculation, at different risk for preeclampsia and in different vascular beds, might be important to detect women susceptible to preeclampsia, by unmasking pre-existing differences, and to enable therapeutic strategies. Pathological microvascular findings after and during preeclampsia and screening strategies for preeclampsia, detected with different assessment methods, are summarized in this chapter.

Introduction

The features of preeclampsia include elevated blood pressure and proteinuria with edema and coagulation abnormalities in a high-resistance circulation [1]. The placenta and its impaired remodeling of the spiral arteries due to abnormal trophoblast invasion lead to excessive release of syncytiotrophoblast microparticles that generate endothelial dysfunction in preeclampsia [2].

Therefore, vasoactive substances, such as soluble fms-like tyrosine kinase-1, are released into the maternal circulation, resulting in reduced nitric oxide bioavailability, vasoconstriction throughout the microvasculature, increased peripheral resistance and hypertension [3–5]. The microvasculature is known to be responsive to vascular endothelial growth factor, which is decreased in preeclampsia [4, 6].

However, the extent to which microvascular dysfunction results from endothelial dysfunction, sympathetic influence, neuronal or myogenic disturbance, increased permeability or microangiopathy, at different levels of risk for preeclampsia and in different vascular beds, remains uncertain.

Postpartum Analysis of the Microcirculation in Preeclampsia

Ramsey et al. demonstrated for the first time, using laser Doppler flowmetry in vivo, that microvascular function in response to acetylcholine and sodium nitroprusside was reduced 15–25 years after preeclampsia [7]. Hence, impaired microvascular function of the forearm skin, which was associated with insulin resistance, may predispose to coronary heart disease [7]. Skin microvascular hyperemic response after reactive hyperemia, assessed with laser Doppler flowmetry on the finger, was not different between women 23 years after preeclampsia and controls [8]. Rather, microvascular response correlated with insulin resistance and other cardiovascular risk factors [8]. This indicates chronically impaired microvascular function and an increased risk of cardiovascular disease several years after preeclampsia [8].

Although several months after preeclampsia acetylcholine-mediated skin microvascular response, assessed with laser Doppler flowmetry on the finger, was increased, this mechanism may reflect an underlying microangiopathy, which defines enhanced sympathetic vasoconstrictor activity and is potentially a compensatory response to the macrovascular endothelial dysfunction observed years after preeclampsia [9]. Besides an enhanced acetylcholine-mediated micro-vasodilatation of the forearm skin several months after preeclampsia, which was not different between mild, early-onset or severe preeclampsia, there was an increased 30-year and lifetime risk for cardiovascular disease [10].

Conversely, acetylcholine-mediated microvascular response, analyzed with the same method, returned to normal levels 6 weeks postpartum, when preeclampsia occurred after bilateral uterine arterial notching at 18–20 weeks gestation [6]. That supports the two-year resolution hypothesis of preeclampsia, which suggests that vascular changes that still occur after preeclampsia seem to have recovered two years later. Accordingly, microvascular dysfunction, e.g. stiffening and narrowing of retinal vessels during preeclampsia, assessed with Dynamic Vessel Analyzer under the influence of flickering light, partly resolves after preeclampsia and thereby also supports this resolution hypothesis [11]. However, structural rarefaction of skin capillaries, assessed with video microscopy, persisted 5–15 weeks after preeclampsia, which is analogous with similar observations in essential hypertension and could offer an explanation for the underlying mechanisms behind the increased long-term cardiovascular risk observed in women who suffered from preeclampsia [12].

When microvascular endothelial dysfunction was revealed with EndoPAT in mothers and their offspring 5–8 years after a preeclampsia that was accompanied by small-for-gestational-age infants and high concentrations of inflammatory and antiangiogenic maternal biomarkers, such as high-sensitivity C-reactive protein and soluble fms-like tyrosine kinase, the concept of transgenerational risk of cardiovascular disease after preeclampsia is supported [4]. Therefore, prophylactic lifestyle changes could be offered to both individuals, to reduce their cardiovascular risk [4].

Furthermore, preeclampsia itself seems to be a risk factor for several cardiovascular complications, based on the evidence of impaired coronary flow reserve and increased intima-media thickness in the coronary microvasculature in women without cardiovascular risk factors 5 years after preeclampsia [13]. Chronic inflammation and oxidative stress may contribute to this microvascular endothelial dysfunction in preeclampsia, assessed with transthoracic echocardiography [13]. This possibly early manifestation of inflammation-driven atherosclerosis of the coronary microvasculature may increase the risk for future coronary artery disease after preeclampsia [13]. Therefore, additional coronary risk factors should be changed once an increased coronary artery disease risk is detected with coronary flow reserve [13].

Analysis of the Microcirculation after the Onset of Preeclampsia

Ex-vivo, acetylcholine-induced relaxation of subcutaneous arteries from preeclamptic women was attenuated, which may account for enhanced pressor sensitivity and peripheral vascular resistance and therefore provides direct evidence of endothelial dysfunction in preeclampsia [14].

Laser Doppler evaluation of the finger skin revealed microvascular endothelial dysfunction in nonobese women with normotensive intrauterine growth restriction (IUGR), which was demonstrated by enhanced acetylcholine-mediated vasodilatation [2]. This may cause endothelial cell damage in the fetal umbilical placental microcirculation with a consequent reduction in fetoplacental blood flow, due to distinct expression of endothelial genes and adhesion molecules as well as adenosine and nitric oxide synthase involvement [15–17]. Therefore, it is suggested that microvascular maternal endothelial dysfunction leads to both intrauterine growth restriction and preeclampsia, depending on the absence (IUGR) or presence (preeclampsia) of metabolic syndrome [2].

In women diagnosed with preeclampsia, the acetylcholine-mediated microvascular response, assessed with laser Doppler flowmetry of the forearm skin, was enhanced [18]. This suggests an intact microvascular endothelial relaxation response to nitric oxide in preeclampsia [18]. The increased endothelial cell activation may relate to other factors which are released by the preeclamptic endothelium in response to acetylcholine, including enhanced vascular permeability and coagulation [18].

A similar enhancement in capillary flux was observed in the skin over the ankle in women with preeclampsia and gestational hypertension, using laser Doppler flowmetry without iontophoresis [1]. These postural-induced vascular changes indicate a disturbed venoarteriolar reflex, due to a persistent vasoconstriction, which is possibly mediated by sympathetic overactivity [1]. Hence, the additional postural-induced vasoconstrictive stimulus may result in reflex ischemic vasodilatation, similar to vascular changes leading to cutaneous edema in preeclampsia or cerebral encephalopathy in eclampsia [1, 19]. An intact venoarteriolar reflex usually results in an arteriolar constriction to counteract the increased capillary filtration [19].

However, finger skin laser Doppler flowmetry without iontophoresis was not altered in preeclampsia during venous occlusion [20]. On the contrary, nailfold capillaroscopy with polarization spectral imaging revealed a similar disturbance in venoarteriolar reflex during venous occlusion, in preeclamptic women [20]. The discrepancy between both methods may be explained by the fact that laser Doppler flowmetry measures the flow in both these nutritive capillaries and in the thermoregulatory plexus at a greater depth [20].

Several different types of video microscopy in various sites have been used to assess different aspects of the microcirculation in preeclamptic women. When looking at capillary density most studies using intravital video microscopy found no or little decline in basal capillary density but a significant reduction in maximal capillary density in the skin of preeclamptic women as compared to normotensive pregnant women [12, 21–23]. Basal capillary density represents the number of capillaries, which are open and perfused at the time of measurement, and is often referred to as functional capillary density. Maximal capillary density is obtained by additionally recruiting the nonperfused capillaries by venous congestion. It represents the structural or total capillary density. Using a noninvasive side-stream dark field imaging device in the sublingual microcirculation, Cornette et al. did not observe any significant difference in perfused vessel density for either large vessels (arterioles and venules) or capillaries between severe preeclamptic women and healthy controls [24]. These findings are analogous to the previous observations in the skin, where differences were only observed after recruitment by venous congestion.

When assessing changes in vessel diameters and appearance, subtle changes in the microcirculation of preeclamptic women are described, such as reduced conjunctival venular diameters, an increased percentage in tortuous and dilated nailfold capillaries and reduced change in venous capillary limb diameters after venous congestion [23, 25]. When assessing microvascular flow, using either capillaroscopy and polarization spectral imaging in the nailfold or sidestream dark field imaging in the sublingual microcirculation, no differences in capillary blood cell velocity, microvascular flow index or heterogeneity of flow could be observed between preeclamptic and healthy pregnant controls [19, 20, 24, 26]. Nevertheless, a significantly greater decrease in red cell velocity after venous occlusion suggests an impaired veno-arteriolar reflex at the nutritive level of the skin microvasculature [20, 26]. Despite major changes in macrovascular hemodynamic parameters, blood pressure reduction in severe preeclamptic women with a hypertensive crisis did not affect sublingual microvascular perfusion [27].

An impaired venoarteriolar reflex of the skin in women with preeclampsia, which apparently can be preferably demonstrated with postural laser Doppler flowmetry of the ankle or capillaroscopy of the finger, represents impaired sympathetic vasoconstriction, or may alternatively indicate a down-regulation of smooth muscle cell receptors by sympathetic overactivity [1, 19, 20].

Despite the absence of significant differences in sublingual microvascular perfusion between preeclamptic women and healthy pregnant controls, impaired capillary perfusion, with reduced perfused vessel density, reduced microcirculatory flow index and increased heterogeneity of capillary perfusion, was observed in women with HELLP (hemolysis, elevated liver enzymes, and low platelets) syndrome [24, 28].

The disturbed microvascular reactivity, due to an increased peripheral resistance, seems to be a characteristic of preeclampsia, which is otherwise indicated by a delayed rise in peripheral deep body temperature after cooling of the leg [29]. Although upregulation of Angiotensin II receptors of the smooth muscle cells is suggested to cause an enhanced forearm vasoconstrictor response to Angiotensin II, assessed with strain-gauge plethysmography, this is improbably caused by reduced microvascular nitric oxide activity, since forearm vasoconstrictor response to NG-monomethyl-L-arginine, a nitric oxide synthase inhibitor, was not altered [3, 30]. Therefore, in preeclampsia, L-arginine supplementation may not be of value due to the fact that other factors, including raised endothelin levels, alterations in the ratio of thromboxane A_2 to prostacyclin, sympathetic overactivity and increased levels of tumor necrosis factor-α, might be responsible for the increased systemic vascular resistance, which is also reflected by reduced vasodilator response to acetylcholine [3, 30, 31].

Furthermore, raised tumor necrosis factor-α levels correlate with increased microvascular filtration capacity, using Filtrass strain-gauge plethysmography on the arm, and may contribute to increased microvascular permeability in preeclampsia [31]. Therefore, reactive oxygen species, released by extensively infiltrating neutrophils, may cause enhanced Angiotensin II-mediated vasoconstriction in omental arteries from women with

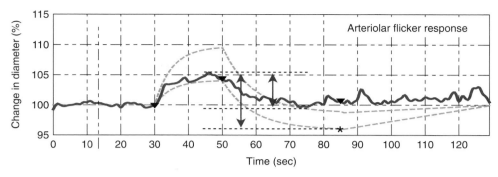

Figure 10.1 This sum curve of a dynamic retinal flicker analysis of a woman with preeclampsia demonstrates that the arteriolar flicker-induced dilatation is within the normal ranges (dashed green lines), but the typical arteriolar constriction component (asterisk) is missing, and thereby, the arteriolar amplitude is lower (short blue double-headed arrow) than in normal pregnancy (long blue double-headed arrow). (A black and white version of this figure will appear in some formats. For the color version, please refer to the plate section.)

preeclampsia as a crucial mechanism for systemic hypertension [32]. Thus, the suggested general vasospasm, particularly in severe preeclampsia, may also be evidenced by low capillary hydrostatic pressure in subcutaneous tissue, assessed with wick-in-needle technique, as opposed to mild preeclampsia [33].

Due to the increased microvascular permeability in preeclampsia, vasoactive factors, such as endothelin-1 and nitric oxide, are also able to access the retinal vascular smooth muscle cells directly [31]. Retinal vessels lack sympathetic innervation and exhibit autoregulation over a wide range of perfusion pressure changes that include metabolic and myogenic processes, to maintain retinal blood flow [11]. Hence, it is suggested that in preeclampsia the vasoconstrictive effect of endothelin-1 may be counteracted by a strong nitric oxide-mediated vasodilatation [3, 9]. Endothelium-derived oxygen species, which are abundant in preeclampsia, induce further vasoconstriction in pre-contracted ophthalmic arteries and thus may contribute to further progression of diseases involving altered blood flow and vascular tone, such as hypertension [32, 34]. Retinal glia cells can be stimulated by flickering light, using a Dynamic Vessel Analyzer that causes a flow and nitric oxide-mediated dilatation of retinal vessels by neurovascular coupling, with a subsequent arteriolar constriction [11]. In preeclampsia the autoregulatory competence of the retinal microvasculature seems to be preserved, due to an unchanged flicker-induced dilatation of retinal vessels, but the reduced arteriolar amplitude as a result of the absent arteriolar constriction component (Figure 10.1) indicates pre-aged and stiffened microvessels with dysfunctional endothelium [11]

These opposing mechanisms may lead to arteriolar narrowing and reduced arteriolar-to-venular ratio, vasospastic edema with choroidal, retinal and nerve fiber layer thickening and most severely to hypertensive retinopathy [34, 35]. Furthermore, transient blindness or blurred vision in preeclampsia may also result from petechial hemorrhages with focal edema in the occipital cortex, due to vasospasm, disturbed microvascular autoregulation with further disease progression and increased capillary permeability [35]. These retinal microvascular alterations are possibly compensated by increased mean arterial pressure.

Additionally, preeclampsia is associated with microvascular endothelial dysfunction, indicated by a reduced ratio between peak laser Doppler flux during reactive hyperemia and local hyperthermia on the forearm skin [36]. The ratio reflects maximum endothelium-dependent to maximum reachable endothelium-independent vasodilatation [36]. Microvascular endothelial dysfunction could also be demonstrated in preeclampsia with sleeping-disordered breathing, using EndoPAT [37]. This device evaluates endothelial microvascular function by assessing changes in finger pulse wave amplitude.

Analysis of the Microcirculation Prior to the Onset of Preeclampsia

Prior to the onset of preeclampsia, EndoPAT analysis did not provide additional information in women with an increased risk for preeclampsia [38]. Although arteriolar and venular narrowing occurs in the 1st and 2nd trimester, before the onset of preeclampsia in the retinal microcirculation, which is easily and noninvasively investigable using a fundus camera, this suggests that microvascular disturbance precedes rather than results from the increase of blood pressure and therefore possibly unmasks pre-existing differences in women with preeclampsia [5]. Structural rarefaction of skin capillaries, assessed with video microscopy, preceded the onset of the clinical symptoms and has the potential to be used as a marker for the prediction of preeclampsia [12, 21].

However, several weeks after bilateral uterine arterial notching at 18–20 weeks gestation, microvascular response to acetylcholine and to sodium nitroprusside, analyzed with laser Doppler flowmetry on the forearm, was increased prior to preeclampsia [6]. This endothelium-dependent and -independent reaction suggests enhanced sensitivity to nitric oxide and involvement of other endothelium-derived substances, such as nitric oxide, prostacyclin and endothelium-derived hyperpolarizing factor, to offset the impaired placental perfusion [6].

Although preeclampsia may arise from a maternal predisposition to metabolic syndrome or endothelial dysfunction [2], it is uncertain whether microvascular alterations are a cause or consequence of preeclampsia, due to the lack of prepregnancy studies. However, these microvascular findings preceded the clinical onset of preeclampsia, potentially serve as markers and suggest the implication of the microcirculation in the pathophysiology of preeclampsia. Therefore, the early detection of microvascular alterations in women with an increased risk for preeclampsia may allow the application of certain targeted therapies, prior to the development of preeclampsia [6]. For instance, methyldopa reduces microvascular resistance in preeclampsia, measured in the central retinal artery [39].

Conclusion

Summarizing, it is hypothesized that in preeclampsia a pre-existing endothelial dysfunction and a consequently increased permeability enable vasoactive substances and inflammatory mediators to access the smooth muscle cells, which results in a disturbed microvascular reactivity and autoregulation that also affects the placenta. Nitric oxide production is assumed to be unaffected.

Beyond the persistent peripheral vasoconstriction, due to sympathetic overactivity, the microcirculation exhibits blood flow regulative competence to counteract the impaired macrovascular endothelial function. The disruption of this microvascular autoregulatory competence, with further disease progression and the resulting atherosclerotic changes, which are partially genetically determined, indicate an increased risk for future cardiovascular disease.

The analysis of the microcirculation, at different risk for preeclampsia and in different vascular beds, might be important to detect women susceptible to preeclampsia, by unmasking pre-existing differences in early gestation and to enable therapeutic strategies. Therefore, further studies are needed.

Key Points

- It is hypothesized that in preeclampsia a pre-existing endothelial dysfunction and a consequently increased permeability enable vasoactive substances and inflammatory mediators to access the smooth muscle cells, which results in a disturbed microvascular reactivity and autoregulation.
- The disruption of this microvascular autoregulatory competence indicates an increased risk for future cardiovascular disease.
- The analysis of the microcirculation in different vascular beds might be important to detect women susceptible to preeclampsia.

References

1. Foong LC, Chong YS, Chua S, Johnson P, De Swiet M. Impaired vasoconstriction in pregnancy-induced hypertension assessed using doppler fluximetry. *Obstet Gynecol*, 2000;**95**(4):491–5.

2. Koopmans CM, Blaauw J, van Pampus MG, Rakhorst G, Aarnoudse JG. Abnormal endothelium-dependent microvascular dilator reactivity in pregnancies complicated by normotensive intrauterine growth restriction. *Am J Obstet Gynecol*, 2009;**200**(1):66 e1–6.

3. Anumba DO, Robson SC, Boys RJ, Ford GA. Nitric oxide activity in the peripheral vasculature during normotensive and preeclamptic pregnancy. *Am J Physiol*, 1999;**277**(2 Pt 2):H848–54.

4. Kvehaugen AS, Dechend R, Ramstad HB, Troisi R, Fugelseth D, Staff AC. Endothelial function and circulating biomarkers are disturbed in women and children after preeclampsia. *Hypertension*, 2011;**58**(1):63–9.

5. Lupton SJ, Chiu CL, Hodgson LA, et al. Changes in retinal microvascular caliber precede the clinical onset of preeclampsia. *Hypertension*, 2013;**62**(5):899–904.

6. Khan F, Blech JJ, MacLeod M, Mires G. Changes in endothelial function precede the clinical disease in women in whom preeclampsia develops. *Hypertension*, 2005;**46**(5):1123–8.

7. Ramsay JE, Stewart F, Greer IA, Sattar N. Microvascular dysfunction: a link between pre-eclampsia and maternal coronary heart disease. *BJOG*, 2003;**110**(11):1029–31.

8. Spaan JJ, Houben AJ, Musella A, Ekhart T, Spaanderman ME, Peeters LL. Insulin resistance relates to microvascular reactivity 23 years after preeclampsia. *Microvasc Res*, 2010;**80**(3):417–21.

9. Blaauw J, Graaff R, van Pampus MG, et al. Abnormal endothelium-dependent microvascular reactivity in recently preeclamptic women. *Obstet Gynecol*, 2005;**105**(3):626–32.

10. Murphy MS, Vignarajah M, Smith GN. Increased microvascular vasodilation and cardiovascular risk following a pre-eclamptic pregnancy. *Physiol Rep*, 2014;**2**(11).

11. Brueckmann A, Seeliger C, Lehmann T, Schleußner E, Schlembach D. Altered retinal flicker response indicates

microvascular dysfunction in women. *Hypertension*, 2015;**66**(4):900–5.

12. Nama V, Manyonda IT, Onwude J, Antonios TF. Structural capillary rarefaction and the onset of preeclampsia. *Obstet Gynecol*, 2012;**19**(5):967–74.

13. Ciftci FC, Caliskan M, Ciftci O, et al. Impaired coronary microvascular function and increased intima-media thickness in preeclampsia. *J Am Soc Hypertens*, 2014;**8** (11):820–6.

14. McCarthy AL, Woolfson RG, Raju SK, Poston L. Abnormal endothelial cell function of resistance arteries from women with preeclampsia. *Am J Obstet Gynecol*, 1993;**168**(4):1323–30.

15. Escudero C, Sobrevia L., A hypothesis for preeclampsia: adenosine and inducible nitric oxide synthase in human placental microvascular endothelium. *Placenta*, 2008;**29**(6):469–83.

16. Dunk CE, Roggensack AM, Cox B, et al. A distinct microvascular endothelial gene expression profile in severe IUGR placentas. *Placenta*, 2012;**33**(4):285–93.

17. Wang X, Athayde N, Trudinger B. Microvascular endothelial cell activation is present in the umbilical placental microcirculation in fetal placental vascular disease. *Am J Obstet Gynecol*, 2004;**190** (3):596–601.

18. Davis KR, Ponnampalam J, Hayman R, Baker PN, Alrulkumaran S, Donnelly R. Microvascular vasodilator response to acetylcholine is increased in women with pre-eclampsia. *BJOG*, 2001;**108**(6):610–4.

19. Rosén L, Ostergren J, Fagrell B, Stranden E. Skin capillary blood cell velocity in preeclampsia. The effect of plasma expansion. *Int J Microcirc Clin Exp*, 1989;**8** (3):237–44.

20. Vollebregt KC, Boer K, Mathura KR, de Graaff JC, Ubbink DT, Ince C. Impaired vascular function in women with pre-eclampsia observed with orthogonal polarisation spectral imaging. *BJOG*, 2001;**108**(11):1148–53.

21. Antonios TF, Nama V, Wang D, Manyonda IT. Microvascular remodelling

in preeclampsia: quantifying capillary rarefaction accurately and independently predicts preeclampsia. *Am J Hypertens*, 2013;**26**(9):1162–9.

22. Hasan KM, Manyonda IT, Ng FS, Singer DR, Antonios TF. Skin capillary density changes in normal pregnancy and pre-eclampsia. *J Hypertens*, 2002;**20**(12): 2439–43.

23. Rusavy Z, Pitrova B, Korecko V, Kalis V. Changes in capillary diameters in pregnancy-induced hypertension. *Hypertens Pregnancy*, 2015;**34**(3):307–13.

24. Cornette J, Herzog E, Buijs EA, et al. Microcirculation in women with severe pre-eclampsia and HELLP syndrome: a case-control study. *BJOG*, 2014;**121**(3): 363–70.

25. Houben AJ, de Leeuw PW, Peeters LL, Configuration of the microcirculation in preeclampsia: possible role of the venular system. *J Hypertens*, 2007;**25**(8):1665–70.

26. Rosén L, Ostergren J, Fagrell B, Stranden E. Mechanisms for edema formation in normal pregnancy and preeclampsia evaluated by skin capillary dynamics. *Int J Microcirc Clin Exp*, 1990;**9**(3):257–66.

27. Cornette J, Buijs EA, Duvekot JJ. et al. Haemodynamic effects of intravenous nicardipine in severe pre-eclamptic women with a hypertensive crisis. *Ultrasound Obstet Gynecol*, 2016;**47**(1):89–95.

28. Sarmento SG, Santana EF, Campanharo FF. et al. Microcirculation Approach in HELLP Syndrome Complicated by Posterior Reversible Encephalopathy Syndrome and Massive Hepatic Infarction. *Case Rep Emerg Med*, 2014;**2014**:389680.

29. Miyamoto S, Shimokawa H, Touno A, Kurokawa T, Nakano H. Characteristics of changes in blood circulation induced by cold stimulation in pre-eclamptic women. *Int J Gynaecol Obstet*, 1988;**27**(2):159–64.

30. Bowyer L, Brown MA, Jones M. Forearm blood flow in pre-eclampsia. *BJOG*, 2003;**110**(4):383–91.

31. Anim-Nyame N, Gamble J, Sooranna SR, Johnson MR, Steer PJ. Microvascular

permeability is related to circulating levels of tumour necrosis factor-alpha in pre-eclampsia. *Cardiovasc Res*, 2003;**58**(1): 162–9.

32. Mishra N, Nugent WH, Mahavadi S, Walsh SW. Mechanisms of enhanced vascular reactivity in preeclampsia. *Hypertension*, 2011;**58**(5):867–73.

33. Oian P,and Maltau JM. Calculated capillary hydrostatic pressure in normal pregnancy and preeclampsia. *Am J Obstet Gynecol*, 1987;**157**(1):102–6.

34. Abu Samra K. The eye and visual system in the preeclampsia/eclampsia syndrome: What to expect? *Saudi J Ophthalmol*, 2013;**27**(1):51–3.

35. Dinn RB, Harris A, Marcus PS. Ocular changes in pregnancy. *Obstet Gynecol Surv*, 2003;**58**(2):137–44.

36. Beinder E, Schlembach D. Skin flux during reactive hyperemia and local hyperthermia in patients with preeclampsia. *Obstet Gynecol*, 2001;**98**(2):313–8.

37. Yinon D, Lowenstein L, Suraya S. et al. Pre-eclampsia is associated with sleep-disordered breathing and endothelial dysfunction. *Eur Respir J*, 2006;**27**(2): 328–33.

38. Carty DM, Neisius U, Rooney LK, Dominiczak AF, Delles C. Pulse wave analysis for the prediction of preeclampsia. *J Hum Hypertens*, 2014;**28** (2):98–104.

39. Hung JH, Yen MY, Pan YP, Hsu LP. The effect of methyldopa on retinal artery circulation in pre-eclamptic gravidae. *Ultrasound Obstet Gynecol*, 2000;**15**(6): 513–9.

Chapter

11

How to Assess Arterial Function?

Helen Perry, Carmel McEniery and Asma Khalil

Summary

Today, many noninvasive techniques exist to evaluate arterial function via waveform analysis, assessment of endothelial function and large artery stiffness. Flow-mediated dilatation and venous occlusion plethysmography are used for endothelial function assessment. Regional large artery stiffness can by estimated by pulse wave velocity measurement, whereas ultrasound or MRI are used for assessment at the local level. Arterial waveform analysis is mostly performed with tonometry devices. This chapter gives a brief summary of the techniques that are considered safe for usage in pregnancy.

Introduction

Research on arterial function has grown in prominence in recent years, particularly in relation to pregnancy and complications of pregnancy. This is largely due to emerging evidence that various aspects of arterial function such as endothelial function, central blood pressure and large artery stiffness predict cardiovascular outcomes in a variety of patient groups and in the general population. Furthermore, the development of non-invasive, automated and operator-independent techniques and equipment have made the task of assessing arterial function much simpler to perform in both the research and routine clinical settings. Traditional 'gold standard' techniques such as invasive cardiac catheterization are not feasible on a large scale, least of all in a pregnant population. This chapter will focus on the available techniques to assess three major aspects of arterial function:

- Endothelial function
- Large artery stiffness
- Arterial waveform characteristics

Before undertaking measurements of arterial function, it is important to have a basic understanding of the arterial tree. In humans, the arterial tree originates at the aorta and has many branches, which decrease in diameter until reaching the smallest arterioles, which then branch into capillaries. Blood is pumped in a forward direction from the left ventricle around the arterial tree. When using any of the methods to assess arterial function, it is important to consider factors that may influence the results, both when repeating measurements in the same subject and when comparing populations in epidemiological studies. The main factors that can have an effect on the results are listed in Table 11.1.

Table 11.1 Factors that can influence arterial function measurements [1]

Factor	Recommended Management
Room Temperature	Controlled environment kept at 22°C +/–1°C
Rest	At least 10 mins in recumbent position
Time of day	Similar time of day for repeat measurements
Smoking, eating, drinking	Refrain for at least 3 hours before measurements, particularly caffeinated beverages
Alcohol	Refrain for 10 hours before measurements
Position	Should be documented. Ideally supine
Cardiac arrhythmia, White Coat Hypertension	Be aware of effect on recordings

Endothelial Function

The endothelium which lines the internal surface of the arteries responds to changes in the hemodynamic signals by releasing a number of vasodilatory or vasoconstrictive substances. Continuous balance and adjustment of these substances maintains the vascular hemostasis, and any disruption results in endothelial injury. Nitrous Oxide (NO) is a key endothelial vasodilator, and reduced NO bioavailability leads to endothelial injury and dysfunction. Endothelial dysfunction is considered a primary etiology for the development of athero-sclerosis as well as the earliest detectable process in the development of atherosclerosis-related cardiovascular disease. For this reason, much interest has been given to the techniques and applications of measuring endothelial function. The techniques described below have all been used in research and clinical settings outside of pregnancy [2–4]. Studies using flow-mediated dilatation in pregnant populations have shown enhanced endothelial function in apparently healthy pregnancies, as early as 10 weeks, while in preeclamptic pregnancies endothelial function was found to be impaired [5, 6].

Flow-mediated Dilatation

Assessment of endothelial function via flow-mediated dilatation (FMD) has been proposed to represent a functional bioassay for endothelium-derived NO bioavailability. An FMD test works by measuring the percentage difference in arterial diameter during vasodilation following an initial period of vasoconstriction. It requires a high-frequency linear vascular ultrasound system, with both 2D and color Doppler settings, as well as an internal ECG monitor so that each image frame of blood flow can be synchronized to the cardiac cycle. The test is typically performed with the subject supine. A baseline longitudinal image of the brachial artery with clear anterior and posterior intimal interfaces between the lumen and vessel wall is first acquired and baseline recordings of arterial diameter and blood flow velocity are obtained. Then, arterial occlusion is created by a forearm blood pressure cuff placed distal to the ultrasound probe and inflated to suprasystolic pressure (≥25–50 mmHg above systolic arterial pressure) for a standardized length of time (usually 5 minutes). Subsequent cuff deflation induces a brief high-flow state through the brachial artery (reactive hyperemia) and the resulting increase in shear stress causes endothelium-dependent vasodilation. The longitudinal image of the artery is recorded continuously from 30 seconds before to 2 minutes after cuff deflation. Various analyses can be performed with the data, and FMD is calculated as a percentage change using the peak diameter in response to reactive hyperemia in relation to the baseline diameter [3].

Venous Occlusion Plethysmography

Venous occlusion plethysmography measures total forearm blood flow, the majority of which is through skeletal muscle. The hands are generally excluded from the study (by wrist cuff occlusion) as they receive most blood flow through skin, have many arteriovenous shunts and generally have different physiology to the rest of the forearm. Venous occlusion plethysmography works on the underlying principle that if venous return from the arm is obstructed and arterial inflow continues unimpeded, the forearm swells at a rate proportional to the rate of arterial inflow [4]. The procedure is generally carried out in the following way: a wrist cuff is inflated to suprasystolic pressure and 60 seconds allowed before measurements commenced. A second cuff is placed around the upper arm and inflated to about 40 mmHg (higher than venous pressure but lower than diastolic pressure) at intervals of 10 seconds with 5 seconds deflation. This allows venous emptying while not impeding arterial inflow. The arms are positioned above the heart using pads and cushions. A strain gauge is placed around the widest part of the arm and the changes in circumference (which reflect changes in forearm volume) are measured. Due to the ischemia created by the wrist cuff, there is a time limit to the measurements [7].

This test is most useful when comparing dose-response relationships of different drugs within a single study, and results can be expressed as absolute or percentage changes in blood flow or ratio of blood flow (infused/control arm) or even as calculated resistance. When comparing recordings between different subjects, results can be difficult to interpret due to variations in arterial pressure, initial forearm blood flow and forearm size. Indeed, an individual's forearm blood flow can vary in different settings and throughout the day, possibly in relation to the Circadian Rhythm [8, 9].

Examples of the available devices, parameters recorded, their strengths and their limitations can be found in Table 11.2.

Arterial Stiffness

Arterial stiffness is dictated by the molecular, cellular and histological structure of the arterial wall and this varies throughout the arterial tree. As a general rule, in healthy, younger people, peripheral vessels have higher levels of arterial stiffness than central vessels. This can be reversed with aging or in disease, where the central vessels often become less elastic than the peripheral vessels [1].

The concept of peripheral vessels being stiffer is central to the most widely accepted model of the arterial tree: the propagative model. This model considers a visco-elastic tube which allows generation of a forward pressure wave which travels along the tube. At the various branching points and toward the end of the tube, where resistance is higher, retrograde waves are generated. The higher the arterial stiffness, the greater the velocity of the pulse wave and the retrograde wave. The differences in stiffness at peripheral and central vessels leads to a difference in amplification of the pressure wave, and amplification will be greater in the peripheral vessels [1]. For this reason, peripheral and central pulse pressure will differ and should not be used interchangeably.

Table 11.2 Examples of existing noninvasive devices for the assessment of arterial function

Method	Examples of Devices	Measurements Recorded	Strengths	Limitations	Evidence in Pregnancy
Endothelial Function					
Flow-mediated Dilatation	Ultrasound	Blood flow velocity, flow-mediated dilatation	Results can be compared between different subjects	Operator dependent, thorough subject preparation required	Prospective cohort studies assessing relationship with preeclampsia and fetal growth. Postnatal assessment of women with gestational diabetes [23–25]
Venous Occlusion Plethysmography	N/A	Forearm blood flow	Best for dose-relationship testing of a drug in a single subject	Not easily comparable between different subjects due to the variables affecting forearm blood flow	Postnatal case-control studies in women with preeclampsia [26,27]
Arterial Stiffness					
Tonometry +ECG	SphygmoCor® CPV (AtCor Medical)	Aortic pulse wave velocity (PWV) from transit-time delay between carotid-femoral measurements	Good intra-observer variability in one study	Could be technically challenging	Cross-sectional studies in preeclampsia /women at risk of preeclampsia and normal pregnancy [28–30]
Piezoelectrical sensors (mechano-transducer)	Complior® (ALAM Medical)		Good correlation with SphygmoCor in nonpregnant population [31]	Could be technically challenging	No studies found
Oscillometric distension	Vicorder® (SMT Medical)		Good intra-observer variability in one study		Comparison to SphygmoCor in second trimester [32]

Method	Device	Measures	Advantages	Disadvantages	Studies
Brachial Cuff Oscillometric Technique	Arteriograph® (TensioMed)	Aortic pulse wave velocity (PWV)	Operator independent, validated against invasive technique in nonpregnant population. Measures AIx and PWV simultaneously		Large longitudinal study in women at risk of developing preeclampsia, First trimester screening studies for preeclampsia and gestational diabetes. [18–20]
Echo tracking	ARTSENS®	Vessel wall diameter changes using ultrasound	Direct measure (not transfer/ model dependent)	Requires technical expertise/operator dependent	No studies found
Waveform Reflection					
Radial tonometry +transfer function	SphygmoCorCP® (AtCor Medical)	Aortic waveform, central systolic pressure, augmentation index (AIx), central pulse pressure (CPP)	High observer agreement in small studies Acceptable to patient	Operator dependent Relies on transfer function	Longitudinal study, case-control studies, cross-sectional studies in population at risk of preeclampsia [14, 28–30]
Brachial Cuff	Arteriograph® (TensioMed)	Aortic waveform central systolic pressure and augmentation index (AIx)	Operator independent, validated against invasive technique. Measures AIx and PWV simultaneously		Large longitudinal study in women at risk of developing preeclampsia, First trimester screening studies for preeclampsia and gestational diabetes. [18–20]

Table 11.2 (cont.)

Method	Examples of Devices	Measurements Recorded	Strengths	Limitations	Evidence in Pregnancy
	SphygmoCor XCEL® (AtCor Medical)	Pulse wave analysis, central systolic pressure, AIx, CPP	Operator independent, nonpregnant reference ranges available Acceptable to patient	Limited validation studies	Conference presentation of first trimester measurements in women at risk of preeclampsia. [33]
	BP+® (USCOM)	Central and peripheral BP, arterial stiffness augmentation index, pulse rate variability	Operator independent Acceptable to patient	Limited validation studies	None found

Several small studies evaluating pulse wave velocity in pregnancy and a systematic review of 23 studies evaluating the effect of preeclampsia on arterial stiffness have reported that women with preeclampsia have elevated arterial stiffness both during and after pregnancy [10].

Systemic arterial stiffness can only be measured using models, and will not be covered in detail here. Regional and local arterial stiffness can be measured at various sites along the arterial tree using noninvasive measures. Examples of the methods used are outlined below.

Regional

Pulse wave velocity (PWV) measurements are generally regarded as the most straightforward and easily reproducible measures of arterial stiffness. Aortic PWV, as measured by the carotid-femoral velocity, is considered as the 'gold standard,' as the thoracic and abdominal aorta make the largest contribution to arterial buffering actions and therefore the pathophysiological process of arterial stiffness. However, other sites are also used. The PWV is calculated by obtaining waveforms at two different sites and calculating the time delay (Δt) between the feet of the two waveforms. The distance between the two sites needs to be accurately recorded and measurements can be more difficult to obtain in conditions such as obesity, pregnancy and large bust size. Waveforms can be obtained using pressure, distension or Doppler methods. Once the waveform has been obtained, Δt is calculated using the foot-to-foot method, as in Figure 11.1.

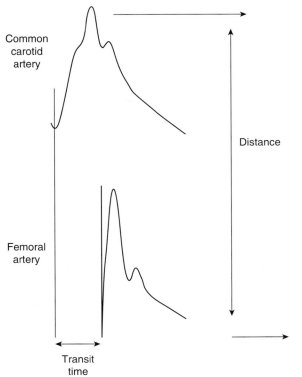

Figure 11.1 Foot-to-foot measurement of carotid-femoral pulse wave velocity

The available pressure sensor methods include the Complior® System (Colson, France); this uses dedicated mechanotransducers applied to the skin and the measurements can be obtained at the carotid-femoral, carotid-brachial and femoral-dorsalis sites. The SphygmoCor® system (AtCor, Sydney, Australia) uses an applanation tonometer to obtain both a proximal (e.g. carotid) and distal (e.g. radial/femoral) pulse sequentially and measures the transit time between the two sites in relation to the R-wave of an ECG which is monitored simultaneously. The Vicorder® (Skidmore Medical Limited, Bristol, United Kingdom) device uses an oscillometric distension technique to obtain simultaneous volumetric pressure recordings from a sensor placed over the carotid artery and a thigh cuff placed over the femoral artery. A neck pad which is only inflatable over several centimeters is placed around patient's neck, and a cuff is around the patient's upper right thigh. Both carotid and femoral cuffs are inflated to 65 mmHg and the corresponding oscillometric signal from each cuff is obtained in real time. Once the operator is satisfied with the waveform quality, the test is terminated and an algorithm of the two waveforms is analyzed to produce Δt [11]. The Arterigraph® device (TensioMed, Budapest, Hungary) uses an oscillometric technique with an upper arm cuff. By inflating to suprasystolic pressure, it occludes the brachial artery, excluding its characteristics (such as wall movement) from the recording, meaning the recorded waveform is reflective of the central systemic circulation. The Arteriograph® calculates the aortic PWV by measuring the jugular-symphasis measurement to represent the aortic length. As well as being validated against tonometry methods such as SpygmoCor®, the Arteriograph® has also been validated in nonpregnant population against cardiac catheterization for the measurement of the aortic PWV [12].

Local

Local arterial stiffness can be measured with ultrasound devices. MRI has been used in the research setting, and while it offers the advantage of being able to measure deep arteries like the aorta, it is not practical for large scale studies or clinical use. Local arterial stiffness can be measured in two ways with ultrasound: using video-image analysis, or with echo-tracking devices.

In video-image analysis, a bi-dimensional ultrasound system is used to measure vessel diameter in diastole and the stroke changes in diameter. Echo-tracking devices use a radiofrequency signal to obtain measurements of vessel diameter with much greater precision than video-analysis devices. The precision for echo-tracking devices in determining change in diameter is $1\,\mu m$ versus $\sim 150\,\mu m$ for video-analysis. The other advantage of echo-tracking devices is that the intima-media thickness can be calculated, which can be used to determine the elastic properties of a vessel.

Examples of the available devices, parameters recorded, their strengths and their limitations can be found in Table 11.2.

Arterial Waveform Characteristics (Reflection)

The arterial waveform is composed of a forward pressure wave created by the ventricular contraction and a reflected wave. The reflection occurs at the periphery, usually at branch points or where there is an area of impedance mismatch. In elastic vessels, where the PWV is low, the reflected waves arrive back at the aortic root during diastole. However, in stiffer arteries, with higher PWV, the reflected wave arrives back earlier, adding to the forward wave and therefore augmenting systolic blood pressure. This can be quantified as the

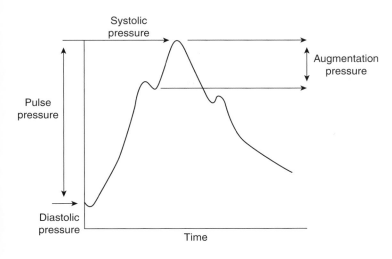

Figure 11.2 The arterial waveform complex

augmentation index (AIx), defined as a difference between the second and first systolic peaks, presented as a percentage of the pulse pressure. A recorded arterial waveform also gives measures of the central pulse pressure and the central systolic pressure. Along with the AIx, these parameters can be interpreted as a measure of arterial function. The waveform and associated measurements are shown in Figure 11.2.

Central (aortic) systolic blood pressure has been shown to independently predict cardiovascular outcomes and may even have a superior predictive value compared with brachial pressure. The central AIx and central pulse pressure are independent predictors for all-cause mortality in end-stage renal disease [13]. A large longitudinal study using the SphygmoCor® radial tonometry system in normal pregnancies has described the longitudinal changes in the AIx during pregnancy, reporting a reduction in the second trimester followed by a rise in the third trimester [14]. A number of techniques are available to perform pulse wave analysis, including newer cuff-based devices, which are operator-independent and simple to use.

The arterial pressure waveform should be measured and analyzed at the central level (i.e. the ascending aorta) as this reflects the true left ventricular load imposed on the vessels. Aortic pressure waveform can be recorded either from the common carotid or radial arteries. Both measurements can be performed noninvasively using a high fidelity probe such as the Millar strain-gauge transducer (SPT-301, Millar Instruments). For radial measurements, it is necessary to apply a transfer function to restore representation of the aortic waveform. Carotid measurements require a higher degree of expertise whereas radial tonometry is easier to perform, making it popular in practice. One consideration when calculating aortic pressure waveform from radial measurements using a transfer function is that the transfer function assumes that all arterial properties at both sites are the same for all patients under all conditions, which is obviously not the case. Despite this, several studies have reported good accuracy (>90%) when compared to aortic measurements [15, 16, 17]. Using an oscillometric technique with an upper arm cuff, the Arteriograph® device (TensioMed, Hungary) calculates the waveform parameters, including the AIx and central BP. As well as being validated against tonometry methods such as the SpygmoCor®, the Arteriograph® has also been validated against cardiac catheterization for measures of AIx and central systolic BP [12]. It has also been studied in large pregnant populations, including those with normal pregnancies, hypertensive disorders and gestational diabetes [18, 19, 20].

Newer technologies (e.g. SphygmoCor XCEL)® use brachial cuff-based measurements and then convert them to aortic values using a transfer function. This has been validated against the existing SphygmoCor® tonometry technology with good initial results [21]. BP+ (USCOM) is a similar device and has undergone comparison to radial tonometry in adults with initially promising results [22].

Examples of the available devices, parameters recorded, their strengths and their limitations can be found in Table 11.2.

Conclusion

Arterial function can be measured with several noninvasive devices and has increasingly been shown to be abnormal in pathological pregnancies such as those affected by preeclampsia. Future work is now required to validate them, create reference ranges for these different devices in pregnancy and establish their diagnostic and/or predictive values.

Key Points

- Arterial function can be assessed by evaluation of large artery stiffness, endothelial function and waveform analysis.
- Several noninvasive methods exist for arterial function assessment, which are safe to use in pregnancy.
- Most technologies now require validation and establishment of normal reference ranges before they can be introduced for general clinical application during pregnancy.

References

1. Laurent S, Cockcroft J, Van Bortel L, et al. Expert Consensus Document on Arterial Stiffness: methodological issues and clinical applications. *Eur Heart J* 2006;**27**: 2588–605.

2. Green D. Point: flow-mediated dilation does reflect nitric oxide-mediated endothelial function. *J Appl Physiol* 2005; **99**:1233–1234; discussion 1237–8.

3. Verma S, Buchanan MR, Anderson TJ. Endothelial function testing as a biomarker of vascular disease. *Circulation* 2003;**108**: 2054–9.

4. Harris RA, Nishiyama SK, Wray DW, and Richardson RS. Ultrasound Assessment of Flow-Mediated Dilation. *Hypertension* *2010*;**55**:1075–85, originally published April 14, 2010.

5. Savvidou, MD, Kametas, NA, Donald, AE, Nicolaides, KH. Non-invasive assessment of endothelial function in normal pregnancy. *Ultrasound Obstet Gynecol* 2000;**15**:502–7.

6. Savvidou, MD, Hingorani AD, Tsikas D, Frölich JC, Vallance P, Nicolaides KH. Endothelial dysfunction and raised plasma concentrations of asymmetric dimethylarginine in pregnant women who subsequently develop pre-eclampsia. *The Lancet*, 2003;**361**(9368):1511–17.

7. Wilkinson I, Webb D. Venous occlusion plethysmography in cardiovascular research: methodology and clinical applications. *Br J ClinPharmacol* 2001;**52**: 631–46.

8. Whitney RJ. The measurement of volume changes in human limbs. *J Physiol (Lond).* 1953;**121**:1–27.

9. Benjamin N, Calver A, Collier J, Robinson B, Vallance P, Webb D. Measuring forearm blood flow and interpreting the responses to drugs and mediators. *Hypertension* 1995;**25**:918–23.

10. Hausvater A, Giannone T, Sandoval YH, et al. The association between preeclampsia and arterial stiffness. *J Hypertens.* 2012; **30**:17–33.

11. Panza JA, Epstein SE, Quyyumi AA. Circadian variation in vascular tone and its relation to alpha sympathetic vasoconstriction. *N Engl J Med* 1991;**325**: 986–90.

12. Horváth IG1, Németh A, Lenkey Z, et al. Invasive validation of a new oscillometric device (Arteriograph) for measuring augmentation index, central blood pressure and aortic pulse wave velocity. *J Hypertens* 2010;**28**:2068–75.

13. London GM, Blacher J, Pannier B et al. Arterial wave reflections and survival in end-stage renal failure. *Hypertension* 2001;**38**:434–8.

14. Khalil A, Jauniaux E, Cooper D, Harrington K. Pulse wave analysis in normal pregnancy: a prospective longitudinal study. *PLoS ONE* 2009; **4**: e6134

15. van Leeuwen-Segarceanu EM, Tromp WF, Bos WJ, Vogels OJ, Groothoff JW, van der Lee JH.Comparison of two instruments measuring carotid-femoral pulse wave velocity: Vicorder versus SphygmoCor. *J Hypertens* 2010;**28**: 1687–91.

16. Karamanoglu M, O'Rourke MF, Avolio AP, et al. An analysis of the relationship between central aortic and peripheral upper limb pressure waves in man. *Eur Heart J* 1993;**14**:160–167.

17. Chen-Huan C, Nevo E, Fetics B, et al. Estimation of central aortic pressure waveform by mathematical transformation of radial tonometry pressure. *Circulation* 1997;**95**:1827–36.

18. Khalil A, Garcia-Mandujano R, Maiz N, Elkhouli M, Nicolaides KH. Longitudinal changes in maternal hemodynamics in a population at risk for pre-eclampsia. *Ultrasound Obstet Gynecol* 2014;**44**:197–204.

19. Khalil A, Akolekar R, Syngelaki A, Elkhouli M, Nicolaides KH. Maternal hemodynamics at 11–13 weeks' gestation and risk of pre-eclampsia. *Ultrasound Obstet Gynecol* 2012;**40**:28–34.

20. Khalil A, Garcia-Mandujano R, Chiriac R, Akolekar R, Nicolaides KH. Maternal hemodynamics at 11–13 weeks' gestation in gestational diabetes mellitus. *Fetal Diagn Ther* 2012;**31**:216–20.

21. Hwang MH, Yoo JK, Kim HK, et al. Validity and reliability of aortic pulse wave velocity and augmentation index determined by the new cuff-based SphygmoCorXcel. *J Hum Hypertens* 2014;**28**:475–81.

22. Park CM, Korolkova O, Davies JE, et al. Arterial pressure: agreement between a brachial cuff-based device and radial tonometry. *J Hypertens.* 2014;**32**(4): 865–72.

23. Praciano De Sousa PC, GurgelAlves JA, Bezerra ME, et al. Brachial artery flowmediated dilation and pulsatility index change as independent predictors for hypertensive disorders in the second trimester of pregnancy. *Eur J ObstetGynecolReprod Biol.* 2016;**200**: 94–7.

24. Iacobaeus C, Kahan T, Jörneskog G, Bremme K, Thorsell M, Andolf E. Fetal growth is associated with first-trimester maternal vascular function. *Ultrasound Obstet Gynecol.* 2016 Oct;**48**(4):483–90.

25. Brewster S, Floras J, Zinman B, Retnakaran R. Endothelial function in women with and without a history of glucose intolerance in pregnancy. *J Diabetes Res.* 2013;2013:382670.

26. Lampinen KH, Rönnback M, Groop PH, Kaaja RJ. A relationship between insulin sensitivity and vasodilation in women with a history of preeclamptic pregnancy. *Hypertension.* 2008;**52**(2):394–401.

27. Agatisa PK, Ness RB, Roberts JM, Costantino JP, Kuller LH, McLaughlin MK. Impairment of endothelial function in women with a history of preeclampsia: an indicator of cardiovascular risk. *Am J Physiol Heart Circ Physiol.* 2004;**286**(4): H1389–93.

28. Savvidou MD, Kaihura C, Anderson JM, Nicolaides KH. Maternal arterial stiffness in women who subsequently develop pre-eclampsia. Berger JS, ed. *PLoS ONE.* 2011;**6** (5):e18703.

29. Macedo ML, Luminoso D, Savvidou MD, McEniery CM, Nicolaides KH. Maternal wave reflections and arterial stiffness in normal pregnancy as assessed by applanation tonometry. *Hypertension.* 2008;**51**:1047–51.

30. Kaihura C, Savvidou MD, Anderson JM, McEniery CM, Nicolaides KH. Maternal arterial stiffness in pregnancies affected by preeclampsia. *Am J Physiol Heart Circ.* 2009;**297**(2): H759–H764.

31. Stea F, Bozec E, Millasseau S, Khettab H, Boutouyrie P, Laurent S. Comparison of the Complior Analyse device with Sphygmocor and Complior SP for pulse wave velocity and central pressure assessment.*J Hypertens.* 2014;**32**(4):873–80.

32. Everett TR, Mahendru A, McEniery CM, Lees CC, Wilkinson IB. A comparison of SphygmoCor and Vicorder devices for measuring aortic pulse wave velocity in pregnancy. *Artery Research,* 2012;**6**(2): 92–6.

33. Lan P, Keehn L, Milne L, McNeill K, Chowienczyk P, Sinha MD. Pulse wave analysis and the risk of early-onset pre-eclampsia. *Pregnancy Hypertension.* 2016;**5**:1:26.

Chapter 12

How to Do a Maternal Venous Doppler Assessment

Wilfried Gyselaers

Summary

Doppler sonography can be used for vascular studies, at both the arterial and venous side of the circulation. Due to the large anatomical variability of the venous compartment, the typical physiologic properties of venous hemodynamics, the many physiologic variables interfering with venous return and current technological limitations to measure velocities in the lower range, the methodology to assess veins differs completely from arterial Doppler measurements. This chapter summarizes the practical aspects, possibilities and limitations of a reported protocol for venous Doppler studies in pregnant women.

Introduction

Methods to study venous hemodynamics have been reviewed extensively by Pang [1]. Mean circulatory filling pressure techniques and intravascular ultrasound imaging have been used under experimental conditions. The constant cardiac output reservoir technique and blood pool scintigraphy require the application of major cardiac surgery and radioactive tracers respectively. Only plethysmography and the in vivo microscopic measurement of dorsal hand vein diameter can be used safely in pregnant women, but both methods are technically difficult and not readily available in most prenatal clinics, labor wards or maternity units. Apart from this, the physiologic behavior of peripheral veins does not always reflect what happens in the central or splanchnic veins [2, 3].

As most obstetricians are familiar with obstetric ultrasound scanning and Doppler sonography, this method is a simple, noninvasive and accessible tool to investigate venous hemodynamics, in both nonpregnant and pregnant subjects.

Practical Aspects of Venous Doppler Sonography

Because of high intra- and interobserver variation reported for Doppler-derived measurements [4], methodologic standardization is needed, especially when potentially confounding factors are to be excluded, such as respiratory movements, orthostasis and muscle contractions. A standardized Duplex ultrasound examination has been reported, which enables the acquisition of reproducible data for renal interlobar and hepatic vein impedance index (defined as [Maximum flow velocity (MxV) – Minimum flow velocity (MnV)]/MxV) (5). After oral informed consent, all women have a conventional ultrasound scan together with a Doppler flow examination of both kidneys and liver. All examinations are performed using a 3.5- to 7-MHz probe, which is normally used for obstetric ultrasound scanning. The scanner is also equipped with a lead for registration of the maternal electrocardiogram

(a) (b)

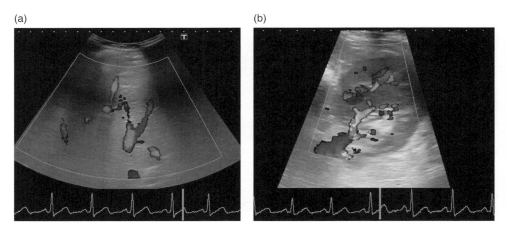

Figure 12.1 Color Doppler images of intrahepatic and intrarenal vasculature. (A black and white version of this figure will appear in some formats. For the color version, please refer to the plate section.)

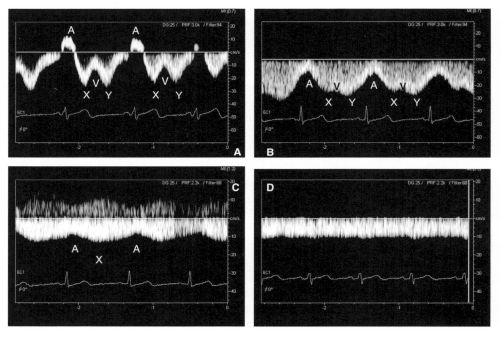

Figure 12.2 Different types of venous Doppler wave forms, as commonly seen in the hepatic and renal veins.

(ECG), and thus the ECG-signal is depicted simultaneously with the Doppler waves (Figures 12.1 & 12.2).

Examinations are performed at random intervals throughout the day, irrespective of food intake [6]. All women are examined in the supine position, despite the potential risk for compression of the vena cava with subsequent reduction of cardiac output and the supine hypotension syndrome [7]. The reason for this is that the central veins play a fundamental role in the control of cardiac output, and sensitivity for compression of these veins may be an important physiologic variable in the evaluation of the venous contribution to the maternal circulation and uteroplacental-fetal blood supply in normal and pathologic pregnancies.

The reproducibility of this methodology is evaluated in a subset of women [5]. For this group, measurements were performed twice on the same individual by two or more investigators, and the inter- and intraclass correlation coefficient (ICC) was calculated using maximum likelihood estimation for the linear mixed model [8, 9]. Next to this, the impact of an increasing number of repeat samples per kidney was examined by calculating the means and standard deviations of 2, 3, 4, 5 and 6 consecutive measurements per kidney, and by estimation of the intraclass correlation (MIXED procedure, SAS) [10]. From this, in the reported setting, a mean value of three consecutive measurements allows obtaining reproducible Doppler flow indices at the level of renal interlobar and hepatic veins [5].

Both kidneys and liver are scanned in the transverse plane, as illustrated in Figure 12.3 [11]. The anteroposterior diameter (mm) of the midpolar intrarenal pyelon is measured at the level just above the renal hilus. The interlobar arteries and veins are identified using color Doppler flow mapping. The impact of breathing movements on the ultrasound image is demonstrated to every patient and the relevance of holding breath during Doppler measurements is explained and demonstrated. Once the patient is familiar with the instructions of the ultrasonographer, the examination is performed according to a standard protocol: 1) A simultaneous Doppler signal of both interlobar arteries and veins is required for unequivocal identification of the examined vessels; 2) The real-time ultrasound image in combined B-D mode is frozen after visualization of at least 2–3 similar Doppler flow patterns during interrupted breathing; 3) The direction of the Doppler beam is adjusted according to the axis of the examined vessel when necessary, which normally should not exceed 30°; 4) Venous peak velocity (PV) and presystolic velocity (PSV) are plotted and VI is calculated automatically (PV – PSV/PV): VI is the venous Doppler equivalent of the arterial resistance index (RI); 5) For every woman, three consecutive measurements are performed for each kidney, for the reasons explained above.

In the liver, the right, left and middle branches of the hepatovenous tree are identified using color Doppler flow mapping and differentiated from hepatic arteries and the portal system [12]. Again, the impact of breathing movements on the ultrasound image is demonstrated and the woman is instructed. The same protocol as explained above is performed: 1) Doppler signals are sampled at three different locations from the craniocaudal midportion in the liver, preferably one sample of each of the main branches; 2) The real-time ultrasonic B-image and Doppler signal are visualized simultaneously and the scanning image is frozen after visualization of at least two to three similar Doppler waveforms during interrupted breathing; 3) As the direction of the Doppler beam is mostly parallel with the examined vessels, Doppler angle correction is rarely needed. If so, the axis of adjustment normally does not exceed 30°; 4) Velocities of the HV Doppler wave characteristics A, X, V and Y are measured (see Figure 4.1). For the monophasic or flat Doppler waveforms, where Doppler wave characteristics cannot easily be identified, venous maximum velocity (MxV) and minimum velocity (MnV) can be considered to represent the equivalents of X and Y and of A and V, respectively (see Figure 4.2). 5) For every woman, each of three consecutive measurements is recorded. After the scan, mean values of the three measured values of A-, X-, V- and Y-velocities are calculated and these results are registered in the database.

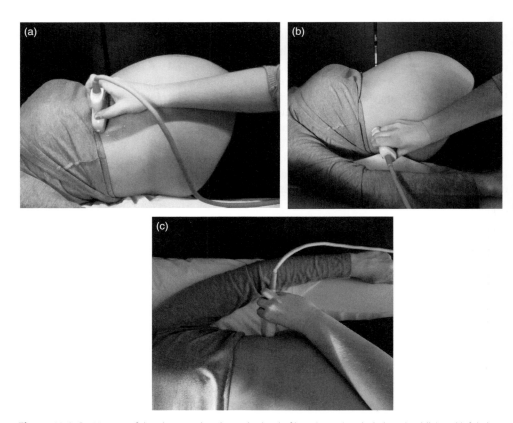

Figure 12.3 Positioning of the ultrasound probe at the level of liver (upper), right kidney (middle) and left kidney (bottom). (A black and white version of this figure will appear in some formats. For the color version, please refer to the plate section.)

For each of the veins, the time interval between the ECG P-wave and the corresponding venous Doppler A-wave (PA in milliseconds) can be measured (13) (see Figure 4.2). As the heart rate increases with advancing gestation, all measured PA-intervals should be expressed relative to the ECG-wave duration measured between consecutive R signals (RR interval) in milliseconds. Three consecutive intrarenal and hepatic venous pulse transit times (PTT) – labeled as PA/RR – are measured at each location and stored in the database.

Improving the Reproducibility of Venous Doppler Sonography

It has been demonstrated that the reproducibility of maternal venous Doppler sonography benefits from three inferences: 1) the use of repeated measures; 2) the addition of the maternal ECG; and 3) training [14].

The inter- and intraobserver intraclass correlation (ICC) of single venous impedance index values is low at around 0.35 [5]. ICC markedly improves to > 0.7 when mean values of three consecutive measurements are used [15]. This improvement is also illustrated by Bland–Altman analysis: the correlation range for renal interlobar vein impedance index is –0.22, 0.20 for single measurements, and decreases to –0.14, 0.12 after repeated measurements [14].

Because of the natural variation in the shape of venous Doppler waves, the identification of different wave characteristics and subsequent calculation of the venous impedance index may sometimes be very difficult. The maternal ECG can easily be used as a guiding reference for correct measurement of venous Doppler flow values [16]. For this, the ultrasound scanner needs an ECG lead, which allows depicting the ECG simultaneously with the Doppler wave pattern at the screen. Intraobserver correlation coefficient of renal interlobar vein Doppler measurements increased to > 0.80 with ECG-assistance [14].

As reported for many other measurements in ultrasound and/or Doppler sonography, intra- and interobserver correlation coefficients markedly improve from > 0.70 to > 0.9 after intensive training [14]. Training in venous Doppler sonography should include both the practical performance of the scanning technique as well as the correct interpretation of the Doppler wave characteristics.

Limitations and Pitfalls of Venous Doppler Sonography

Doppler sonography of the venous system is not as straightforward as at the level of heart and/or arteries. As explained above, venous Doppler wave patterns are influenced by many physiologic variables, such as breathing movements, gravity, external compression, muscle contractions, intraluminal valves, etc. [6] Next to this, interindividual anatomical variations are much more pronounced in the venous than in the arterial compartment [17].

Some specific diseases or organ pathologies can also influence the shape of venous Doppler waves and the value of venous flow measurements, such as chronic liver disease, portal hypertension or liver transplantation [18], renal tumor [19] or hydronephrosis [20], autoimmune vasculitis, etc. It should be emphasized that these diseases may interfere with the correct interpretation of venous Doppler measurements, with abnormal values present in perfectly normal pregnancies, and apparently normal values found during gestational hypertensive disease. The latter can also partially be explained by the dynamic character of venous vascular physiology, which is responsible for fluctuating values of venous impedance index [11]. These observations indicate that abnormal venous Doppler flow measurements do not necessarily reflect a state of disease, or vice versa. Serial measurements and longitudinal observations may help to distinguish normal from pathologic venous hemodynamic function [21].

Key Points

- The methodology to perform a venous Doppler assessment differs from arterial Doppler measurements, due to the large anatomical variability of the venous compartment, the typical physiologic properties of venous hemodynamics, the many physiologic variables interfering with venous return and current technological limitations in measuring velocities in the lower range.
- Venous Doppler sonography benefits from training, the simultaneous use of a maternal ECG and performing repeated measures.

- Patient specific conditions and disease may interfere with venous Doppler measurements, and should be taken into account before performing this assessment.

References

1. Pang CC. Measurement of body venous tone. *J Pharmacol Toxicol Methods*. 2000;**44**(2):341–60.

2. Pang CC. Autonomic control of the venous system in health and disease: effects of drugs. *Pharmacol Ther*. 2001;**90**(2–3):179–230.

3. Gelman S. Venous function and central venous pressure: a physiologic story. *Anesthesiology*. 2008;**108**(4):735–48.

4. Lui EY, Steinman AH, Cobbold RS, Johnston KW. Human factors as a source of error in peak Doppler velocity measurement. *J Vasc Surg*. 2005;**42**(5):972–9.

5. Gyselaers W, Molenberghs G, Van Mieghem W, Ombelet W. Doppler measurement of renal interlobar vein impedance index in uncomplicated and preeclamptic pregnancies. *Hypertens Pregnancy*. 2009;**28**(1):23–33.

6. Teichgraber UK, Gebel M, Benter T, Manns MP. Effect of respiration, exercise, and food intake on hepatic vein circulation. *J Ultrasound Med*. 1997;**16**(8):549–54.

7. Kinsella SM, Lohmann G. Supine hypotensive syndrome. *Obstet Gynecol*. 1994;**83**(5 Pt 1):774–88.

8. Verbeke G MG. Linear Mixed Models for Longitudinal Data. 2nd edn. New York: Springer; 2001.

9. Laenen A, Vangeneugden T, Geys H, Molenberghs G. Generalized reliability estimation using repeated measurements. *Br J Math Stat Psychol*. 2006; **59**(Pt 1):113–31.

10. SAS Institute Inc. SAS/IML software: Changes and enhancements through release. 1995. Cary, NC.

11. Gyselaers W, Mullens W, Tomsin K, Mesens T, Peeters L. Role of dysfunctional maternal venous hemodynamics in the pathophysiology of pre-eclampsia: a review. *Ultrasound Obstet Gynecol*. 2011;**38**(2):123–9.

12. Gyselaers W, Molenberghs G, Mesens T, Peeters L. Maternal hepatic vein Doppler velocimetry during uncomplicated pregnancy and pre-eclampsia. *Ultrasound Med Biol*. 2009;**35**(8):1278–83.

13. Tomsin K, Mesens T, Molenberghs G, Gyselaers W. Venous pulse transit time in normal pregnancy and preeclampsia. *Reprod Sci*. 2012;**19**(4):431–6.

14. Staelens AS, Tomsin K, Oben J, Mesens T, Grieten L, Gyselaers W. Improving the reliability of venous doppler flow measurements: relevance of combined ECG, training and repeated measures. *Ultrasound Med Biol*. 2014;**40**(7):1722–8.

15. Mesens T, Tomsin K, Molenberghs G, Gyselaers W. Reproducibility and repeatability of maternal venous Doppler flow measurements in renal interlobar and hepatic veins. *Ultrasound Obstet Gynecol*. 2010;**36**(1):120–1.

16. Gyselaers W. Hemodynamics of the maternal venous compartment: a new area to explore in obstetric ultrasound imaging. *Ultrasound Obstet Gynecol*. 2008;**32**(5):716–7.

17. Spentzouris G, Zandian A, Cesmebasi A, et al. The clinical anatomy of the inferior vena cava: a review of common congenital anomalies and considerations for clinicians. *Clin Anat*. 2014;**27**(8):1234–43.

18. Kruskal JB, Newman PA, Sammons LG, Kane RA. Optimizing Doppler and color flow US: application to hepatic sonography. *Radiographics*. 2004;**24**(3):657–75.

19. Helenon O, Correas JM, Chabriais J, Boyer JC, Melki P, Moreau JF. Renal vascular Doppler imaging: clinical benefits

of power mode. *Radiographics*. 1998;**18**(6): 1441–54; discussion 55–7.

20. Bateman GA, Cuganesan R. Renal vein Doppler sonography of obstructive uropathy. *AJR Am J Roentgenol*. 2002;**178**(4):921–5.

21. Mesens T, Tomsin K, Oben J, Staelens A, Gyselaers W. Maternal venous hemodynamics assessment for prediction of preeclampsia should be longitudinal. *J Matern Fetal Neonatal Med*. 2015;**28**(3): 311–5.

Chapter 13

Noninvasive Techniques for Measuring Cardiac Output During Pregnancy

Victoria L. Meah, Eric J. Stöhr and John R. Cockcroft

Summary

Cardiac output is considered an important indicator of cardiac function during pregnancy. Due to the risks associated with the use of invasive methods, noninvasive cardiac output assessment is preferred within the obstetric population. Cardiac output can be measured using different noninvasive techniques, such as echocardiography, cardiac magnetic resonance imaging, inert gas rebreathing, bioimpedance/bioreactance, and finger plethysmography, all of which are discussed within this chapter. Some considerations of each method in relation to cardiac output measurement in the parturient are also discussed. Recommendations for noninvasive cardiac output assessment during pregnancy are provided.

Introduction

Cardiac output (CO) is reflective of the peripheral blood flow demand and the convective O_2 delivery, and hence is considered by many gynecologists and obstetricians as an important indicator of cardiac function during pregnancy. The measurement of CO and its change across pregnancy can be extremely useful when assessing cardiovascular (dys)function. In many areas of research, thermodilution performed with pulmonary artery catheterization (PAC) is considered as the practical gold-standard measurement of CO and has historically been used to determine the accuracy of new techniques. However, in the clinical diagnostic or therapeutic setting this technique is not feasible. As PAC is highly invasive, it is not desirable during pregnancy, and in nearly all situations, noninvasive techniques are preferred for use within the obstetric population. Therefore, this chapter will provide a synopsis of those common noninvasive methods for measurement of maternal CO that are frequently used in practice. At the end of this chapter, considerations of their use in relation to the parturient are discussed.

Techniques

Echocardiography

Since its initial use by Edler and Hertz [1], the use of cardiac ultrasound ("echocardiography") has become the most widely used diagnostic tool to differentiate normal from abnormal cardiac structure and function [2]. During pregnancy, echocardiography is the preferred screening method to assess maternal cardiac function due to its lack of radiation exposure, good availability, good mobility and relatively high temporal resolution [3]. Within echocardiography, multiple techniques exist that allow for the quantification of CO during pregnancy. For example, it is important to distinguish two-dimensional and three-dimensional

Table 13.1 Overview of different echocardiographic techniques used during pregnancy

Name of technique	Image acquisition	Modality	Dimension	Recommended use?
Teichholz	Parasternal long-axis	M-mode	1-D	no
Suprasternal Doppler	Suprasternal notch (jugulum)	Doppler	1-D	yes
Single plane	Apical 4-chamber	B-mode	2-D	yes
Simpson's biplane	Apical 4-chamber & 2-chamber	B-mode	2-D	yes
Triplane	Apical 4-chamber, 2-chamber & long-axis	Multiple B-mode	2-D	yes
LV outflow tract	Parasternal long-axis & Doppler on apical 4-chamber	B-mode & Doppler	2-D	yes
3-D	Apical 4-chamber	B-mode	3-D	yes

"brightness-mode imaging," which also enable the visualization of the structure of the heart, from those echocardiographic modalities such as Doppler and M-mode that provide a quantitative indication of cardiac function without being able to determine morphological adaptation of the maternal heart. Table 13.1 provides an overview of these modalities. In all techniques, it is important to adhere to general principles of data acquisition, such as consistent frame rates, imaging depth, acoustic windows (i.e. measurement locations on the chest) and position of the parturient. Appropriate training and experience are essential to ensure reliable and valid CO measurements. It is strongly recommended that the different echocardiographic techniques, or indeed any other method to measure CO, should not be used interchangeably. This section will briefly introduce the different echocardiographic techniques that can be used to determine CO during pregnancy.

Teichholz

The Teichholz method [4] is probably one of the oldest techniques, though now rarely used. For this reason, the description of its use will be brief. The Teichholz method is a one-dimensional approach, which measures the change in left ventricular (LV) dimension between the end-diastolic and end-systolic state from a parasternal long-axis view. While validated against invasive techniques and useful for many years [5], its limitation is that the volume of the LV is estimated from a single measurement plane, therefore not accounting for interindividual differences in LV shape or – more importantly – for a nonuniform adaptation of the maternal heart. Due to the structural cardiac adaptations known to occur during pregnancy, geometric assumptions of calculations of CO may not be valid [6]. It is worth mentioning that the M-mode approach has the advantage that the frame rates are higher than in any other technique, and therefore fast-moving structures such as cardiac valves can be examined with high accuracy [7]. As for its use in quantifying CO, it is preferable to seek alternative approaches first, and only use it if no other options are available.

Single Plane B-mode (4-chamber Area)

The single plane B-mode 4-chamber view is an improvement compared with the Teichholz technique. It is a two-dimensional (area) approach and takes into account the shape of the LV along its entire length. The area-change from end-diastolic to end-systolic state is used to estimate LV volumes and calculate stroke volume (see Figure 13.1a). Multiplied by the prevailing heart rate, CO can be estimated. Its disadvantage is that the LV shape is only viewed from one plane, which means that asymmetric morphology in other areas remains undetected. This technique is preferable over the Teichholz technique, but the Simpson's (modified) biplane approach discussed in the following section presents a further improvement.

Simpson's (Modified) Biplane

The technical basis of the Simpson's (modified) biplane technique is based upon the single plane approach referred to previously. Here, a second plane is added to the single plane 4-chamber image (a so-called 2-chamber image; see Figure 13.1b) and, together with a validated formula, the two end-diastolic areas and end-systolic areas result in an improved estimation of stroke volume and CO. Of course, this technique can also not fully eliminate the presence of asymmetric wall morphologies as it is based upon two planes out of a total of 360°. Occasionally in pregnant women, it may not be possible to obtain high-quality images from the left lateral window typically used to collect 4- and 2-chamber images. This is caused by changes in body habitus during pregnancy as a result of the gravid uterus and the enlargement of breast tissue. Under such circumstances, other approaches are needed and the LV outflow tract method may be a welcome alternative. However, at present the Simpson's (modified) biplane technique is considered robust. A potential limitation of this approach and the single plane 4-chamber method are low frame rates. Provided frame rates are > 40–50 frames per second, a good estimate of CO can be achieved (see Echocardiography section for important technical considerations). Overall, this technique has many advantages and should be used preferentially over many other approaches [8].

Triplane

The triplane analysis is a further extension of the Simpson's (modified) biplane approach. It has been enabled by advances in ultrasound transducer technologies, which now enable the simultaneous acquisition of three single apical planes, evenly distributed / interspersed by 60 degrees (see Figure 13.2). This is an important improvement from the separate acquisition of the Simpson's (modified) biplane method and its semiautomatic analysis helps the investigator to obtain valid numbers in a relatively short time. It should be mentioned that this technique will likely require additional training. It is essential to ensure standardization of all three imaging planes to allow for optimal measurement; however, this can be challenging to achieve in the displaced maternal heart, especially when acoustic windows are limited (see section on Simpson's (Modified) Biplane). This technique is very promising as it removes some of the error inherent to other echocardiographic measurements and allows volumetric estimations within the same cardiac cycle.

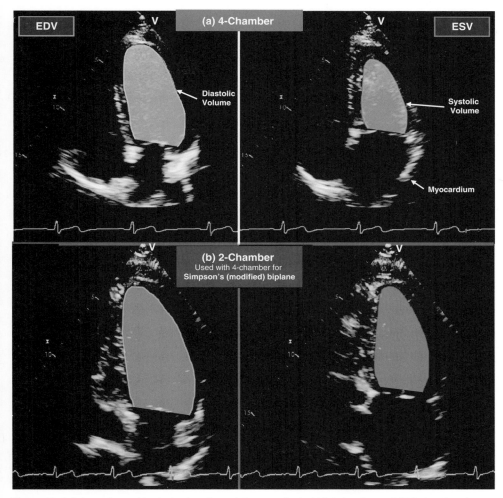

Figure 13.1 Echocardiographic single plane B-mode images of apical (a) 4-chamber and (b) 2-chamber views. The 4-chamber view can be used on its own to calculate cardiac output through estimation of stroke volume by measuring the area-change between end-diastolic (EDV) and end-systolic volumes (ESV) of the left ventricle, shown on the figure by yellow and green areas, respectively. The Simpson's (modified) biplane method uses EDV and ESV measurements from both the 4- and 2-chamber images, which increases the reliability and validity of cardiac output estimations as it may account for some interindividual variation in cardiac asymmetry. (A black and white version of this figure will appear in some formats. For the color version, please refer to the plate section.)

Emerging 3D Modalities

In recent years, 3-D echocardiography has become commercially available and has received remarkable interest because it may overcome most of the limitations previously mentioned in relation to other echocardiographic methods. For the quantification of CO, 3-D echocardiography does not appear to be superior to standardized 2-D Simpson's (modified) biplane measurements as low frame rates of acquisition (20–30 frames per second) currently introduce some error. Undoubtedly, 3-D echocardiography will be

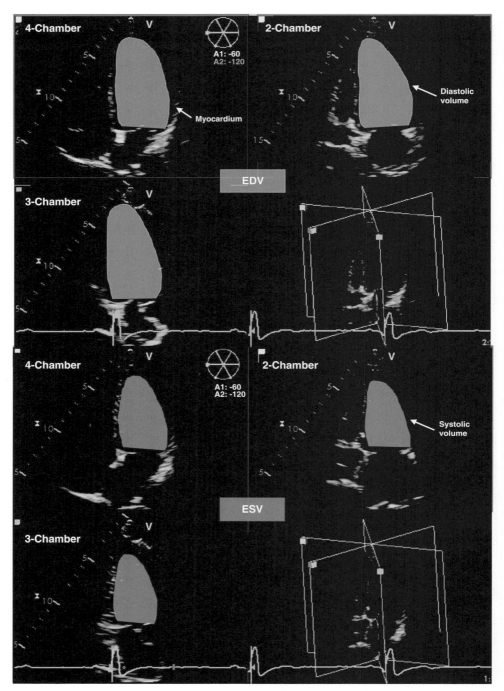

Figure 13.2 Echocardiographic triplane images of apical 4-chamber, 2-chamber and 3-chamber views collected from the same cardiac cycle. Stroke volume is estimated using the area-change between end-diastolic (EDV) and end-systolic (ESV) volumes (shown by yellow and green areas, respectively), in each of the three planes of the left ventricle. (A black and white version of this figure will appear in some formats. For the color version, please refer to the plate section.)

the measurement tool of the future, and practitioners are advised to become familiar with the method while its accuracy improves as a result of technical advancements.

LV Outflow Tract

As mentioned previously, it is possible for the apical 4-chamber and 2-chamber windows to be obstructed and an alternative approach may be required. In this case, the combined measurements of the aortic diameter and aortic blood flow velocity are a useful option. The so-called LV outflow tract measurement is the composite of a measurement of the aortic diameter obtained from a parasternal long-axis view and a Doppler signal from an apical 5-chamber window. Although the 5-chamber view is located on the patient's chest in the same or a similar place as the 4-chamber and 2-chamber views, it only requires good representation of a small area (the aortic outflow tract) and may therefore be an appropriate choice (see Figure 13.3). Once the aortic diameter and velocity time integral have been estimated, a formula allows for the calculation of stroke volume. An assumption of this measurement is that aortic diameter stays constant throughout the cardiac cycle, which is debatable and may introduce error [8]. Overall, this technique is the second choice after the Simpson's (modified) biplane approach.

Suprasternal Doppler

As the name suggests, the suprasternal Doppler approach is a Doppler approach, but without the guidance from 2-D ultrasound imaging (B-mode imaging). It is widely used in pregnancy and has been validated in some devices [9]. As such, it is recommended and has proven useful as a diagnostic and monitoring tool. A small methodological shortfall is

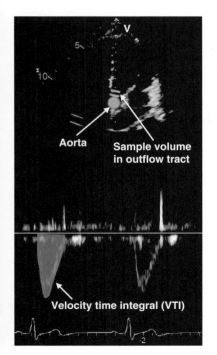

Figure 13.3 Echocardiographic image showing a Doppler signal of the left ventricular aortic outflow tract (LVOT) from an apical 5-chamber window. To collect this Doppler signal, a sample volume (indicated by the yellow lines) is placed within the aortic outflow tract just prior to the aortic valve (blue circle). The velocity time integral (VTI) is then calculated by tracing the Doppler waveform obtained at the LVOT (indicated by the red trace). Stroke volume is calculated by applying the equation: LVOT VTI x cross-sectional area of the aorta ($CSA = \pi r^2$), where aortic diameter is obtained from a separate parasternal long-axis view image. (A black and white version of this figure will appear in some formats. For the color version, please refer to the plate section.)

the aforementioned lack of visualization of the heart itself, which would help to confirm the exact location of the Doppler sample within the aorta. Absolute values are not as accurate as those from other ultrasound techniques as the aortic diameter required for the calculation of CO is not known, but estimated from a height-dependent equation that does not account for changes in aortic diameter during pregnancy. In addition, increased aortic blood flow and velocity as a result of the increased circulating blood volume during gestation, and upward and leftward displacement of the heart by the gravid uterus, may also affect the measurement of CO from suprasternal Doppler [10]. Some technical training is recommended to achieve competency in the use of suprasternal Doppler devices; however, once completed, it offers reproducible results [11]. Overall, this is a reliable technique that is time efficient and easy to apply in practice and may be useful in the quantification of longitudinal changes in CO across pregnancy.

Cardiac Magnetic Resonance Imaging (MRI)

The use of MRI to measure CO in pregnancy is very similar to that of some of the echocardiographic approaches. Similar to Simpson's (modified) biplane, triplane and 3-D echocardiography, MRI images are acquired and LV end-diastolic and end-systolic contours are manually (or semiautomatically) traced. However, with MRI this occurs on short-axis views (in contrast to longitudinal views in Simpson's (modified) biplane, triplane and 3-D echocardiography). The contours of the separate short-axis slices are then stacked and summated, which ultimately results in the calculation of stroke volume (see Figure 13.4). While highly accurate, it is questionable whether pregnant women without the suspicion of other cardiac abnormalities should undergo a lengthy, physically challenging (repeated breath-holds) and relatively expensive procedure to assess CO. However, it has to be acknowledged that for pregnancy research purposes, the accuracy of MRI is appealing and is certainly considered a valid and reliable method. In contrast to echocardiography, cardiac MRI is not affected by changes in ventricular geometry and physical changes of pregnancy. While no adverse reports of cardiac MRI in the parturient are known, concerns regarding the effects of teratogenicity and acoustic damage on the developing fetus have been noted [3]. It is recommended that cardiac MRI should be avoided in the first trimester (until after fetal organogenesis), and should only be used when other techniques cannot provide adequate diagnostic information. A contrast medium can be used in cardiac MRI to enhance the resolution of images. Gadolinium is a commonly used contrast agent that is assumed to cross the fetal blood placental barrier. Although long-term risks of exposure to the developing fetus are unknown, free gadolinium ions are toxic and have been associated with increased risk of nephrogenic systemic fibrosis in adults with renal insufficiency. Therefore, the use of gadolinium-based MRI is controversial during pregnancy.

Inert Gas Rebreathing

Inert gas rebreathing is a method based on the Fick principle involving the rebreathing of blood soluble and insoluble gases from which CO is calculated through measurement of their relative levels. The Fick principle states that blood flow is proportional to the arteriovenous oxygen difference across an organ. Therefore, the rate of disappearance of the blood soluble gas from the alveolar space is proportional to pulmonary blood flow, and this is equivalent to CO in the absence of intrapulmonary shunts. The blood insoluble gas is used

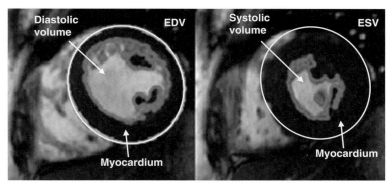

Figure 13.4 Magnetic resonance imaging (MRI) of the myocardium from a short-axis view. Stroke volume is estimated using the area-change between end-diastolic (EDV) and end-systolic (ESV) volumes of the left ventricle on multiple stacked images from the short-axis view.
Image kindly provided by Dr. Jonathan Rodrigues, Clinical Research Fellow in Cardiac Imaging, NIHR Bristol Cardiovascular Biomedical Research Unit, Bristol Heart Institute.
(A black and white version of this figure will appear in some formats. For the color version, please refer to the plate section.)

to estimate lung volume from which the blood soluble gas disappears. The concentrations of gases are measured at the rebreathing valve through use of a gas analyzer. The measurement must be conducted either for a determined duration or at a set breathing frequency, and the accuracy of this method depends on the ability of the individual to perform the rebreathe maneuver correctly. The accuracy of the rebreathing method may be affected by increased carbon dioxide production and high CO states [12], both of which are known to be increased in the parturient. Overall, this is a safe technique that has been used previously in pregnancy [13].

Bioimpedance and Bioreactance

Bioimpedance techniques detect changes in electrical resistance induced by vascular blood flow across the cardiac cycle. Standard systems apply a high-frequency electrical current of known amplitude across the thorax and measure the resulting changes in voltage. The impedance, or ratio between voltage and amplitude, is proportional to the amount of fluid in the thorax, and the rate of change in impedance relates to the blood flow in the aorta from which stroke volume (SV), and therefore CO is estimated. The electrical current is transferred through skin electrodes on the thorax, which are attached in equipment-dependent locations. Algorithms within systems adjust outputs to account for individual vascular flow; however, clinical validation studies continue to show conflicting accounts of the reliability of this technique [14]. Accuracy of CO measurement can be affected by the placement of electrodes, patient movement and variations in body size, electrocautery and arrhythmia. Bioimpedance can also be affected by changes in hematocrit, intrathoracic fluid, and peripheral edema. all of which are known to alter across the course of gestation [6, 15].

Bioreactance is a variation of the impedance technique, in which equipment analyzes the frequency variations of a delivered oscillating current across the thorax. The analysis of frequency, as opposed to amplitude modulation used in bioimpedance, results in a reduced signal-to-noise ratio and, therefore, an improvement in the accuracy of CO measurement. Bioreactance is considered a more reliable technique than bioimpedance for the measurement of CO as it is less affected by placement of electrodes, patient movement and variable environments [15]. Both methods are easily applicable, mobile and relatively low cost, making them attractive for routine use. It should be noted that despite the clear advantages of their practical use, neither bioimpedance nor bioreactance have been validated for use during gestation, and therefore their accuracy must be considered [16]. Assumptions about these techniques may not be valid in conditions of low flow, i.e. during high-resistance disease states such as gestational hypertension or preeclampsia, and therefore may not be suitable for use in clinical pregnant populations [17, 18].

Finger Plethysmography

Finger plethysmography allows for continuous, noninvasive measurement and monitoring of blood pressure and CO. This technique is based upon finger arterial pressure pulse contour analysis. Devices assess pulse pressure using photoelectric plethysmography in combination with a volume-clamp technique through an inflatable finger cuff. A volume-clamp technique refers to when the diameter of an artery under a cuff wrapped around the finger is kept constant. Changes in arterial diameter are detected by an infrared photo-plethysmograph built into the finger cuff and are impeded by an inflatable air bladder to maintain the correct clamped diameter. Blood pressure and heart rate are derived from the stored pressure trace. CO is derived through analysis of the pulse contour using aortic characteristic impedance, compliance and estimated cardiac afterload [19]. Due to its potential of beat-by-beat continuous measurements of blood pressure, CO and other hemodynamic parameters, this method may be particularly useful in the monitoring of hypertensive disorders during pregnancy [20]. However, the accuracy of plethysmography has been contested in states of changing vascular resistance. While healthy pregnancy is associated with a low-resistance, high-volume state, this may be reversed in manifestations of preeclampsia to a high-resistance, low-volume state. Therefore, the clinical application of such devices for monitoring CO during pregnancy may not be appropriate [21]. Peripheral edema, a common issue experienced during pregnancy, may also influence the reliability of finger plethysmography in the measurement of CO. Some devices require the input of physical characteristics (i.e. weight) to determine individual aortic pressure-area relationships, and these algorithms may be invalid during pregnancy due to changes in body habitus and remodeling of the aorta as a result of gestation. Consequently, this technique may be best used to monitor blood pressure in the parturient.

Benefit of Measuring Cardiac Output During Exercise

While an understanding of resting CO is important, a dynamic evaluation of the maternal cardiovascular system will likely provide greater insight into potential maladaptive responses. Pregnancy has been described as a continuous physiological stress test for the maternal cardiovascular system, but this unique process can be accompanied by clinical disorders that arise solely during gestation and consequently revert postpartum. Previous studies have demonstrated the potential of exercise-testing to unmask cardiac abnormalities that are otherwise undetected at rest [22]. It is hypothesized that dysfunction identified during a physiological challenge, such as exercise, may precede the clinical manifestation of disease and could allow the earlier detection and treatment of cardiovascular issues during pregnancy [23]. Measurement of CO during exercise is possible using echocardiography, cardiac MRI, inert gas rebreathing and finger plethysmography. Increased heart rate and body movement associated with exercise presents additional challenges to the accuracy of each method. Additional technical training may be necessary to acquire reliable and valid results.

Summary

In this chapter, different noninvasive techniques for the measurement of CO in the parturient have been presented and discussed. An overview of these noninvasive techniques is provided in Table 13.2. Each method requires a specific approach, and some methods are preferred over others. In general, a robust, cost-efficient and safe method is the Simpson's (modified) biplane technique. Other approaches, such as the LV outflow tract method, suprasternal Doppler and occasionally MRI are also appropriate for CO measurements in an obstetric population. The limitations of the aforementioned and other techniques discussed within this chapter should be acknowledged in relation to pregnancy. The authors advise the reader to consult published guidelines prior to practical implementation of any technique.

Key Points

- Echocardiography is the most commonly used noninvasive method to estimate CO in pregnant women.
- New emerging techniques for CO measurement are cardiac MRI, inert gas rebreathing, bioimpedance or -reactance technologies and finger plethysmography.
- All methods have technology-specific possibilities and limitations, which may also differ between pregnant and nonpregnant individuals.
- A dynamic evaluation of the maternal cardiovascular system during exercise will likely provide greater insight into normal and potentially maladaptive responses.

References

1. Singh S, Goyal A. The origin of echocardiography: a tribute to Inge Edler. *Tex Heart Inst J.* 2007;**34**(4):431–8.

2. Oxborough D. A practical approach to transthoracic echocardiography. *Brit J Cardiac Nurs.* 2008;**3**:163–9.

3. Regitz-Zagrosek V, Blomstrom Lundqvist C, Borghi C, et al. ESC Guidelines on the management of cardiovascular diseases during pregnancy: the Task Force on the Management of Cardiovascular Diseases during Pregnancy of the European Society of Cardiology (ESC). *Eur Heart J.* 2011;**32** (24):3147–97.

4. Teichholz LE, Kreulen T, Herman MV, Gorlin R. Problems in echocardiographic volume determinations: echocardiographic-angiographic correlations in the presence of absence of asynergy. *Am J Cardiol.* 1976;**37**(1):7–11.

5. Kronik G, Slany J, Mosslacher H. Comparative value of eight M-mode echocardiographic formulas for determining left ventricular stroke volume. A correlative study with thermodilution and left ventricular single-plane cineangiography. *Circulation.* 1979;**60**(6):1308–16.

6. van Oppen AC, Stigter RH, Bruinse HW. Cardiac output in normal pregnancy: a critical review. *Obstet Gynecol.* 1996;**87**(2): 310–8.

Table 13.2 Overview of noninvasive techniques of cardiac output measurement during pregnancy

Modality	Name	Advantages	Disadvantages	References
Echocardiography	Teichholz	• High temporal resolution	• No visual verification of anatomical location; • 1-dimensional so unable to account for cardiac asymmetry	[3, 15, 24]
Echocardiography	Single plane	• Accounts for some anatomical asymmetry • End-diastolic and end-systolic volumes can be estimated	• Only 2-dimensional for a 3-dimensional structure	
Echocardiography	Simpson's (modified) biplane	• Accounts for more anatomical asymmetry; • End-diastolic and end-systolic volumes can be estimated	• Data obtained from different images and therefore different cardiac cycles	
Echocardiography	Triplane	• Accounts for most of the anatomical symmetry • End-diastolic and end-systolic volumes can be estimated; • Within-beat data	• Difficult to perform measurements; • Additional training required	
Echocardiography	3-D	• Potentially accounts for all anatomical asymmetry • End-diastolic and end-systolic volumes can be estimated • Within-beat data	• Low temporal resolution • Stitching artifacts • Difficult to perform measurements	
Echocardiography	LV outflow tract	• Good accuracy due to incorporation of blood velocities • Easy to measure in individuals in whom biplane or triplane images are difficult	• Data obtained from different images and therefore different cardiac cycles	

Method		Advantages	Disadvantages	References
Echocardiography	Suprasternal Doppler	• Easy use • Accurate velocity measurements	• No visual verification of anatomical location • No measurement of aortic diameter	[9]
Magnetic resonance imaging (MRI)		• High spatial resolution • Possible to account for anatomical asymmetry due to stacking of images	• Relatively low temporal resolution	[25, 26]
Rebreathing	Inert gas rebreathing	• Safe noninvasive method	• Variation in breathing patterns can influence results	[27, 28]
Impedance	Bioimpedance	• Easily applicable, mobile and low cost noninvasive method	• Measurement affected by electrode placement, patient movement and variable environments	[15, 18]
	Bioreactance	• Measurement more reliable than bioimpedance due to lower signal-to-noise ratio	• Assumptions of technique may not be valid in high-resistance disease states	[15, 17]
Finger plethysmography		• Continuous beat-by-beat monitoring	• Influenced by algorithms based on patient physical characteristics which may not be valid during pregnancy	[29]

7. Feigenbaum H. Role of M-mode technique in today's echocardiography. *J Am Soc Echocardiogr.* 2010;**23**(3):240–57; 335–7.

8. Melchiorre K, Sharma R, Thilaganathan B. Cardiac structure and function in normal pregnancy. *Curr Opin Obstet Gynecol.* 2012;**24**(6):413–21.

9. McNamara H, Barclay P, Sharma V. Accuracy and precision of the ultrasound cardiac output monitor (USCOM 1A) in pregnancy: comparison with three-dimensional transthoracic echocardiography. *Br J Anaesth.* 2014;**113**(4):669–76.

10. Poppas A, Shroff SG, Korcarz CE, et al. Serial assessment of the cardiovascular system in normal pregnancy. Role of arterial compliance and pulsatile arterial load. *Circulation.* 1997;**95**(10):2407–15.

11. Dey I, Sprivulis P. Emergency physicians can reliably assess emergency department patient cardiac output using the USCOM continuous wave Doppler cardiac output monitor. *Emerg Med Australas.* 2005;**17**(3): 193–9.

12. Marik PE. Noninvasive cardiac output monitors: a state-of the-art review. *J Cardiothorac Vasc Anesth.* 2013;**27**(1): 121–34.

13. Mahendru AA, Everett TR, Wilkinson IB, Lees CC, McEniery CM. A longitudinal study of maternal cardiovascular function from preconception to the postpartum period. *J Hypertens.* 2014;**32**(4):849–56.

14. Jhanji S, Dawson J, Pearse RM. Cardiac output monitoring: basic science and clinical application. *Anaesthesia.* 2008;**63**(2):172–81.

15. Staelens AS, Bertrand PB, Vonck S, Malbrain MLNG, Gyselaers W. Non-invasive methods for maternal cardiac output monitoring. *Fetal Matern Med Rev.* 2015:1–17.

16. Wallenburg HC. Maternal haemodynamics in pregnancy. *Fetal Matern Med Rev.* 1990;**2**(01):45–66.

17. Keren H, Burkhoff D, Squara P. Evaluation of a noninvasive continuous cardiac output monitoring system based on thoracic bioreactance. *Am J Physiol Heart Circ Physiol.* 2007;**293**(1):H583–9.

18. Easterling TR, Benedetti TJ, Carlson KL, Watts DH. Measurement of cardiac output in pregnancy by thermodilution and impedance techniques. *Br J Obstet Gynaecol.* 1989;**96**(1):67–9.

19. Dyson KS, Shoemaker JK, Arbeille P, Hughson RL. Model flow estimates of cardiac output compared with Doppler ultrasound during acute changes in vascular resistance in women. *Exp Physiol.* 2010;**95**(4):561–8.

20. Rang S, de Pablo Lapiedra B, van Montfrans GA, Bouma BJ, Wesseling KH, Wolf H. Modelflow: a new method for noninvasive assessment of cardiac output in pregnant women. *Am J Obstet Gynecol.* 2007;**196**(3):235 e1–8.

21. Elvan-Taspinar A, Uiterkamp LA, Sikkema JM, et al. Validation and use of the Finometer for blood pressure measurement in normal, hypertensive and pre-eclamptic pregnancy. *J Hypertens.* 2003;**21**(11):2053–60.

22. Gibbons RJ, Balady GJ, Beasley JW, et al. ACC/AHA Guidelines for Exercise Testing. A report of the American College of Cardiology/American Heart Association Task Force on Practice Guidelines (Committee on Exercise Testing). *J Am Coll Cardiol.* 1997;**30**(1):260–311.

23. Meah VL, Cockcroft J, Stöhr EJ. Maternal cardiac twist pre-pregnancy: potential as a novel marker of pre-eclampsia. *Fetal Matern Med Rev.* 2013;**24**(4):289–95.

24. Armstrong WF, Ryan T. *Feigenbaum's Echocardiography.* 7th edn: Lippincott Williams & Wilkins; 2009.

25. Lorenz CH, Walker ES, Morgan VL, Klein SS, Graham TP, Jr. Normal human right and left ventricular mass, systolic function, and gender differences by cine magnetic resonance imaging. *J Cardiovasc Magn Reson.* 1999;**1**(1):7–21.

26. La Gerche A, Claessen G, Van de Bruaene A, et al. Cardiac MRI: a new gold standard for ventricular volume quantification during high-intensity exercise. *Circ Cardiovasc Imaging.* 2013;**6**(2):329–38.

27. Jakovljevic DG, Nunan D, Donovan G, Hodges LD, Sandercock GR, Brodie DA. Comparison of cardiac output determined by different rebreathing methods at rest and at peak exercise. *Eur J Appl Physiol.* 2008;**102**(5):593–9.

28. Peyton PJ, Bailey M, Thompson BR. Reproducibility of cardiac output measurement by the nitrous oxide rebreathing technique. *J Clin Monit Comput.* 2009;**23**(4):233–6.

29. Schutte AE, Huisman HW, Van Rooyen JM, Oosthuizen W, Jerling JC. Sensitivity of the Finometer device in detecting acute and medium-term changes in cardiovascular function. *Blood Press Monit.* 2003;**8**(5): 195–201.

Techniques of Measuring Plasma Volume Changes in Pregnancy

Anneleen Staelens and Marc Spaanderman

Summary

Restricted plasma volume prior to and during pregnancy has been clinically linked to placental syndrome – that is to say, gestational maternal hypertensive sequellae on the one hand and fetal growth restriction on the other. As most of the plasma volume is localized at the venous side of the vascular system, when having a healthy heart, plasma volume largely reflexes venous reserve capacity to balance alterations in arterial needs. Plasma volume can be measured directly by bleeding, obviously not applicable to human research, or indirectly using dilution or indicator dilution techniques. The latter two techniques require first order kinetics. Moreover, the indicator must be traceable and measurable. Finally, when used in pregnancy, they must be safe for both mother and fetus. More novel bioelectrical impedance techniques claim to be able to estimate whole body extracellular fluid content. The reliability to assess plasma volume, as part of the extracellular volume, by bioimpedance, remains to be elucidated, but when consistent and precise, it has the potency to be highly applicable in daily care.

Introduction

Plasma volume reflects, when corrected for total red blood cell mass, the total size of the whole body intravascular volume. As in unstressed conditions about two-thirds of this volume is localized in the venous compartment, it is a strong indicator of venous volume. As the venous system is roughly 30 times more compliant than the arterial system, the venous compartment primarily serves as a readily available reservoir to balance increased arterial needs. As such, functionally, plasma volume may be viewed as a static marker for venous reserve capacity. Clinically, in normotensive women, low nonpregnant plasma volume relates to several reproductive problems, such as unexplained recurrent miscarriage, preeclampsia, preterm birth and small-for-gestational-age infancy [1, 2]. During pregnancy, as early as in the middle of the last century, but also replicated later, low plasma volume has also been linked to gestational hypertensive disease and fetal growth restriction [3–5]. Whether or not this results from shallow increase in plasma volume, normal increase in pre-existing low plasma volume or loss of volume may vary between subjects and timing of the assessment.

Theoretically, plasma volume can be determined by direct measurement (exsanguination), dilution method, indicator dilution method and bioimpedance. As this chapter focuses on plasma volume measurement prior to and in human pregnancy, we limit to our description to indicator dilution technique and bioimpedance.

Dilution Method

In the nineteenth century, German physician Karl von Vierordt calculated plasma volume in animals by exsanguination without sacrificing them as done earlier by Welkler [6, 7]. Von Vierordt determined the dilution of the erythrocytes when he assumed plasma volume had restored, supposing absent reactive rise in erythrocytes. This reactive endogenous dilution technique is neither precise nor applicable in humans. Alternatively, by rapid infusion of fluid load, exogenous imposed dilution of subjects blood, plasma and blood volume can be assessed, evaluating changes in blood composition prior, during and after completion of the plasma volume expansion [8–10]. As the loss to the interstitial space may be substantial, especially in those with increased capillary leakage, this technique may lead to overestimation of the actual plasma volume. None of these techniques are currently employed.

Indicator Dilution Technique

Opposite to estimation of plasma volume by dilution of the circulatory content, indicator dilution techniques are based on administration of molecules which will be distributed over the circulation. These injected recognizable substances must have certain qualities to allow reliable assessment of plasma volume: first, they must stay in the circulation throughout the measurement without affecting vessel integrity, and, second, they should not disappear due to combined loss as a consequence of binding, disintegration, degradation or renal excretion affecting accountable first-order disappearance. The metabolization pathway and half-life of the indicator has to be known and cannot be too short. Finally, if used throughout pregnancy, they should neither pass into nor be metabolized by the placenta, ensuring safety for the developing fetus and accuracy for the plasma volume assessment. Therefore, tracers preferably have large molecular weight so as to prevent transcapillary escape, should not bind to plasma proteins, vessel wall or other blood components, and disappearance must be the consequence of either renal excretion or hepatogenic metabolization.

With any indicator dilution method, the volume of blood plasma is calculated according to the following equation:

$$Volume_{Plasma} \times concentration\ marker_{t=0} =$$
$$Volume_{Injected\ dye} \times concentration\ marker_{Injected\ dye}$$

To assess the concentration of the injected marker in the circulation at virtual t=0, assuming a first-order disappearance kinetic, after log transforming the measured concentrations of the dye at given time points after injections allowing the dye to distribute over the circulation, by regression analysis, the concentration of the dye at virtual t=0 can be assessed by the intercept of the y axis at t=0.

Albumin

Dyes

Human albumin (molecular weight 66.5kDa) is a large water-soluble globular protein which is abundantly present in blood plasma, where it strongly regulates the colloidal osmotic pressure, as it normally does not easily escape from the circulation. In recent decades, different albumin-binding indicators have been used to measure plasma volume. **T-1825 or Evans Blue** is an azo dye which has a very high affinity for human serum albumin, and this was the most-used plasma indicator dilution marker until the use of radioisotopes was developed. The greatest challenge in measuring Evans Blue concentration is its variable absorbance in turbid plasma. Theoretically, determining of the concentration of the dye with the spectrophotometer at 620 nm would overcome most errors despite turbidity of plasma, residual dye in repeated determinations and hemolysis of samples [11]. Nonetheless, comparison of different analytical strategies in determination of plasma volume using Evans Blue dye revealed no significant differences among the mean plasma volumes obtained with any method in pregnant women [11]. Also the intra- and interassay coefficients of variation were comparably low (<2.8%) irrespective of the method employed [11].

Indocyanine green (cardio-green), another color-dye, has also been used for determining plasma volume. Measurements correlate well with Evans Blue (correlation coefficient r=0.98); however, it is known to be less stable, due to its elimination by the liver with a plasma half-life of only 3 minutes [12]. Multiple adverse reactions, especially in patients with iodide sensitivity, mean that this dye was hardly used.

Iodine

Later, [131]**iodide** (half-life 8d) and [125]**iodide** (half-life 60d) have been developed as radioactive tracers and used as albumin markers. This overcomes the overestimation of plasma fluid seen in dye-albumin measurements in some specific clinical conditions of increased transcapillary leakage such as edema, ascites or proteinuria. Therefore, the International Committee for Standardization in Haematology (ICSH) described radioiodine-labeled human serum albumin as a plasma label as the most reliable and reproducible technique for measuring plasma volume [13]. With this indicator dilution technique, the labeled albumin is injected, and from a contralateral vessel, different venous blood samples are collected: one sample before the injection (t=0), and multiple samples at an exact time interval after the injection. Due to the known clearance rate, an exact plasma volume can be derived from the concentration in the blood samples.

Different studies report comparable results between plasma volume determination with Evans Blue and I-labeled albumin. Mean plasma volume determined by Evans Blue dilution did not differ significantly from that determined by ^{125}I-Human serum albumin in either clear or turbid samples [11]. In addition, both I-isotopes perform comparably in assessment of plasma volume and transcapillary permeability [14].

Dextran

Notwithstanding radioiodine-labeled human serum albumin is seen as the gold standard; however, radioactive substances should better be avoided during pregnancy. Therefore, high-molecular weight dextran may represent an attractive alternative to measure plasma volume as it seems to combine the advantages of ^{125}I-labeled albumin (a long half-life and a distribution space which is less susceptible for transcapillary leakage) with those of the dyes (nonradioactivity).

Dextran-70 can be quantitated by enzymatic determination of glucose, the only degradation product of dextran-70 after hydrolysis [15], and has different advantages for the use during pregnancy: as dextran is relatively rapidly cleared from the plasma, consecutive measurements are possible. Moreover, the disappearance rate of dextran makes it possible to calculate the capillary leakage [16]. This might be of potential interest in hypertensive gestational complications such as preeclampsia.

Next to the systematic error of about 50mL larger distribution space compared to ^{125}I-albumine, good correlations between detran-70 and ^{125}I-albumine in nonpregnant subjects has been found: the mean difference in plasma volume measured with the two indicators was 6%, with an error of 5% in the plasma measurements with dextran-70 [16].

FE-labeled Transferrin

Although radio-iodinated serum albumin is recommended, there are numerous other labeled proteins successfully used to measure plasma volume in humans. ^{59}FE-labeled transferrin has been investigated because of its lower cost against iodine. It has been suggested that the reliability of ^{59}FE-labeled transferrin in comparison with iodinated human serum albumin may be less and depend on iron saturation (and with it first order disappearance kinetics), affecting the fractional clearance rate, which is in general faster than ^{125}I, but especially in iron deficiency [17, 18].

Hydroxyethyl Starch

Hydroxyethyl starch (HES) is a colloid with high in vitro molecular weight (130 kDa), but with a still high in vivo weight (70–80 kDa). It consists of glucose and hydroxyethyl glucose that are interconnected by α–glycosidic bondings. Using HES as a dilution marker was first proposed in 1997 [19]. The HES method for plasma volume estimation is found to be rapid, safe, well tolerated and acceptable for use in pregnant women as it does not cross the placenta [20, 21]. Unlike the other dilution methods, which are based on the dilution of a known quantity of the indicator, plasma volume measurements using HES are based on the increase in plasma glucose concentration after acid hydrolysis [19, 22]. Complete hydrolysis of HES disrupts the α–glycosidic bonds and produces glucose and hydroxyethyl glucose, resulting in a fixed concentration of glucose, which does not change by extending the hydrolysis process. Therefore, the difference of glucose concentration before and after the injection with HES is proportional with the HES concentration in the plasma (Δ glucose $\approx$ concentration$_{HES}$), which is proportional to the quotient of the HES volume injected and the plasma volume (concentration$_{HES}$ $\approx$ volume$_{HES}$ /plasma volume). This results in the following equation:

$$\Delta\ Glucose = k \times \frac{Volume_{HES}}{Plasma\ volume}$$

with k found to be a constant factor of 3082mg% [19]. From this, plasma volume can be calculated as:

$$Plasma\ volume\ (mL) = \frac{3082 \times Volume_{HES}}{\Delta\ Glucose}$$

It is unclear whether this technique can be used after HES has been infused for plasma expansion.

Bioelectrical Impedance Analysis

Technique

A different approach to determine body fluid content can be the use of bioelectrical impedance analysis (BIA). BIA allows the calculation of body composition and volumes by analyzing the changes in frequency [Hz] of an electric input voltage signal going through the body. After applying electrodes on hand and foot, an alternating current flows through physiologic fluids of the body by the movement of ions, passing capacitive and resistive elements. Because water and electrolytes are the determinants of electrical conduction in the body, body fluid content can be evaluated by the BIA technique in which the current flows primarily in the extracellular space at low frequencies, whereas at high frequencies the current flows through intercellular space and extracellular volumes.

In the BIA assessment, several arithmetical choices are made: first, the human body is viewed as cylinder, which comprises different smaller cylinders (arms, legs and thorax), and, second, body composition is supposed homogenous. With respect to fluid content, BIA estimates total body water, which is the sum of intracellular water and extracellular water. The latter consist of interstitial, transcellular and plasma volume.

Benefits and Limitations

Different studies validated the reliability of total body water, intracellular and extracellular water using a bioimpedance technique [23, 24]. They showed that multifrequency impedance is able to accurately predict body water when compared to dilution methods [24].

Whereas the classic methods for plasma volume assessment are expensive and not easy to employ for clinical use, the BIA method is simple and safe. However, there are some concerns regarding the validity of BIA in pregnant women. The body composition is assumed to be homogenous, which is not true for critically ill patients or pregnant women. Full body bioelectrical impedance measurements might be influenced by the amniotic fluid and the fetus when analyzing the "maternal" body composition. Moreover, although plasma volume and extracellular volume relate to each other, edema formation might alter this relation [25, 26].

Measurements in Pregnancy

The increase of total body water and extracellular water volume in normal pregnancies measured with the BIA technique has been reported extensively [25, 27]. As plasma volume is proven to be increased during pregnancy, one may conclude that the measured augmentation of total body water and extracellular water implies an increase of plasma volume. However, concurrent measurement of plasma volume along with BIA during pregnancy has not been done so far.

Therefore, the BIA technique may be a valid technique to measure intracellular and extracellular water, but it is currently not suitable to distinguish between intra- and extravascular fluid in pregnancy.

Conclusion

Plasma volume can be measured indirectly using dilution or indicator dilution techniques. Techniques require first-order kinetics with an indicator that is both traceable and measurable. When used in pregnancy, they must be safe for both mother and fetus, implying no negative effects on maternal vessel wall integrity and absent placental passage. Bioelectrical impedance techniques claim to be able to estimate whole body extracellular fluid content, but the reliability of assessing plasma volume, as part of the extracellular volume, by bioimpedance remains to be elucidated.

Key Points

- Dilution or indicator dilution techniques are considered the methods of choice to measure plasma volume in a research setting. The need for intravascular instillation hampers their introduction in prenatal care.
- Bioelectrical impedance is suggested as an alternative noninvasive technology to estimate intra- and extracellular fluid volumes; however, the reliability of this method remains to be elucidated.

References

1. Scholten RR, Sep S, Peeters L, Hopman MT, Lotgering FK, Spaanderman ME. Prepregnancy low-plasma volume and predisposition to preeclampsia and fetal growth restriction. *Obstet Gynecol*. 2011;**117** (5):1085–93.

2. Donckers J, Scholten RR, Oyen WJ, Hopman MT, Lotgering FK, Spaanderman ME. Unexplained first trimester recurrent pregnancy loss and low venous reserves. *Hum Reprod*. 2012;**27**(9): 2613–8.

3. Freis ED, Kenny JF. Plasma Volume, Total Circulating Protein, and "Available Fluid" Abnormalities in Preeclampsia and Eclampsia. *J Clin Invest*. 1948;**27**(2):283–9.

4. Salas SP, Marshall G, Gutierrez BL, Rosso P. Time course of maternal plasma volume and hormonal changes in women with preeclampsia or fetal growth restriction. *Hypertension*. 2006;**47**(2):203–8.

5. Gallery ED, Hunyor SN, Gyory AZ. Plasma volume contraction: a significant factor in both pregnancy-associated hypertension (pre-eclampsia) and chronic hypertension in pregnancy. *Q J Med*. 1979;**48** (192):593–602.

6. Welker H. *Bestimmungen der Menge des Körperblutes und der Blutfärbekraft, sowie Bestimmungen von Zahl, Maass, Oberfläche und Volumen des einzelnen Blutkörperchens beim Thier und beim Menschen*. Präger Vrtljschr. 1854.

7. Von Vierordt KH. Das Abhängigkeitsgesetz der mittleren Kreislaufszeiten von den mittleren Puls-Frequenzen der Tierarten. *Arch. f. physiol. Heilk. N. F.* 1858;**2**:527.

8. Phillips RA, Yeomans A, Dole VP, Farr LE, Van Slyke DD, Hogan D. Estimation of blood volume from change in blood specific gravity following a plasma infusion. *J Clin Invest*. 1946;**25**:261–9.

9. Valentin G. Versuche über die in dem thierischen Körper enthaltene Blutmenge. *Repert f Anat u Physiol*. 1838;**3**:281.

10. Erlanger J. Blood volume and its regulation. *Physiol Rev*. 1921;**1**:177.

11. Brown MA, Mitar DA, Whitworth JA. Measurement of plasma volume in pregnancy. *Clin Sci (Lond)*. 1992;**83** (1):29–34.

12. Haneda K, Horiuchi T. A method for measurement of total circulating blood volume using indocyanine green. *Tohoku J Exp Med*. 1986;**148**(1):49–56.

13. International Committee for Standardization in Haematology. Recommended methods for measurement of red-cell and plasma volume: International Committee for

Standardization in Haematology. *J Nucl Med.* 1980;**21**(8):793–800.

14. Walker WG, Ross RS, Hammond JD. Study of the relationship between plasma volume and transcapillary protein exchange using I 131-labeled albumin and I 125-labeled globulin. *Circ Res.* 1960;**8**:1028–40.

15. Dubick MA, Wade CE. A review of the efficacy and safety of 7.5% NaCl/6% dextran 70 in experimental animals and in humans. *J Trauma.* 1994;**36**(3):323–30.

16. van Kreel BK, van Beek E, Spaanderman ME, Peeters LL. A new method for plasma volume measurements with unlabeled dextran-70 instead of 125I-labeled albumin as an indicator. *Clin Chim Acta.* 1998;**275**(1):71–80.

17. Najean Y, Dresch C, Ardaillou N, Bernard J. Iron metabolism – a study of different kinetic models in normal conditions. *Am J Physiol.* 1967;**213**(2):533–46.

18. Ricketts C, Cavill I. Measurement of plasma volume using 59Fe-labelled transferrin. *J Clin Pathol.* 1978;**31**(2):196–8.

19. Tschaikowsky K, Meisner M, Durst R, Rugheimer E. Blood volume determination using hydroxyethyl starch: a rapid and simple intravenous injection method. *Crit Care Med.* 1997;**25**(4):599–606.

20. Vricella LK, Louis JM, Chien E, Mercer BM. Blood volume determination in obese and normal-weight gravidas: the hydroxyethyl starch method. *Am J Obstet Gynecol.* 2015;**213**(3):408 e1–6.

21. Soens MA, Birnbach DJ, Ranasinghe JS, van Zundert A. Obstetric anesthesia for the obese and morbidly obese patient: an ounce of prevention is worth more than a pound of treatment. *Acta Anaesthesiol Scand.* 2008;**52**(1):6–19.

22. Forster H, Wicarkzyk C, Dudziak R. Determination of the plasma elimination of hydroxyethyl starch and dextran using improved analytical methods. *Infusionsther Klin Ernahr.* 1981;**8**(2):88–94.

23. De Lorenzo A, Deurenberg P, Andreoli A, Sasso GF, Palestini M, Docimo R. Multifrequency impedance in the assessment of body water losses during dialysis. *Ren Physiol Biochem.* 1994;**17**(6):326–32.

24. De Lorenzo A, Candeloro N, Andreoli A, Deurenberg P. Determination of intracellular water by multifrequency bioelectrical impedance. *Ann Nutr Metab.* 1995;**39**(3):177–84.

25. Valensise H, Andreoli A, Lello S, Magnani F, Romanini C, De Lorenzo A. Multifrequency bioelectrical impedance analysis in women with a normal and hypertensive pregnancy. *Am J Clin Nutr.* 2000;**72**(3):780–3.

26. da Silva EG, Carvalhaes MA, Hirakawa HS, Peracoli JC. Bioimpedance in pregnant women with preeclampsia. *Hypertens Pregnancy.* 2010;**29**(4):357–65.

27. Yasuda R, Takeuchi K, Funakoshi T, Maruo T. Bioelectrical impedance analysis in the clinical management of preeclamptic women with edema. *J Perinat Med.* 2003;**31**(4):275–80.

Chapter

15

Treatment Options for Hypertension in Pregnancy

Lin Fung Foo, Jasmine Tay and Ian Wilkinson

Summary

Hypertensive disorders of pregnancy affect approximately 5–10% of all maternities and are major contributors of maternal and neonatal morbidity and mortality worldwide. This group of disorders encompasses chronic hypertension, as well as conditions that arise de novo in pregnancy: gestational hypertension and preeclampsia. The latter group is thought to be part of the same continuum but with arbitrary division. Research into the etiology of hypertension in pregnancy has largely been focused on preeclampsia, with a majority of studies exploring either pregnancy-associated factors such as placental derived or immunologic responses to pregnancy tissue, or maternal constitutional factors such as cardiovascular health and endothelial dysfunction. The evidence base for the pathophysiology and progression of hypertensive disorders in pregnancy, particularly preeclampsia, is reviewed. Clinical algorithms and pharmacological agents for the management of hypertension in pregnancy are summarized, with a brief focus on postpartum considerations. Novel therapeutic options for the management of preeclampsia are also explored.

Introduction

Hypertensive disorders are the most common medical complication in pregnancy, affecting approximately 5–10% of all maternities. Despite advances in obstetric medicine, it remains the second highest cause of maternal mortality worldwide [1], as well as a major cause of morbidity for the mother and the baby [2, 3]. Hypertension can exist prior to (as chronic hypertension), or develop de novo in pregnancy within two well-defined disorders: preeclampsia or gestational hypertension. Preeclampsia can often develop superimposed on established gestational or chronic hypertension. Analysis of several national databases recording maternal outcomes demonstrate that substandard care in aspects of recognition and blood pressure control can lead to devastating consequences, both for mother and baby [4]. Given the changing demographics of mothers worldwide (toward a trend of older mothers with more chronic health conditions such as obesity and diabetes), it is expected the incidence of hypertensive disorders will continue to increase. Maternity services will need to adapt to provide appropriate diagnosis and timely intervention, ideally with interdisciplinary management by obstetric, cardiac and general medical services. Similarly, there are opportunities for new research in this area to better define mechanisms of pathogenesis, as well as treatment strategies to improve maternal and fetal outcomes.

The Clinical Spectrum of Hypertension in Pregnancy

By convention, the threshold for diagnosis of hypertension in pregnancy is blood pressure levels of ≥140 mmHg systolic or ≥90 mmHg, confirmed by two readings at rest 4 to 6 hours apart. The National High Blood Pressure Education Program (NHBPEP) consensus report [5] has stated that patients with BP readings below the threshold for diagnosis but who have a 30 or 15 mmHg rise in systolic and diastolic pressures respectively be streamlined as high-risk patients at risk of developing a hypertensive disorder in pregnancy. The United Kingdom National Institute of Clinical Excellence (NICE) [6] further divides pregnancy-associated hypertension into risk tiers as below:

Mild: diastolic BP 90–99 mmHg, systolic BP 140–149 mmHg

Moderate: diastolic BP 100–109 mmHg, systolic BP 150–159 mmHg

Severe: diastolic BP 110 mmHg or greater, systolic BP 160 mmHg or greater

A hypertensive emergency or crisis is usually taken to be a systolic reading of >169 mmHg or a diastolic of 109 mmHg, and warrants immediate blood pressure reduction in order to limit end-organ damage [7]. This differs from a situation of hypertensive urgency, where blood pressure reduction should be achieved over a period of a few hours. Readings in pregnancy are labile (especially in the context of preeclampsia, which is often characterized by compartmental fluid shifts), and acutely sensitive to antihypertensive therapy. High blood pressure measurements should therefore be reduced promptly but gradually, with continuous monitoring of maternal and fetal parameters; overzealous reduction leads to a decrease in placental circulation and fetal distress. The recommendation is that diastolic blood pressure should not be reduced by more than 30 mmHg, and that neither should the mean arterial pressure (MAP) be reduced by more than 25%.

There are four categories of hypertensive disorders in pregnancy as described below, and in Figure 15.1. Using terminology recommended by the NHBPEP working group [5], these are categorized into:

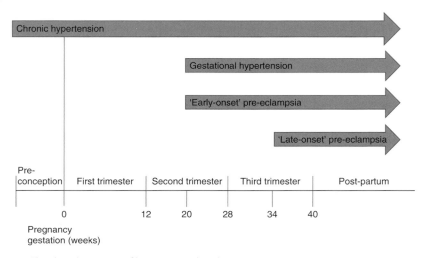

Figure 15.1 The clinical spectrum of hypertensive disorders in pregnancy

- Preeclampsia
- Chronic hypertension of any cause
- Preeclampsia superimposed on chronic hypertension
- Gestational hypertension

It should be noted that despite the distinctions above, it is thought that preeclampsia and gestational hypertension may be a continuum of the same condition but with arbitrary division.

Preeclampsia

Preeclampsia, preeclamptic toxemia (PET) or proteinuric pregnancy-induced hypertension (PPIH) are roughly synonymous terms traditionally describing a syndrome of new-onset hypertension with significant proteinuria ($\geq$300 mg of protein in 24 hours or two urine samples collected more than 4hrs apart with $\geq$1+ proteinuria on stick test) diagnosed in the second half of pregnancy [8]. However, further recognition of the potential inaccuracies in the measurement of proteinuria and the potential for severe maternal complications in pregnancies complicated by de novo hypertension without proteinuria has led to the recommendation that PET be defined as such [9]; the presence of de novo hypertension and the coexistence of one or more of the following new-onset conditions:

1. Proteinuria
2. Other maternal-organ dysfunction such as renal insufficiency, liver involvement, neurological complications including eclampsia or hematological complications
3. Uteroplacental dysfunction including fetal growth restriction

With regards to diagnosing new onset hypertension, it is important to have recordings of blood pressure documented either prepregnancy or in early pregnancy before there has been a physiological decrease in blood pressure. A "normal" baseline blood pressure measured between 16–20 weeks gestation may result in a missed diagnosis of chronic hypertension. The International Society for the Study of Hypertension in Pregnancy (ISSHP) recommends that if a woman presents with hypertension after 20 weeks gestation and an earlier blood pressure is unknown, she should be managed as gestational hypertension or preeclampsia [9].

Incidence rates of PET vary between 3–7%, reports of which can be biased by study population (numbers of primigravidas, body mass index and age). The cause of preeclampsia is not known; however, it is observed to occur most commonly in nulliparous women usually after 20 weeks gestation, and frequently late in the third trimester. There appears to be a genetic predisposition, as the risk of preeclampsia is increased threefold in women with an affected first degree relative.

Rates of PET are reported to vary widely in different ethnic groups, with studies showing black African American women are twice as likely to develop preeclampsia compared to women of Caucasian descent [10]. Ethnic differences for developing hypertension in pregnancy have been found to mirror the development of cardiovascular disease in later life [11]. Outside pregnancy, ethnicity is known to account for higher resting and ambulatory blood pressure in Afro-Caribbean women compared to women of European origin [12]. It is also well understood that nonpregnant black populations do not respond well to antihypertensive treatment with beta-blockers, presumably due to their relatively low cardiac output and high peripheral vascular resistance state when compared to a similar Caucasian population.

Preeclampsia is thought to develop from the interaction of two disease processes: 1) maternal disease (abnormal vasculature, renal or metabolic systems disease) or cardiovascular predisposition; and 2) fetal causes in the form of placental factors. The exact mechanisms of these interactions are not clear; however, it is postulated that varying the influence of both factors can produce two separate phenotypes of preeclampsia: an early-onset phenotype which is associated with poor placentation and fetal growth restriction, and a late-onset phenotype, which is not thought to be related to placental causes [13, 14].

In general, early-onset preeclampsia (generally defined as < 34 weeks) represents 5–20% of all cases, including the most severe manifestations [15]. This form is linked to immune and placental maladaptation and is characterized by early sympathetic dominance in the cardiovascular system, elevated circulating markers of endothelial dysfunction, inadequate trophoblastic invasion of the uterine spiral arteries, and early onset of fetal complications such as iatrogenic preterm birth, and low birth weights [16–18].

In contrast, late-onset PE is the most common, encompassing more than 80% of all cases [15], and is commonly observed on the background of pre-existing maternal morbidities such as chronic hypertension, renal disease and obesity. Fetuses born of a late-onset PE pregnancy have a proportionately higher birth weight when compared to early-onset PE cases [19].

Management

A diagnosis of preeclampsia requires hospital admission, given the disorder's potential to worsen rapidly, and the increased risk of placental abruption, especially when it develops superimposed on chronic hypertension [20]. Delivery remains the only known "cure." At term, induction of labor or delivery is mandated [6]. Attempts to prolong gestation to reduce the risk of neonatal morbidity by optimal blood pressure management should be undertaken if pregnancy is <34 weeks and there is good clinical response to therapy. Gestation is permitted to continue as long as blood pressure is sufficiently controlled, there are no signs on life-threatening maternal complications (such as DIC, HELLP, eclampsia) and fetal monitoring is reassuring.

Following diagnosis, women should receive regular blood pressure recording and monitoring of serum urea and creatinine, uric acid, hemoglobin, platelet count, liver function and coagulation screen if there is thrombocytopenia present. Uterine artery Doppler blood flow examination should be arranged, looking particularly for high-resistance wave forms in the uterine arteries, which is predictive of associated intrauterine growth restriction and placental abruption.

Excessive fluid replacement should be avoided, as this may exacerbate interstitial edema. Urine output as low as 10mls/hour may be acceptable. Thromboprophylaxis with thromboembolic deterrent (TED) stockings and low-molecular-weight heparin should be administered.

There is no pharmacological cure for preeclampsia. Therapy is directed toward managing hypertension. Choices of pharmacological agents for treatment of preeclampsia and other hypertensive disorders in pregnancy are similar, and are therefore elaborated on in a separate section, and summarized in Tables II (a) and II (b).

Table 15.1 Preeclampsia signs, symptoms and clinical investigations

Symptoms
Headache
Nausea & vomiting
Peripheral edema
Rapid weight gain
Generalized lethargy or malaise
Visual disturbances including blindness (from occipital lobe edema)
Right upper quadrant or epigastric pain from liver edema +/- hepatic hemorrhage
Confusion from cerebral edema
Eclamptic convulsion

Signs
Hypertension
Brisk reflexes
Clonus
Retinal edema
Retinal hemorrhage
Pulmonary edema
Oliguria
Jaundice
Fetal growth restriction
Placental abruption

Investigations
Proteinuria
Hematuria from acute tubular necrosis or HELLP syndrome
Thrombocytopenia
Disseminated intravascular coagulopathy

Table 15.2 (a) Pharmacological agents for longer term treatment of hypertension in pregnancy

Drug treatment	Dose, daily (oral)	Notes	Contraindication
β-receptor blockers			
Labetalol	100mg–2.4g 2–3 divided doses/day	– No obvious association with congenital abnormalities – May decrease uteroplacental blood flow & impair fetal response to hypoxic stress – Decreased fetal heart rate described – May be associated with neonatal hypoglycemia at higher doses	– Asthma – Congestive heart failure – Severe maternal bradycardia
Atenolol	25–50mg once/day	– Associated with low birth weights when started in 1st trimester	

Table 15.2 (a) (cont.)

Drug treatment	Dose, daily (oral)	Notes	Contraindication
α-blocker			
Methyldopa	250mg–3g 2–3 divided doses/day	– Drug of choice according to NHBPEP working group – No obvious association with congenital abnormalities with well documented safety profile up to 7.5 years of exposed infants – Associated with mild hypotension in babies in first 2 days of life – May cause autoimmune hemolytic anemia	– Liver disease – Acute porphyria – Caution in depression (methyldopa)
Clonidine	150 mcg–1.5mg 3 divided doses/day	– Comparable safety data to methyldopa but no long-term follow up data	
Calcium channel blockers			
Nifedipine (modified release)	20mg–80mg 2 divided doses/ day	– No obvious association with congenital abnormalities – Side effects include headache and flushing – May inhibit labor – Possible synergistic actions with magnesium sulfate	– Advanced aortic stenosis
Amlodipine	5–10mg Once/day	– No reports in human pregnancy – Breastfeeding not recommended, excretion in milk unknown	
Verapamil	240–480mg 2–3 divided doses/day	– No obvious association with congenital abnormalities	
Angiotensin-Converting-Enzyme (ACE) inhibitors/ Angiotensin Receptor Blockers (ARBs)			

Contraindicated in pregnancy. Links to fetal loss in animals. In human pregnancy, associations with miscarriages, cardiac defects, fetopathy, neonatal anuria, neonatal skull hypoplasia

Table 15.2 (b) Pharmacological agents for acute control of severe hypertension/ hypertensive crisis

Drugs	Dose	Notes
Hydralazine	Bolus: 5mg followed by 5–10mg every 20–30 minutes; or infusion of 0.5–10mg per hour	– Drug of choice from NHBPEP working group – Some association with fetal distress leading to operative deliveries
Labetalol	50mg intravenously over at least 1 minute, repeated after 5 minutes to a maximum dose of 200mg	– Lower incidences of maternal side effects such as acute hypotensive episodes and maternal bradycardia
Nifedipine (short acting)	10–30mg oral dose, repeat in 45 minutes if needed	– Fetal bradycardia associated with acute severe hypotension – Long-acting preparations preferred, short-acting preparations not approved by US FDA or UK BNF for management of hypertension
Nitroprusside	Constant infusion of 0.5–1.5 mcg/kg/minute	– Only considered for life-threatening severe hypertension – Possible cyanide toxicity if used for more than 4 hours – Also risk of cardio neurogenic syncope

Specifically for preeclampsia, the aim should be to reduce blood pressure slowly using oral therapy to a target of 140–150/80–100 mmHg [6]. There is no evidence that tighter control to <140/90 mmHg results in better outcomes, and rapid reduction in blood pressure of >25% mean arterial pressure might lead to maternal end-organ hypoperfusion (e.g. cerebrovascular accident, myocardial infarction) or may affect placental perfusion and fetal growth.

Chronic Hypertension in Pregnancy

Chronic hypertension is diagnosed either by pre-existing medical history, or by a raised blood pressure reading (>140/90 mmHg) in the first half of pregnancy. It complicates approximately 3% of all pregnancies. Occasionally, secondary hypertension may be diagnosed de novo in pregnancy, the most frequent cause being intrinsic renal disease. Other causes such as phaeochromocytoma, primary aldosteronism, Cushing's syndrome and aortic coarctation should be investigated and excluded.

The physiological decline of blood pressure in early pregnancy and the rise in blood pressure later in gestation is exaggerated in women with chronic hypertension. Hence, they may present normotensive at initial pregnancy visits, and be mistakenly diagnosed with gestational hypertension later on in pregnancy.

The major risk of chronic hypertension in pregnancy is the development of super-imposed preeclampsia, the risk of which is five-fold compared to a normotensive individual. On its own, chronic hypertension is also associated with adverse morbidity for mother and fetus: overall risk of developing eclampsia is increased by a factor of 10, there is a threefold increase in stillbirth and a 2.5 fold increase in having a small-for-gestational-age baby [21].

The signs of preeclampsia superimposed on chronic hypertension are the same as in isolated preeclampsia, except that the blood pressure levels start to rise from a higher baseline. In differentiating both conditions, generally with chronic hypertension there is no change in blood pressure from baseline, no increase in maternal plasma urate levels (values below 0.30 mmol/L are unlikely in preeclampsia) and no significant proteinuria.

Management

Prior to conception, the majority of the commonly used antihypertensive drugs is not known to be teratogenic and can therefore be continued. However angiotensin-converting enzymes/angiotensin receptor blockers should be avoided as they are associated with fetal anomalies particularly renal agenesis and first trimester miscarriages [22] [23, 24]. By the 12th week of pregnancy, the decline in blood pressure in normal pregnancy usually means that antihypertensive therapy can be discontinued temporarily until the blood pressure rises again, usually in the third trimester.

Although there are no placebo-controlled trials available, historic data suggest that treating severe chronic hypertension in pregnancy reduces maternal and fetal risks. However, there is no clear evidence that blood pressure reduction reduces the risks of developing preeclampsia [25]. The consensus threshold level for treatment is split between recommended treatment at a level exceeding 160/100 mmHg or 140/90 mmHg. Given potential concerns about excessive BP reduction, careful consideration of individual cases should be practiced. In general, therapy should be initiated if readings approach 160/100 mmHg. The target blood pressure is less clear, but a reasonable guide would be to aim for a blood pressure of 130–150/80–100 mmHg. Choice of drugs is dictated by fetal considera-tions. Methyldopa may be preferred as its fetal effects are more clearly defined than for other antihypertensive therapies.

Unlike preeclampsia, women do not have to be hospitalized in a maternity unit upon diagnosis, as there is inconclusive evidence that it predisposes to placental abruption [26]. Admission and intravenous therapy for uncontrolled severe hypertension (without super-imposed preeclampsia) is rare as blood pressure can usually be reasonably controlled with oral pharmacological agents.

Pregnancy-Induced Hypertension

Pregnancy-induced hypertension (PIH) is hypertension without significant proteinuria that develops after 20 weeks of pregnancy gestation. It is sometimes observed in the context of resolving chronic hypertension in the first and second trimester due to normal physiological changes in pregnancy, followed by an unmasking in the third trimester, leading to a presumptive diagnosis of PIH. Generally, blood pressure of women with PIH is expected to normalize after delivery or in the puerperium. The incidence of PIH increases with gestation, with approximately 50% of cases occurring near term.

There is much about PIH etiology that remains unknown. It is possible that PIH is either within the spectrum of hypertensive disorders in pregnancy and therefore a continuant of preeclampsia, or a separate entity of its own pathology, or, indeed, an exaggerated form of adaptation to cardiovascular changes in pregnancy to maintain placental perfusion as gestation advances.

The majority of women with PIH have good maternal and fetal outcomes. However, PIH can evolve into preeclampsia (diagnosed when significant proteinuria presents) in 15–20% of pregnancies [27]. There are suggestions in the literature that PIH diagnosed prior to 35 weeks is more predictive of subsequent development of preeclampsia as the pregnancy progresses [28]. Identifying this subgroup is significant as these pregnancies are at an increased risk of fetal death, preterm delivery and low birth weight when compared to PIH or unaffected pregnancies [29].

Severe PIH (defined as hypertension of >160/110 on two separate occasions) is associated with increased adverse perinatal outcomes (small for gestational age at birth and prematurity) when compared to preeclampsia with lower blood pressure readings [30]. This is supported by a previous study where high diastolic blood pressures are associated with high perinatal mortality [31].

Management

NICE guidelines recommend the threshold of treatment for PIH as >150/100 (moderate hypertension); this is similar to the threshold for preeclampsia [6]. However, management of well-controlled PIH is frequently undertaken on an outpatient basis as compared to the latter.

Pharmacological Treatment of Hypertensive Disorders in Pregnancy

When choosing an antihypertensive drug for use in pregnancy, the main considerations, aside from efficacy and adverse effects on the mother, are the risk of teratogenicity. This is pertinent to women with chronic hypertension as the greatest risk window is up to 13 weeks gestation when organogenesis is occurring. For this reason, older agents that were widely used before concerns of teratogenicity were raised tend to be the mainstay agents with "proven" safety records, and most antihypertensive agents are unlicensed for use in pregnancy because further safety and efficacy studies have not been performed. Nevertheless, drugs administered in the later stages of pregnancy can still affect fetal growth and well-being, while drugs given close to the time of delivery can have lingering effects on the neonate. Considerations of initiating or continuing a pharmacological agent in pregnancy should therefore include an agent which can be used to prolong the pregnancy for as long as safely possible, with minimal fetal exposure in-utero and with minimal vertical transfer during lactation.

Several national and international guidelines have been published to guide choice of antihypertensive agents in pregnancy (see Al Khaja et al. [32] for a comprehensive review of guideline recommendations).

Oral Treatment for Hypertensive Disorders in Pregnancy

For less severe levels of hypertension, α-methyldopa, calcium channel blockers and B-blockers are universally used routinely as first- and second-line drugs [32].

There is extensive data on the use of methyldopa, a false transmitter and α2-agonist, and there appears to be no fetal or neonatal risk with treatment. Birth weight, neonatal complications and development during the first year were similar in children exposed to methyldopa as in the placebo group [33], as were intelligence and neurocognitive development at 7.5 years of age [34]. Blood pressure control is gradual over 6 to 8 hours, due to the indirect mechanism of action. Compared to methyldopa, labetalol was quicker and more efficient in controlling blood pressure in PIH, with a trend toward lower rates of intervention (Cesarean delivery or induction of labor), reduction in occurrence of proteinuria and better tolerance [35]. Adverse effects of central α2-agonist include a decrease in mental alertness and impaired sleep, leading to a sense of fatigue or depression in some patients. This is particularly pertinent in patients at risk of postpartum depression. Clonidine, a selective α2-agonist, acts similarly and is comparable with methyldopa in safety and efficacy, but of some concern is reported excess of sleep disturbance in neonates that were exposed in-utero [36].

A common first or second line drug is labetalol, which has β1-, β2- and α1-adrenergic blocking receptor properties, and direct action on vasodilation. Peak blood concentrations occur in 1 hour in pregnant patients, and plasma half-life in the third trimester ranges from 1.7 to 5.8 hours. When given in the early stages of PIH, labetalol can slow the progression to preeclampsia. The use of atenolol is controversial as some early studies showed an association with significantly lower birth weight and a significantly higher proportion of small-for-gestational-age babies [37–39]. A meta-analysis of 13 population-based case-control or cohort studies on the use of β-blockers in the first trimester of pregnancy showed no increased odds of all or major congenital anomalies (OR=1.00; 95% confidence interval, 0.91–1.10; 5 studies). However, in analyses examining organ-specific malformations, increased odds of cardiovascular defects (OR=2.01; 95% confidence interval, 1.18–3.42; 4 studies), cleft lip/palate (OR=3.11; 95% confidence interval, 1.79–5.43; 2 studies) and neural tube defects (OR=3.56; 95% confidence interval, 1.19–10.67; 2 studies) were observed [40]. Causality is difficult to establish given the small number of heterogeneous studies.

Calcium channel blockers (CCB) given to pregnant rats have shown an increased prevalence of digital and limb defects; however, a large case-control review in humans has not shown an association with increased prevalence of congenital anomalies in offspring exposed to CCBs in-utero [41–43]. Nifedipine in short-acting (immediate release) and long-acting (extended release, prolonged action) formulations is commonly used for the treatment of acute (crisis) severe hypertension, as well as longer term control of nonsevere hypertension in pregnancy, although short-acting nifedipine has been reported to be associated with maternal hypotensive episodes and fetal distress [44, 45]. Maternal side effects of CCB include tachycardia, palpitations, peripheral edema, headaches and facial flushing [46]. A concern with the use of CCB in preeclampsia relates to the concomitant use of magnesium sulfate to prevent seizures; additive effects between nifedipine and magnesium sulfate were observed in a few cases, leading to neuromuscular blockade, myocardial depression or circulatory collapse [47, 48]. However, a recent evaluation has suggested that they may be used together without increased maternal risk [49].

Contrary to the drug classes above, ACEIs and ARBs are both class D drugs according to FDA classifications, although they are generally treated as absolute contraindications, particularly during the second and third trimesters of pregnancy, because of related fetal toxicity. The use of these agents has been reported in association with miscarriage, in-utero death and congenital malformation, in particular fetal renal failure [50–52]. The cause of associated defects is thought to be related to the fetal hypotension that develops, as well as reduced renal blood flow in the fetus, and disruption of prenatal development of the fetal uropoietic system as a result of suppression of the fetal renin–angiotensin system [52, 53]. The risk of use in the first trimester is unclear and thought to be similar to that of other antihypertensive agents [22], although there has been a reported relative risk of 2.71 for congenital malformation when fetuses were exposed in the first trimester [51]. As such, it is best avoided and women who attend prepregnancy counseling should be switched to an alternate agent.

In patients with chronic hypertension, diuretics which were initiated prepregnancy can be continued through, with an attempt to decrease the dose, and can be used in combination with other agents especially for women with salt-sensitive hypertension. Mild volume contraction with diuretic therapy may lead to hyperuricemia, and in so doing so may invalidate serum uric acid levels as a marker for the diagnosis of preeclampsia. Spironolactone is not recommended because of its antiandrogenic effects noted in animal model embryogenesis, although this was not replicated in a reported clinical case [54].

Intravenous Antihypertensives for Acute Crisis

Hydralazine remains a popular first line choice for the management of hypertensive emergencies in pregnancy, as well as for maintenance therapy. It is a potent arteriolar and veno-dilator, whose mechanism is not known though it relaxes arteriolar vascular smooth muscle, thereby producing a reduction in peripheral vascular resistance and vasodilation. Peak plasma concentration can be reached within 30 minutes, with hypotensive effects lasting up to 8 hours. With parenteral administration, onset of action is within 10 to 20 minutes, and can last up to 4 hours. Hydralazine crosses the placenta freely, and also appears in small amounts in breast milk. Plasma renin activity is increased, which can lead to edema. Vasodilation is not generalized, with minimal venous dilation, and therefore less frequent incidences of postural hypotension. Patients often experience flushing, headache, palpitations and sleep disturbance when given intravenous hydralazine. To date, there are no reports of the teratogenic effects of this drug; however, there is minimal data on its use in the first trimester. The hemodynamic effects of hydralazine are more pronounced in patients with preeclampsia, leading to more cases of fetal distress, when compared to administration in patients with PIH. Similarly, hydralazine has a more dramatic effect when used in PIH compared to patients with chronic hypertension in pregnancy. Therefore, lower doses and gradual control of blood pressure reduction should be employed when administrating hydralazine, depending on the diagnosis.

In a small study of 24 patients receiving hydralazine, it was shown to be associated with more cases of fetal distress requiring delivery by Cesarean section [55]. A larger study, however, observed that hydralazine boluses of up to 5 mg repeated every 15 minutes to achieve a MAP of 125 mmHg can be administered with no significant differences in fetal condition on monitoring between treatment and nontreatment group [56], and with good control of maternal blood pressure provided administrative protocol was adhered to.

Labetalol is another frequent candidate for acute hypertensive crisis in pregnancy. However, the use of intravenous labetalol close to delivery has been associated with a few cases of neonatal bradycardia, hypotonia, respiratory distress, hypoglycemia, circulatory collapse and feeding problems [57, 58]. For severe hypertension, intravenous labetalol has been observed to produce fewer maternal symptoms such as hypotension, palpitations and tachycardia than intravenous hydralazine, but it is more associated with fetal bradycardia [59, 60]. A meta-analysis of 24 trials found no significant difference between parenteral labetalol and hydralazine in either effectiveness or safety profile in the context of use in severe hypertension [61]. Similarly, a systematic review of 15 randomized controlled trials on treatment of severe hypertension in pregnancy and postpartum reported that nifedipine, labetalol and hydralazine achieved similar treatment success in most women, with no differences in adverse maternal or fetal outcomes [62].

Potential Novel Therapies

A majority of clinical trials of new medicinal products on the prevention and treatment of hypertensive disorders in pregnancy have been focused on preeclampsia, based on what is thought to relate to pathophysiology of the disorder (deficiency of nitric oxide bioavailability, oxidative stress, endothelial dysfunction, maternal cardiovascular risk factors).

The regulatory role of oxidative stress in preeclampsia, together with encouraging in vivo data, introduced the hypothesis that antioxidant vitamins might have therapeutic potential. However, clinical trials of vitamins C and E showed no reduction in incidence of preeclampsia for women at risk [63, 64]. This has been confirmed with systematic reviews and meta-analyses of trials evaluating a combination of these vitamins [65, 66]. Importantly, questions relating to safety of administration of vitamins C and E have been raised. The number of stillbirths >24 weeks, the need for magnesium sulfate and/or intravenous antihypertensive therapy, as well as the incidence of gestational hypertension has been observed to be higher in women who received vitamins C and E, compared to placebos [64], despite the daily doses of the combined vitamins being below the maximum dosage recommended by the Institute of Medicine of the United States [67]. It is thought that vitamin E supplementation may favor a pro-inflammatory response (Th1) at the feto-maternal interface, and therefore influences adverse pregnancy outcomes [68]. Hence, vitamin C and E cannot be recommended in the prophylaxis and/or treatment of preeclampsia.

As a deficiency of NO bioavailability and/or abnormal endothelial sensitivity to NO has been described in vivo and ex vivo in preeclampsia, several nitric agents have been tested for the prevention and treatment of preeclampsia. These include organic nitrates, S-nitrosothiols, precursors such as L-arginine and inhibitors of cGMP breakdown. Glyceryl trinitrate (GTN) is a widely used organic nitrate in clinical practice for angina pectoris. The evidence for the use of GTN in pregnancy is limited by the small number of women in trials; however, it has potential as a therapeutic agent in the context of hypertensive disease in pregnancy. Its use in women at risk of developing preeclampsia was first reported in 1994, where a dose-dependent reduction in uterine artery resistance was demonstrated with intravenous GTN infusion without any effect on maternal cardiovascular parameters [69]. However, further studies have shown a significant reduction in maternal blood pressure without significant adverse events [70, 71]. A randomized placebo-controlled trial of low-dose transdermal GTN patches in women with abnormal uterine artery Doppler velocimetry at 24–26 weeks showed that although there was no change in the incidence of preeclampsia, GTN increased the likelihood of a complication-free pregnancy [72].

A similar donor compound to GTN, but without the effect of nitrate drug tolerance, is Pentaerithrityl-tetranitrate (PETN), which enhances the expression of the antioxidant genes heme oxygenase-1 (HO-1) and ferritin heavychain (FeHc) in human endothelial cells. In a

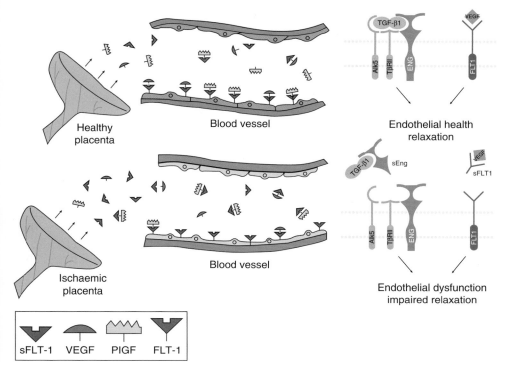

Figure 1.1 Healthy nonischemic placenta secretes normal (balanced) soluble fms-like tyrosine kinase (sFLT) leading to normal levels available for binding to fms-like tyrosine kinase 1 (FLT1) on endothelial cells systemically, leaving healthy and responsive endothelium. Ischemic placenta secretes increased sFLT, which binds circulating factors depleting their availability to FLT1 binding. The result is a dysfunctional endothelial cell leading to maternal systemic vasculopathy.

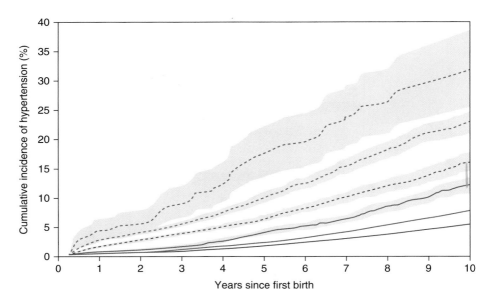

Figure 1.5 Ten-year cumulative incidences of hypertension by years since first pregnancy in women with and without a hypertensive disorder of pregnancy, by age at first delivery, Denmark, 1995-2012. Follow-up began in 1995 or 3 months postpartum, whichever came later; for women with a second pregnancy, follow-up ended at 20 weeks' gestation in the second pregnancy. Unbroken lines: women with no hypertensive disorder of pregnancy in their first pregnancy. Broken lines: women with a hypertensive disorder of pregnancy in their first pregnancy. Gray bands: 95% confidence intervals. Age at delivery: 20-29 years, blue; 30-39 years, green; 40-49 years, red.

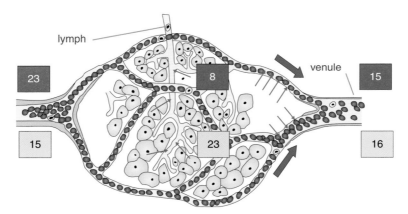

Figure 2.4 Driving forces for transcapillary fluid exchange based on the Starling principle. Hydrostatic and oncotic pressures (mmHg) at the precapillary sphincter, in the capillary bed and at the venular outflow site are listed in red and blue boxes, respectively. Pressure gradients enable serum to leave and re-enter the vascular bed during the passage of blood across the capillary bed.

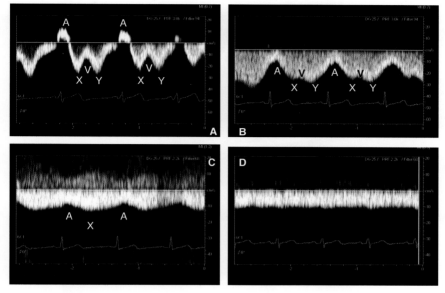

Figure 4.2 Different types of venous Doppler wave forms, as commonly seen in the hepatic and renal veins.

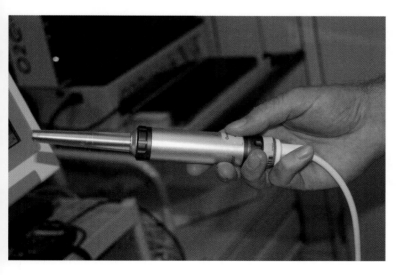

Figure 5.2 IDF probe.

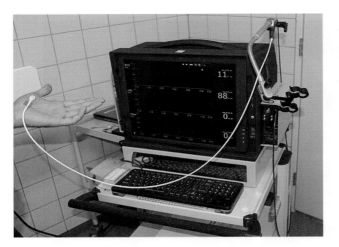

Figure 5.3 O2C monitoring device with glass fiber probe measuring microvascular perfusion on a hand palm.

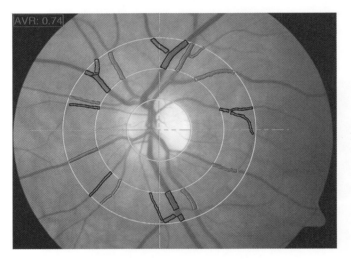

Figure 5.4 This retinal vessel imaging, recorded with a fundus camera (Retinal Vessel Analyzer, Imedos, Jena, Germany), demonstrates the direct measurement of retinal arterioles (red marks) and venules (blue marks) and the consequent automatic calculation of the mean arteriolar (CRAE) and venular (CRVE) diameter as well as the arteriolar-to-venular ratio (AVR).

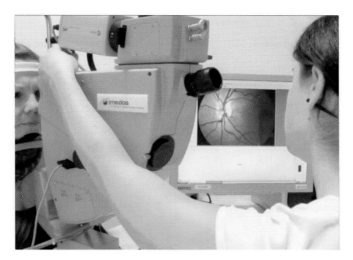

Figure 5.5 The static condition and dynamic behavior of the retinal microvasculature can be noninvasively visualized and analyzed with a fundus camera (Dynamic Retinal Vessel Analyzer, Imedos, Jena, Germany).

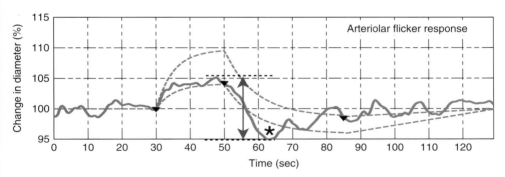

Figure 5.6 This sum curve of a dynamic retinal flicker analysis of a women with normal pregnancy outcome at 34 weeks gestation demonstrates the arteriolar flicker-induced dilatation (second black arrowhead), the physiologic maximum arteriolar constriction (asterisk) and the resulting arteriolar amplitude (blue double-headed arrow) along a normal distribution curve (dashed green lines).

Pressure wave reflection

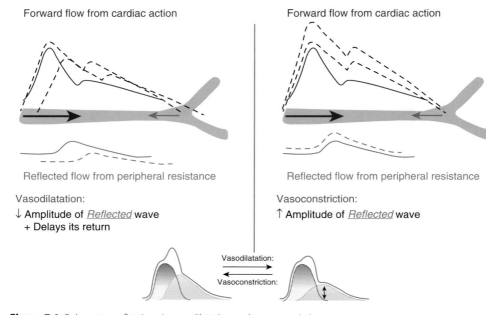

Forward flow from cardiac action

Forward flow from cardiac action

Reflected flow from peripheral resistance

Reflected flow from peripheral resistance

Vasodilatation:
↓ Amplitude of _Reflected_ wave
+ Delays its return

Vasoconstriction:
↑ Amplitude of _Reflected_ wave

Vasodilatation: →

Vasoconstriction: ←

Figure 7.1 Pulse wave reflections in vasodilatation and vasoconstriction.

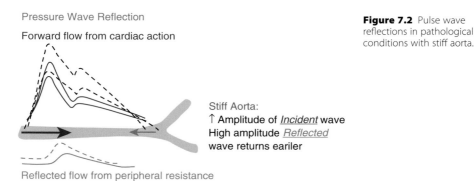

Pressure Wave Reflection

Forward flow from cardiac action

Figure 7.2 Pulse wave reflections in pathological conditions with stiff aorta.

Stiff Aorta:
↑ Amplitude of _Incident_ wave
High amplitude _Reflected_
wave returns eariler

Reflected flow from peripheral resistance

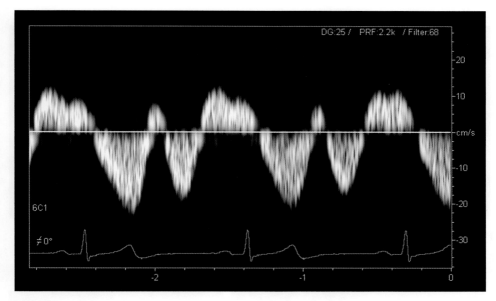

Figure 9.1 An example of tetraphasic hepatic venous Doppler waveforms.

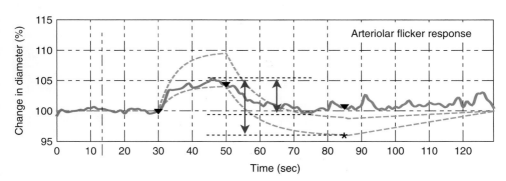

Figure 10.1 This sum curve of a dynamic retinal flicker analysis of a woman with preeclampsia demonstrates that the arteriolar flicker-induced dilatation is within the normal ranges (dashed green lines), but the typical arteriolar constriction component (asterisk) is missing, and thereby, the arteriolar amplitude is lower (short blue double-headed arrow) than in normal pregnancy (long blue double-headed arrow).

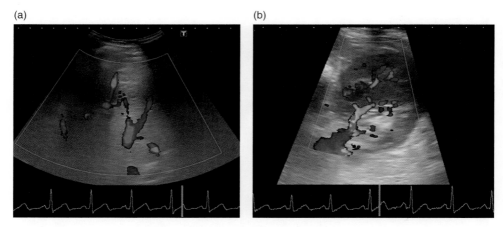

Figure 12.1 Color Doppler images of intrahepatic and intrarenal vasculature.

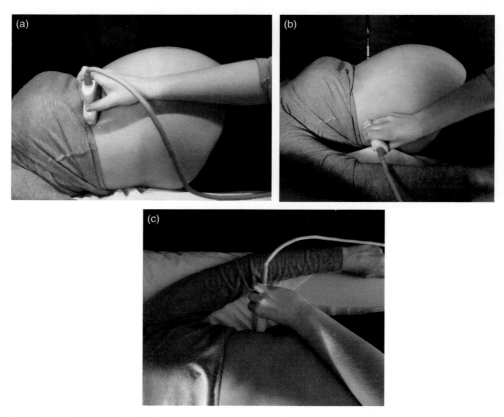

Figure 12.3 Positioning of the ultrasound probe at the level of liver (upper), right kidney (middle) and left kidney (bottom)

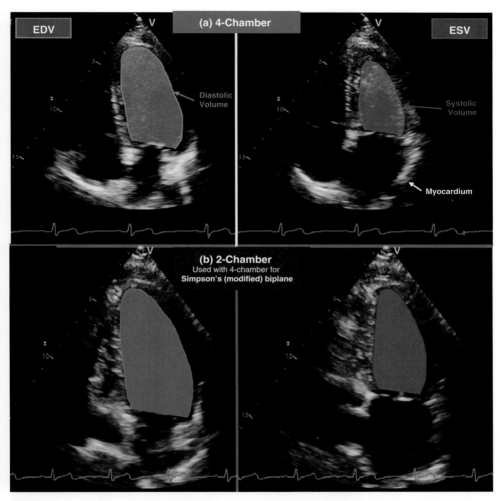

Figure 13.1 Echocardiographic single plane B-mode images of apical (a) 4-chamber and (b) 2-chamber views. The 4-chamber view can be used on its own to calculate cardiac output through estimation of stroke volume by measuring the area-change between end-diastolic (EDV) and end-systolic volumes (ESV) of the left ventricle, shown on the figure by yellow and green areas, respectively. The Simpson's (modified) biplane method uses EDV and ESV measurements from both the 4- and 2-chamber images, which increases the reliability and validity of cardiac output estimations as it may account for some interindividual variation in cardiac asymmetry.

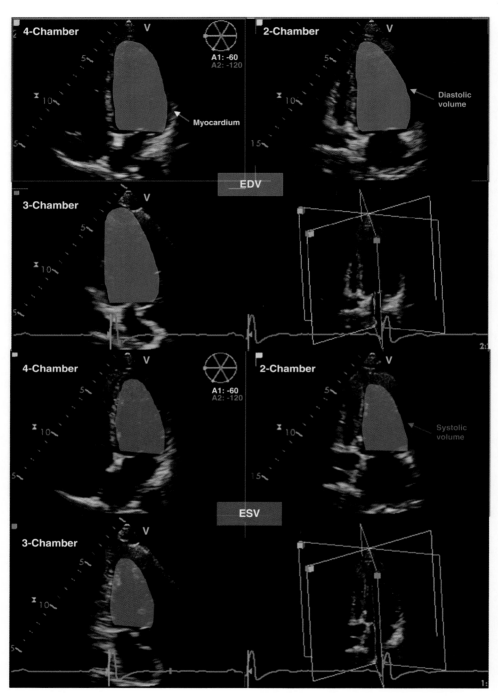

Figure 13.2 Echocardiographic triplane images of apical 4-chamber, 2-chamber and 3-chamber views collected from the same cardiac cycle. Stroke volume is estimated using the area-change between end-diastolic (EDV) and end-systolic (ESV) volumes (shown by yellow and green areas, respectively), in each of the three planes of the left ventricle.

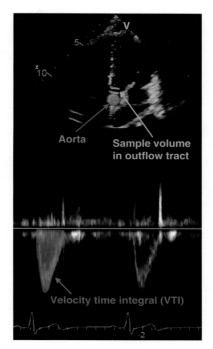

Figure 13.3 Echocardiographic image showing a Doppler signal of the left ventricular aortic outflow tract (LVOT) from an apical 5-chamber window. To collect this Doppler signal, a sample volume (indicated by the yellow lines) is placed within the aortic outflow tract just prior to the aortic valve (blue circle). The velocity time integral (VTI) is then calculated by tracing the Doppler waveform obtained at the LVOT (indicated by the red trace). Stoke volume is calculated by applying the equation: LVOT VTI x cross-sectional area of the aorta ($CSA = \pi r^2$), where aortic diameter is obtained from a separate parasternal long-axis view image.

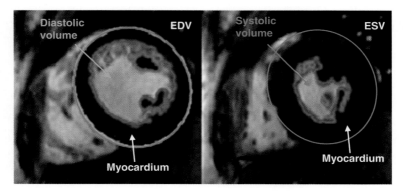

Figure 13.4 Magnetic resonance imaging (MRI) of the myocardium from a short-axis view. Stroke volume is estimated using the area-change between end-diastolic (EDV) and end-systolic (ESV) volumes of the left ventricle on multiple stacked images from the short-axis view.
Image kindly provided by Dr. Jonathan Rodrigues, Clinical Research Fellow in Cardiac Imaging, NIHR Bristol Cardiovascular Biomedical Research Unit, Bristol Heart Institute.

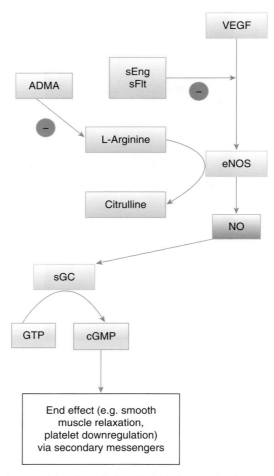

Figure 18.1 Schematic diagram of the effect of NO and soluble factors related to preeclampsia

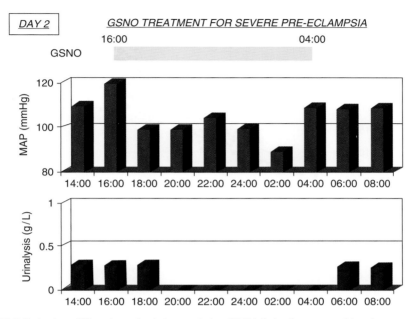

GSNO Continuous Infusion in Severe
PET

DAY 2   GSNO TREATMENT FOR SEVERE PRE-ECLAMPSIA

Figure 18.2 Reduction of BP and proteinuria is seen during GSNO infusion in women with early-onset preeclampsia.

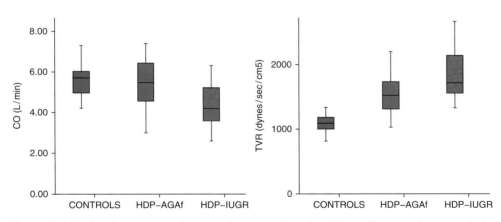

Figure 20.5 E/a diastolic ratio and cardiac output in women affected by HDP classified according to the physio-pathologic phenotypes (p<0.05).

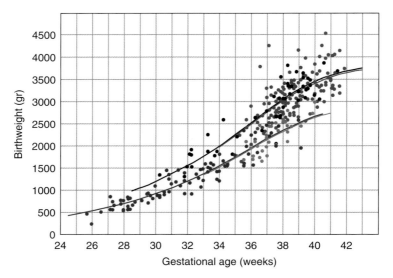

Figure 20.7 Birthweight as a function of gestational age at delivery in HDP-AGAf and HDP-IUGR groups with early (34 weeks of gestation) or late (≥34 weeks of gestation) gestational age at diagnosis [29].
Dark green dots and line: birthweight in HDP-AGAf group <34, and fitted curve.
Light green dots and line: birthweight in HDP-AGAf group ≥ 34, and fitted curve.
Dark red dots and line: birthweight in HDP-IUGR group <34, and fitted curve.
Light red dots and line: birthweight in HDP-IUGR group ≥ 34, and fitted curve.

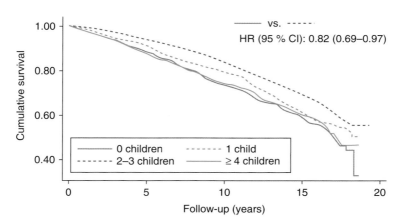

Figure 22.2 Number of children and survival
(Source: Adapted from Kuningas et al. [73]

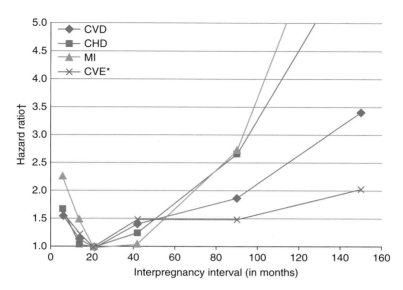

Figure 22.3 Maternal CVD in relation to interpregnancy interval.
(Source: Adapted from Ngo et al. [74])

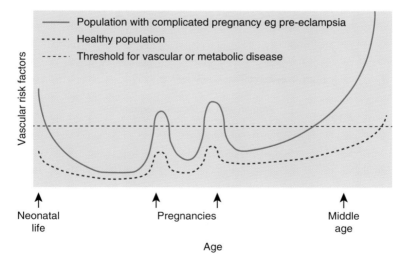

Figure 22.4 Risk of developing vascular disease during life time.
(Source: Adapted from Sattar et al. [75])

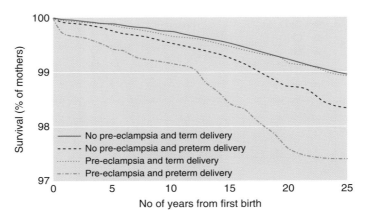

Figure 22.7 Long-term survival of primiparous mothers in relation to preeclampsia and/or preterm delivery. (Source: Adapted from Irgens et al. [78])

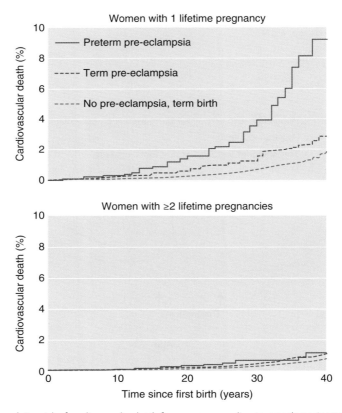

Figure 22.8 Cumulative risk of cardiovascular death for women according to preeclampsia status at first pregnancy and number of lifetime pregnancies. (Source: Adapted from Skjaerven et al. [79])

randomized double-blinded placebo trial, it was shown to significantly decrease the risk for intrauterine growth restriction (IUGR) and/or perinatal death (adjusted relative risk (RR) 0.410; 95% confidence interval, CI, 0.184–0.914), but not the incidence of preeclampsia in at-risk women. Of note, no placental abruption occurred in the PETN treatment arm, compared to five cases in the placebo group. These results suggest that secondary prophylaxis of adverse pregnancy outcome might be feasible in pregnancies exhibiting abnormal placentation using PETN [73].

S-nitrosothiols have a NO group attached to the thiol (RSH) moiety, the former of which can be effectively transferred to endogenous thiols which act as a biological reservoir of NO. The S-nitrosothiol that has been investigated in women with preeclampsia is S-nitrosoglutathione (GSNO). The first reported case of GSNO use was in a woman with severe preeclampsia, with HELLP syndrome. A rapid improvement in the patient's clinical parameters as well as platelet count was observed following infusion with GSNO [74]. A study of GSNO infusion in ten women with severe preeclampsia showed a significant dose-dependent reduction in blood pressure, with no significant effect on fetal circulation [75]. Recently, GSNO infusion administered in women with early-onset preeclampsia was found to reduce augmentation index, a marker of long-term cardiovascular health which has been observed in association with pre-eclampia [76], as well as improve proteinuria and platelet function [77]. GSNO may be a promising therapeutic agent for cases of severe preeclampsia; however, larger studies needed to investigate the safety and efficacy as well as clinical end points for both mother and baby. GSNO is metabolized in vivo by GSNO reductase and a reversible GSNO reductase inhibitor compound; N6022 has been shown to improve endothelial function in vivo, and holds potential to be studied in the context of preeclampsia.

A large trial based in Mexico investigating the use of L-arginine (a NO precursor) showed that supplementation of a combination of L-arginine and antioxidants reduced the incidence of preeclampsia when compared to placebo (30.2% vs. 12.7%). However, these results should be interpreted with caution, as the effects of L-arginine alone were not studied. Furthermore, the study population reported an exceptionally high recurrence rate of preeclampsia (30%), compared with up to approximately 5–16% recurrence risk observed in other countries [78–81], therefore results may not be generalizable or applicable to other obstetric populations. Of note, a small study of intravenous infusion of L-arginine in pregnant women showed a significant reduction in blood pressure, and this effect was more pronounced in those with preeclampsia [82].

Preeclampsia has many pathophysiological similarities as well as risk factors with adult cardiovascular disease. This includes dyslipidemia. Given the encouraging evidence of the beneficial effects of statins on the prevention of cardiovascular events in humans, several trials have tested the effect of pravastatin in rodent models of preeclampsia. Treatment with pravastatin significantly reduced maternal sFlt-1 levels, lowered blood pressure and prevented kidney injury in rats [83–86]. In addition, pravastatin also exerts protective effects on the endothelium and ameliorates preeclampsia symptoms by increasing the release of nitric oxide [85, 87]. Pravastatin is currently being tested in the first human randomized placebo-controlled trial (StAmP) in the UK, for which multicentre recruitment has been completed in 2014.

Several other compounds have been trialed in animal and early phase clinical studies, though none has been shown to be of therapeutic efficacy. These include phosphodiesterase inhibitors (thought to enhance nitric oxide pathway signaling) such as sildenafil, and hormones which are thought to contribute to vasodilatory actions in pregnancy, such as relaxin.

Postpartum Considerations

Postpartum hypertension is frequently preceded by prepregnancy (chronic), antenatal (PIH/ PE) and/or intrapartum hypertension. However, it could also manifest de novo in the postpartum period as preeclampsia. A particular difficulty in the postpartum period is the ability to accurately quantify proteinuria due to contamination of vaginal lochia. It is also important to consider other relevant factors which might have contributed to an elevated blood pressure, such as pain, anxiety and drug use.

NICE guidelines recommend checking blood pressure within 6 hours of delivery in all normotensive women without underlying medical problems and having had an uncomplicated pregnancy and delivery [88]. A further blood pressure check is recommended on day five postpartum to pick up those with late-onset postpartum hypertension. Identifying and treating hypertension appropriately is important as adverse complications such as eclampsia; intracranial hemorrhage, aortic dissection and reversible cerebral vasoconstriction syndrome are closely associated with inadequate treatment of systolic hypertension. This is reflected in the "Top ten recommendations" from the United Kingdom Confidential Enquiries into Maternal and Child Death consensus report, which states that systolic blood pressures above 150–160 require urgent and effective treatment [89].

In women with known postpartum hypertension, NICE recommends blood pressure checks every other day after discharge [6]. Further close follow up (at least weekly blood pressure checks) will allow their medications to be titrated appropriately according to their blood pressure readings. In women with chronic hypertension, consider restarting prepregnancy treatment if appropriate.

There is limited data on use of antihypertensives in the postnatal period as there are no studies on neonatal effects of maternally administered antihypertensive drugs. Safety in breastfeeding remains one of the main considerations. Pharmacological factors that increase drug levels in breast milk include high lipid solubility and low maternal plasma protein binding capacity. Even so, level of the neonate's exposure to these drugs will be affected by the dosage, frequency of administration and bioavailability of the medication [90]. In the United Kingdom, none of the commonly used antihypertensive medications are licensed for use in breastfeeding. However, most clinicians prescribe according to general consensus among the NICE guidelines development group [6]. Labetalol, atenolol, nifedipine and amlodipine are widely used in the postpartum period, with once-daily formulation preferred by some clinicians to improve compliance. Postpartum use of methyldopa is not encouraged as it has been linked with sedation and depression. Conversely, although angiotensin-converting enzyme inhibitors and angiotensin receptor blockers are contraindicated in pregnancy, Enalapril may be considered for use in breastfeeding, with evidence suggesting minimal detectable levels in the infant [91]. Labetalol is one of the most widely used antihypertensives postpartum. It is excreted in breast milk with peak milk concentration within 3 hours of the dose [92].

It is generally accepted that any hypertension and proteinuria should have resolved by 6 weeks postpartum [5]. In the long term, a proportion of women with postpartum hypertension will require drug treatment beyond this period – this is influenced by risk factors such as BMI, age, ethnicity and pre-existing medical conditions. Women under the age of 40 years with a blood pressure of >140/90 should be investigated for secondary causes, including renal disease (chronic kidney disease, renal artery stenosis), endocrine disorders (Conn's syndrome, Cushing's syndrome) and neurological disorders [93].

Some women have persisting proteinuria beyond 6 weeks postpartum, which could be due to underlying renal disease not previously diagnosed. Therefore, persistent unresolved proteinuria of >2+ on urine dipstick should prompt a referral to renal physicians for further investigation and management.

Women who develop hypertension in pregnancy and the postpartum period have increased risk of complications in future pregnancies. This includes preeclampsia, fetal growth restriction and preterm delivery. Women with previous PIH have a 16–47% recurrence rate of developing PIH in her subsequent pregnancy, and a 2–7% risk of developing preeclampsia. In women who had preeclampsia, a recurrence rate of developing PIH and preeclampsia in the next pregnancy has been quoted as 13–53% and 16% respectively [6]. Risk factors for recurrence include onset of preeclampsia at early gestation, persistent hypertension at week 5 postpartum and presence of chronic hypertension pre-pregnancy [5].

The use of low-dose aspirin in women at increased risk of preeclampsia has been extensively investigated as preventive therapy. Low-dose aspirin reduces the risk of preeclampsia by 17%, the risk of fetal or neonatal death by 14% and the relative risk of preterm birth by 8% [94]. The NICE guidelines recommend aspirin 75mg/day daily from the 12th week till delivery in women who had at least two moderate risk factors (first pregnancy, age >40 years, pregnancy interval >10 years, BMI >35 kg/m^2 at booking visit, family history of preeclampsia and multiple pregnancies) or at least one high-risk factor (hypertensive disorder in a previous pregnancy, chronic kidney disease, autoimmune disease, antiphospholipid syndrome, diabetes mellitus or chronic hypertension) [6].

Key Points

- There is no pharmacological cure for preeclampsia. Therapy is directed toward reducing blood pressure slowly using oral therapy to a target of 140–150/80–100 mmHg.
- Preconception blood pressure control can be managed with a majority of antihypertensive drugs, with the exception of angiotensin-converting enzymes and angiotensin receptor blockers which are linked to congenital abnormalities.
- In the United Kingdom, none of the commonly used antihypertensive medications are licensed for use in breastfeeding; most clinicians prescribe according to general consensus among the NICE guidelines development group.
- Novel therapies for prevention and treatment of preeclampsia, such as replacing nitric oxide bioavailability, have not been proven to show significant clinical benefit and more research is needed to explore these therapies.

References

1. Say L, Chou D, Gemmill A, et al. Global causes of maternal death: a WHO systematic analysis. *Lancet Glob Health*, 2014;**2**(6):e323–33.

2. Lindheimer MD, Taler SJ, Cunningham FG. ASH position paper: hypertension in pregnancy. *J Clin Hypertens (Greenwich)*, 2009;**11**(4):214–25.

3. Lo JO, Mission JF, Caughey AB. Hypertensive disease of pregnancy and maternal mortality. *Curr Opin Obstet Gynecol*, 2013;**25**(2):124–32.

4. Foo L, Bewley S, Rudd A. Maternal death from stroke: a thirty year national retrospective review. *Eur J Obstet Gynecol Reprod Biol*, 2013;**171**(2):266–70.

5. National High Blood Pressure Education Program Working Group on High Blood Pressure in Pregnancy. Report of the National High Blood Pressure Education Program Working Group on High Blood Pressure in Pregnancy. *Am J Obstet Gynecol*, 2000;**183**(1):S1–S22.

6. NICE. *National Institute for Health and Clinical Excellence: (CG107) Hypertension in pregnancy: the management of hypertensive disorders during pregnancy.* 2011: London.

7. Paruk F, Moodley J. Untoward effects of rapid-acting antihypertensive agents. *Best Pract Res Clin Obstet Gynaecol*, 2001;**15**(4):491–506.

8. Redman C. Hypertension, in *Medical disorders in obstetric practice*, M.de Swiet, Editor. 2002, Blackwell Publishing Company.159–197.

9. Tranquilli AL, Dekker G, Magee L, et al. The classification, diagnosis and management of the hypertensive disorders of pregnancy: A revised statement from the ISSHP. *Pregnancy Hypertens*, 2014;**4**(2):97–104.

10. Sibai BM, Ewel M, Levine RJ, et al. Risk factors associated with preeclampsia in healthy nulliparous women. The Calcium for Preeclampsia Prevention (CPEP) Study Group. *Am J Obstet Gynecol*, 1997;**177**(5):1003–10.

11. Ghosh G, Grewal J, Männistö T, et al. Racial/ethnic differences in pregnancy-related hypertensive disease in nulliparous women. *Ethn Dis*, 2014;**24**(3):283–9.

12. Chaturvedi N, McKeigue PM, Marmot MG. Resting and ambulatory blood pressure differences in Afro-Caribbeans and Europeans. *Hypertension*, 1993;**22**(1):90–6.

13. Valensise H, Novelli GP, Vasapollo B. Pre-eclampsia: One name, two conditions – the case for early and late disease being different. *Fetal Matern Med Rev*, 2014;**24**:32–7.

14. Ferrazzi E, ST, Aupont JE. The evidence for late-onset pre-eclampsia as a maternogenic disease of pregnancy. *Fetal Matern Med Rev*, 2013; **24**(1):18–31.

15. Huppertz, B. Placental origins of preeclampsia: challenging the current hypothesis. *Hypertension*, 2008; **51**(4):970–5.

16. Sibai B, Dekker G, Kupferminc M. Pre-eclampsia. *Lancet*, 2005;**365**(9461):785–99.

17. Levine RJ, Lam C, Qian C, et al. Soluble endoglin and other circulating antiangiogenic factors in preeclampsia. *N Engl J Med*, 2006;**355**(10):992–1005.

18. Levine RJ, Maynard SE, Qian C, et al. Circulating angiogenic factors and the risk of preeclampsia. *N Engl J Med*, 2004;**350**(7):672–83.

19. Xiong X, Demianczuk NN, Saunders LD, Wang FL, Fraser WD. Impact of preeclampsia and gestational hypertension on birth weight by gestational age. *Am J Epidemiol*, 2002;**155**(3):203–9.

20. Ananth CV, Peltier MR, Kinzler WL, Smulian JC, Vintzileos AM. Chronic hypertension and risk of placental abruption: is the association modified by ischemic placental disease? *Am J Obstet Gynecol*, 2007;**197**(3):273 e1–7.

21. Haelterman E, Bréart G, Paris-Llado J, Dramaix M, Tchobroutsky C. Effect of uncomplicated chronic hypertension on the risk of small-for-gestational age birth. *Am J Epidemiol*, 1997;**145**(8):689–95.

22. Walfisch A, Al-maawali A, Moretti ME, Nickel C, Koren G. Teratogenicity of angiotensin converting enzyme inhibitors or receptor blockers. *J Obstet Gynaecol*, 2011;**31**(6):465–72.

23. Piper JM, Ray WA, Rosa FW. Pregnancy outcome following exposure to angiotensin-converting enzyme inhibitors. *Obstet Gynecol*, 1992;**80**(3 Pt 1):429–32.

24. Rosa FW, Bosco LA, Graham CF, Milstien JB, Dreis M, Creamer J. Neonatal anuria with maternal angiotensin-converting enzyme inhibition. *Obstet Gynecol*, 1989;**74** (3 Pt 1):371–4.

25. Kincaid-Smith P, Bullen M, Mills J. Prolonged use of methyldopa in severe hypertension in pregnancy. *Br Med J*, 1966;**1**(5482):274–6.

26. Ananth CV, Savitz DA, Bowes WA, Luther ER. Influence of hypertensive disorders and cigarette smoking on placental abruption and uterine bleeding during pregnancy. *Br J Obstet Gynaecol*, 1997;**104** (5):572–8.

27. Romero-Arauz JF, Ortiz-Diaz CB, Leaños-miranda A, Martinez-Rodriguez OA. Progression of gestational hypertension to preeclampsia. *Ginecol Obstet Mex*, 2014;**82** (4):229–35.

28. Anumba DO, Lincoln K, Robson SC. Predictive value of clinical and laboratory indices at first assessment in women referred with suspected gestational hypertension. *Hypertens Pregnancy*, 2010;**29**(2):163–79.

29. Villar J, Carroli G, Wojdyla D, et al. Preeclampsia, gestational hypertension and intrauterine growth restriction, related or independent conditions? *Am J Obstet Gynecol*, 2006;**194**(4):921–31.

30. Buchbinder A, Sibai BM, Caritis S, et al. Adverse perinatal outcomes are significantly higher in severe gestational hypertension than in mild preeclampsia. *Am J Obstet Gynecol*, 2002;**186**(1):66–71.

31. Steer PJ, Little MP, Kold-Jensen T, Chapple J, Elliott P. Maternal blood pressure in pregnancy, birth weight, and perinatal mortality in first births: prospective study. *BMJ*, 2004;**329**(7478):1312.

32. Al Khaja KAJ, Sequeira P, Alkhaja AK, Damanhori AH. Drug treatment of hypertension in pregnancy: a critical review of adult guideline recommendations. *J Hypertens*, 2014;**32** (3):454–63.

33. Mutch LM, Moar VA, Ounsted MK, Redman CW. Hypertension during pregnancy, with and without specific hypotensive treatment. II. The growth and development of the infant in the first year of life. *Early Hum Dev*, 1977;**1**(1):59–67.

34. Cockburn J, Moar VA, Ounsted M, Redman CW. Final report of study on hypertension during pregnancy: the effects of specific treatment on the growth and development of the children. *Lancet*, 1982;**1**(8273):647–9.

35. el-Qarmalawi AM, Morsy AH, al-Fadly A, Obeid A, Hashem M. Labetalol vs. methyldopa in the treatment of pregnancy-induced hypertension. *Int J Gynaecol Obstet*, 1995. **49**(2):125–30.

36. Huisjes HJ, Hadders-Algra M, Touwen BC. Is clonidine a behavioural teratogen in the human? *Early Hum Dev*, 1986. **14**(1):43–8.

37. Chobanian AV, Bakris GL, Black HR, et al. The Seventh Report of the Joint National Committee on Prevention, Detection, Evaluation, and Treatment of High Blood Pressure: the JNC 7 report. *JAMA*, 2003;**289**(19):2560–72.

38. Butters L, Kennedy S, Rubin PC. Atenolol in essential hypertension during pregnancy. *BMJ*, 1990;**301**(6752):587–9.

39. Lip GY, Beevers M, Churchill D, Shaffer LM, Beevers DG. Effect of atenolol on birth weight. *Am J Cardiol*, 1997;**79**(10):1436–8.

40. Yakoob MY, Bateman BT, Ho E, et al. The risk of congenital malformations associated with exposure to beta-blockers early in pregnancy: a meta-analysis. *Hypertension*, 2013;**62**(2):375–81.

41. Sorensen HT, Czeizel AE, Rockenbauer M, Steffensen FH, Olsen J. The risk of limb deficiencies and other congenital abnormalities in children exposed in utero

to calcium channel blockers. *Acta Obstet Gynecol Scand*, 2001;**80**(5):397–401.

42. Danielsson BR, Reiland S, Rundgvist E, Danielson M. Digital defects induced by vasodilating agents: relationship to reduction in uteroplacental blood flow. *Teratology*, 1989;**40**(4):351–8.

43. Scott WJ, Jr., Resnick E, Hummler H, Clozel JP, Bürgin H. Cardiovascular alterations in rat fetuses exposed to calcium channel blockers. *Reprod Toxicol*, 1997;**11**(2–3):207–14.

44. Brown MA, Buddle ML, Farrell T, Davis GK. Efficacy and safety of nifedipine tablets for the acute treatment of severe hypertension in pregnancy. *Am J Obstet Gynecol*, 2002;**187**(4):1046–50.

45. Impey L. Severe hypotension and fetal distress following sublingual administration of nifedipine to a patient with severe pregnancy induced hypertension at 33 weeks. *Br J Obstet Gynaecol*, 1993;**100**(10):959–61.

46. Papatsonis DN, Lok CA, Bos JM, Geijn HP, Dekker GA. Calcium channel blockers in the management of preterm labor and hypertension in pregnancy. *Eur J Obstet Gynecol Reprod Biol*, 2001;**97**(2):122–40.

47. Ben-Ami M, Giladi Y, Shalev E. The combination of magnesium sulphate and nifedipine: a cause of neuromuscular blockade. *Br J Obstet Gynaecol*, 1994;**101**(3):262–3.

48. Ales K. Magnesium plus nifedipine. *Am J Obstet Gynecol*, 1990;**162**(1):288.

49. Magee LA, Miremadi S, Li J, et al. Therapy with both magnesium sulfate and nifedipine does not increase the risk of serious magnesium-related maternal side effects in women with preeclampsia. *Am J Obstet Gynecol*, 2005;**193**(1):153–63.

50. Vasilakis-Scaramozza C, Aschengrau A, Cabral HJ, Jick SS. Antihypertensive drugs and the risk of congenital anomalies. *Pharmacotherapy*, 2013;**33**(5):476–82.

51. Cooper WO, Hernandez-Diaz S, Arbogast PG, et al. Major congenital malformations after first-trimester exposure to ACE inhibitors. *N Engl J Med*, 2006;**354**(23):2443–51.

52. Quan A, Fetopathy associated with exposure to angiotensin converting enzyme inhibitors and angiotensin receptor antagonists. *Early Hum Dev*, 2006;**82**(1):23–8.

53. Alwan S, Polifka JE, Friedman JM. Angiotensin II receptor antagonist treatment during pregnancy. *Birth Defects Res A Clin Mol Teratol*, 2005;**73**(2):123–30.

54. Groves TD, Corenblum B. Spironolactone therapy during human pregnancy. *Am J Obstet Gynecol*, 1995;**172**(5):1655–6.

55. Spinnato JA, Sibai BM, Anderson GD. Fetal distress after hydralazine therapy for severe pregnancy-induced hypertension. *South Med J*, 1986;**79**(5):559–62.

56. Paterson-Brown S, Robson SC, Redfern N, Walkinshaw SA, de Swiet M. Hydralazine boluses for the treatment of severe hypertension in pre-eclampsia. *Br J Obstet Gynaecol*, 1994;**101**(5):409–13.

57. Davis RL, Eastman D, McPhillips H, et al. Risks of congenital malformations and perinatal events among infants exposed to calcium channel and beta-blockers during pregnancy. *Pharmacoepidemiol Drug Saf*, 2011;**20**(2):138–45.

58. Olsen, KS, Beier-Holgersen R. Hemodynamic collapse following labetalol administration in preeclampsia. *Acta Obstet Gynecol Scand*, 1992;**71**(2):151–2.

59. Magee LA, Cham C, Waterman EJ, Ohlsson A, von Dadelszen P. Hydralazine for treatment of severe hypertension in pregnancy: meta-analysis. *BMJ*, 2003;**327**(7421):955–60.

60. Vigil-De Gracia P, Lasso M, Ruiz E, Vega-Malek JC, de Mena FT, Lopez JC. Severe hypertension in pregnancy: hydralazine or labetalol. A randomized clinical trial. *Eur J Obstet Gynecol Reprod Biol*, 2006;**128**(1–2):157–62.

61. Duley L, Henderson-Smart DJ, Meher S. Drugs for treatment of very high blood pressure during pregnancy. *Cochrane Database Syst Rev*, 2006;**3**:CD001449.

62. Firoz T, Magee LA, MacDonnell K, et al. Oral antihypertensive therapy for severe hypertension in pregnancy and postpartum: a systematic review. *BJOG*, 2014;**121**(10):1210–8; discussion 1220.

63. Rumbold AR, Crowther CA, Haslam RR, Dekker GA, Robinson JS. Vitamins C and E and the risks of preeclampsia and perinatal complications. *N Engl J Med*, 2006;**354**(17):1796–806.

64. Poston L, Briley AL, Seed PT, Kelly FJ, Shennan AH. Vitamin C and vitamin E in pregnant women at risk for pre-eclampsia (VIP trial): randomized placebo-controlled trial. *Lancet*, 2006;**367**(9517):1145–54.

65. Conde-Agudelo, A, Romero R, Kusanovic JP, Hassan SS. Supplementation with vitamins C and E during pregnancy for the prevention of preeclampsia and other adverse maternal and perinatal outcomes: a systematic review and metaanalysis. *American Journal of Obstetrics and Gynecology*, 2011;**204**(6):503.

66. Basaran, A, Basaran M, Topatan B. Combined vitamin C and E supplementation for the prevention of preeclampsia: a systematic review and meta-analysis. *Obstet Gynecol Surv*, 2010;**65**(10):653–67.

67. Romero, R, Garite TJ. Unexpected results of an important trial of vitamins C and E administration to prevent preeclampsia. *Am J Obstet Gynecol*, 2006;**194**(5):1213–4.

68. Banerjee, S, Chambers AE, Campbell S. Is vitamin E a safe prophylaxis for preeclampsia? *Am J Obstet Gynecol*, 2006;**194**(5):1228–33.

69. Ramsay B, De Belder A, Campbell S, Moncada S, Martin JF. A nitric oxide donor improves uterine artery diastolic blood flow in normal early pregnancy and in women at high risk of pre-eclampsia. *Eur J Clin Invest*, 1994;**24**(1):76–8.

70. Manzur-Verástegui S, Mandeville PB, Gordillo-Moscoso A, Hernández-Sierra JF, Rodríguez-Martínez M. Efficacy of nitroglycerine infusion versus sublingual nifedipine in severe pre-eclampsia: a randomized, triple-blind, controlled trial.

Clin Exp Pharmacol Physiol, 2008;**35**(5–6):580–5.

71. Cetin A, Yurtcu N, Guvenal T, Imir AG, Duran B, Cetin M. The effect of glyceryl trinitrate on hypertension in women with severe preeclampsia, HELLP syndrome, and eclampsia. *Hypertens Pregnancy*, 2004;**23**(1):37–46.

72. Lees C, Valensise H, Black R, et al. The efficacy and fetal-maternal cardiovascular effects of transdermal glyceryl trinitrate in the prophylaxis of pre-eclampsia and its complications: a randomized double-blind placebo-controlled trial. *Ultrasound Obstet Gynecol*, 1998;**12**(5):334–8.

73. Schleussner E, Lehmann T, Kähler C, Schneider U, Schlembach D, Groten T. Impact of the nitric oxide-donor pentaerythrityl-tetranitrate on perinatal outcome in risk pregnancies: a prospective, randomized, double-blinded trial. *J Perinat Med*, 2014;**42**(4):507–14.

74. de Belder A, Lees C, Martin J, Moncada S, Campbell S. Treatment of HELLP syndrome with nitric oxide donor. *Lancet*, 1995;**345**(8942):124–5.

75. Lees C, Langford E, Brown AS, et al. The effects of S-nitrosoglutathione on platelet activation, hypertension, and uterine and fetal Doppler in severe preeclampsia. *Obstet Gynecol*, 1996;**88**(1):14–9.

76. Khalil A, Akolekar R, Syngelaki A, Elkhouli M, Nicolaides KH. Maternal hemodynamics at 11–13 weeks' gestation and risk of pre-eclampsia. *Ultrasound Obstet Gynecol*, 2012;**40**(1):28–34.

77. Everett TR, Wilkinson IB, Mahendru AA, et al. S-Nitrosoglutathione improves haemodynamics in early-onset pre-eclampsia. *Br J Clin Pharmacol*, 2014;**78**(3):660–9.

78. Hernandez-Diaz S, Toh S, Cnattingius S. Risk of pre-eclampsia in first and subsequent pregnancies: prospective cohort study. *BMJ*, 2009;**338**:b2255.

79. Basso O, Christensen K, Olsen J. Higher risk of pre-eclampsia after change of partner. An effect of longer interpregnancy intervals? *Epidemiology*, 2001;**12**(6):624–9.

80. Hargood JL, Brown MA. Pregnancy-induced hypertension: recurrence rate in second pregnancies. *Med J Aust*, 1991;**154**(6):376–7.

81. Trogstad L, Skrondal A, Stoltenberg C, Magnus P, Nesheim BI, Eskild A. Recurrence risk of preeclampsia in twin and singleton pregnancies. *Am J Med Genet A*, 2004;**126**A(1):41–5.

82. Facchinetti F, Longo M, Piccinini F, Neri I, Volpe A. L-arginine infusion reduces blood pressure in preeclamptic women through nitric oxide release. *J Soc Gynecol Investig*, 1999;**6**(4):202–7.

83. Cindrova-Davies T. The therapeutic potential of antioxidants, ER chaperones, NO and H2S donors, and statins for treatment of preeclampsia. *Front Pharmacol*, 2014;**5**:119.

84. Fox KA, Longo M, Tamayo E, et al. Effects of pravastatin on mediators of vascular function in a mouse model of soluble Fms-like tyrosine kinase-1-induced preeclampsia. *Am J Obstet Gynecol*, 2011;**205**(4):366 e1–5.

85. Kumasawa K, Ikawa M, Kidoya H, et al. Pravastatin induces placental growth factor (PGF) and ameliorates preeclampsia in a mouse model. *Proc Natl Acad Sci U S A*, 2011;**108**(4):1451–5.

86. Ahmed A, Singh J, Khan Y, Seshan SV, Girardi G. A new mouse model to explore therapies for preeclampsia. *PLoS One*, 2010;**5**(10):e13663.

87. Redecha P, van Rooijen N, Torry D, Girardi G. Pravastatin prevents miscarriages in mice: role of tissue factor in placental and fetal injury. *Blood*, 2009;**113**(17):4101–9.

88. NICE. *National Institute for Health & Clinical Excellence: (CG37) Routine post-natal care of women and their babies.* 2006.

89. Cantwell R, Clutton-Brock T, Cooper G, et al. Saving Mothers' Lives: Reviewing maternal deaths to make motherhood safer: 2006–2008. The Eighth Report of the Confidential Enquiries into Maternal Deaths in the United Kingdom. *BJOG*, 2011;**118** Suppl 1:1–203.

90. Podymow T, August P, Umans JG. Antihypertensive therapy in pregnancy. *Semin Nephrol*, 2004;**24**(6):616–25.

91. Redman CWG, Kelly JG, Cooper WD. The excretion of enalapril and enalaprilat in human breast-milk. *European Journal of Clinical Pharmacology*, 1990;**38**(1):99.

92. Lunell NO, Kulas J, Rane A. Transfer of labetalol into amniotic fluid and breast milk in lactating women. *Eur J Clin Pharmacol*, 1985;**28**(5):597–9.

93. Bramham K, Nelson-Piercy C, Brown MJ, Chappell LC. Postpartum management of hypertension. *BMJ*, 2013;**346**:f894.

94. Duley L, Henderson-Smart DJ, Meher S, King JF. Antiplatelet agents for preventing pre-eclampsia and its complications. *Cochrane Database Syst Rev*, 2007; **2**: CD004659.

Aspirin

Shireen Meher

Summary

Inadequate vascular adaptation during pregnancy can result in persistent vasoconstriction, excessive thrombosis and inflammation, and poor placentation. This increases the risk of gestational vascular complications such as preeclampsia and fetal growth restriction. Acetylsalicylic acid, or aspirin, is well known for its ability to prevent clotting and suppress inflammation. It is postulated that these effects may improve placentation and endothelial dysfunction; therefore, aspirin has been widely advocated for prevention of preeclampsia and its complications. Evidence from randomized trials (RCTs) shows that aspirin has small but consistent benefits in reducing preeclampsia and improving perinatal outcome. The exact mechanism by which aspirin improves pregnancy outcomes remains unclear, and this has fueled the debate over which women are most likely to benefit from aspirin, and what is the optimal dose and time to start therapy.

This chapter reviews the pharmacological properties of aspirin, and mechanisms by which it may improve the pathophysiology of uteroplacental insufficiency. The current evidence base is presented, and unresolved issues around aspirin therapy are discussed.

Aspirin

Aspirin was introduced in 1897 as an anti-inflammatory agent, and its inhibitory effect on platelet function was recognized in 1967. It is one of the most commonly prescribed medications around the world, particularly for cardiovascular disease, because of its ability to prevent clotting.

Mechanism of Action

Aspirin acts by inhibiting the synthesis of cyclic prostanoids from their precursor arachidonic acid, by irreversibly inactivating the cyclooxygenase enzymes (COX-1 and COX-2) (Figure 16.1) [1].

Prostanoids mediate cellular functions and play a role in the regulation of inflammation, platelet aggregation, vascular tone and blood flow (Figure 16.1). The prostanoid thromboxane A2 (TXA2) is produced by platelets and causes platelet aggregation and vasoconstriction. In contrast, the prostanoid prostacyclin (PGI2), produced by vascular endothelial cells, induces vasodilatation and inhibits platelet aggregation. Although aspirin inhibits production of both TXA2 and PGI2, the antithrombotic effect of TXA2 inhibition predominates over PGI2 inhibition [2]. This may be because COX inhibition in platelets is irreversible, whereas vascular endothelial cells can regenerate COX. A lower dose of aspirin or controlled-release preparation results in preferential inhibition of platelet COX over

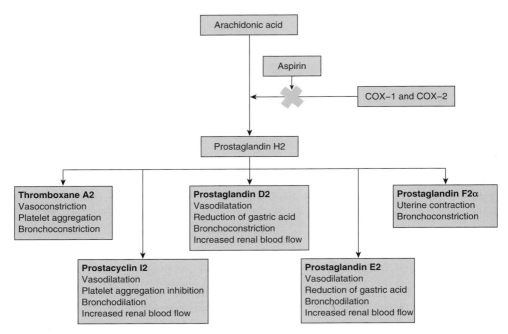

Figure 16.1 Prostanoid synthesis and function

endothelial COX, and this differential effect has the advantage of enhancing the antithrombotic effects of aspirin by preserving endothelial PGI2 production.

Aspirin has also been demonstrated to act through mechanisms that are independent of the COX pathway. It facilitates platelet inhibition by neutrophils, through a nitric oxide/cGMP-dependent process [1]. Aspirin can act as an antioxidant by directly scavenging hydroxyl radicals and preventing oxidation of proteins. It has also been shown to inhibit nuclear factor-kB (NFκ B) activation, a gene transcription factor that plays a key role in regulating the expression of cytokines, chemokines, adhesion molecules, pro-inflammatory enzymes and apoptosis [3].

2.2 Pharmacological Properties

Aspirin is rapidly absorbed from the upper gastrointestinal tract, with peak plasma concentrations in 40 minutes. Platelet inhibition can be demonstrated within 60 minutes [2]. Although the plasma half-life of aspirin is only 20 minutes, its effects last for the duration of the life of the platelet, which is around 10 days. After a single dose of aspirin, platelet activity recovers daily by 10% as a result of platelet turnover. However, normal hemostasis has been demonstrated even if 20% of platelets have normal COX activity [4].

The dose of aspirin required to effectively stop TXA2 production in healthy individuals is 100 mg [5]. Lower doses lead to a dose-dependent effect but the effect of repeated daily doses is cumulative. Outside pregnancy, therapeutic benefits of aspirin have been demonstrated with doses ranging from 30 to 1500 mg daily; higher doses increase the risk of gastrointestinal side effects without additional benefits [2]. During pregnancy, lower doses

(50 to 150 mg daily) have been used due to concerns about potential risk of bleeding in the mother and baby, as aspirin crosses the placenta [6].

Rationale for Use of Aspirin in Preventing Preeclampsia and its Complications

Pathophysiology of Preeclampsia

Preeclampsia is characterized by the development of hypertension and either proteinuria or other end-organ dysfunction after 20 weeks of gestation. Clinical features result from microangiopathy of target organs, including the brain, liver, kidney and placenta. Fetal complications from placental involvement include fetal growth restriction and perinatal death. The underlying cause of preeclampsia is unclear, but the pathophysiology is thought to involve both placental hypoxia and increased maternal susceptibility from genetic factors, immune maladaptation and systemic disease [7].

During early placental development in normal pregnancy, the extravillous cyto-trophoblast from the fetus invades the uterine spiral arteries of the decidua basalis and myometrium. The cytotrophoblast replaces the endothelial lining of spiral arteries by pseudovasculogenesis, or vascular mimicry where adhesions molecules expressed in the cytotrophoblast are downregulated to adopt an endothelial cell phenotype [8]. This process transforms the spiral arteries from small caliber vessels into large diameter, high capacitance vessels that allow increased placental blood flow to the fetus. The first wave of trophoblast invasion is complete by around 10 weeks gestation, transforming arterioles in the decidua basalis, and a second wave that starts at 14–15 weeks transforms their myometrial segments. Active endovas-cular trophoblast has been seen up to 22 weeks [9].

In preeclampsia, these vascular adaptations may be patchy or fail to extend into the myometrium, leading to placental hypoperfusion. The molecular basis for abnormal pla-cental development remains unknown. Pseudovasculogenesis has been demonstrated to be impaired; cytotrophoblasts fail to mimic the vascular adhesion phenotype, and are unable to invade the myometrial spiral arterioles effectively. Angiogenic proteins are also important in the regulation of placental vascular development [8]. The soluble receptor for vascular endothelial growth factor (sFlt-1) is an endogenous anti-angiogenic protein that, along with antiangiogenic protein soluble endoglin (sEng), impairs vasculogenesis by binding to proangiogenic proteins vascular endothelial growth factor (VEGF) and placental growth factor (PIGF).

Placental ischemia is thought to trigger the release of certain factors into maternal circulation that leads to endothelial cell dysfunction. Several pathways have been proposed, including endothelial cell membrane damage from oxidative stress, cytokines, syncitiotro-phoblast fragments from placental tissue and antiangiogenic growth factors [7, 8].

Endothelial cell dysfunction leads to vasoconstriction, derangement of the coagulation system and intravascular volume contraction. Hypertension occurs secondarily to diffuse vasoconstriction, with reduced vasodilators PGI2 and nitric oxide, increased vasoconstric-tors TXA2 and endothelin, increased responsiveness of endothelium to the vasopressor Angiotensin II and norepinephrine, and increased sympathetic tone in blood vessels. There is widespread activation of the coagulation system with alteration of the TXA2:PGI2 ratio, and platelet activation and consumption. Injured endothelial cells leak fluid into the extravascular interstitial space, causing edema and a reduction in circulating blood volume. Plasma volume contraction, which may be by as much as 40%, leads to reduced organ perfusion and damage [7, 8].

Effect of Aspirin on Pathophysiology of Preeclampsia

Effect of Aspirin on Platelet and Endothelial Function

Controlled studies and RCTs have consistently shown that low-dose aspirin can selectively inhibit TXA2 activity in maternal circulation, and this also correlates with improved pregnancy outcomes.

Aspirin 50 mg daily inhibited more than 90% of platelet TXA2 production, and significantly decreased the urinary excretion of TXA2, but not PGI2 metabolites in an RCT [10]. Another RCT showed that the mean ratio of serum TXA2 to serum metabolites of PGI2 after three weeks of treatment decreased by 35% in the aspirin group but increased by 51% in the placebo group [11]. The incidence of preeclampsia was also reduced in women taking aspirin. Benigni et al. also found that women randomized to aspirin had lower serum and urinary metabolites of TXA2 compared to the placebo group, while the metabolites of prostacyclin remained unchanged. This correlated with longer pregnancies and higher birthweights in the newborns of women taking aspirin [12].

Effect of Aspirin on Placentation

Whether aspirin has a direct effect on placentation is unclear. To investigate the impact of aspirin on placental development, studies have evaluated trophoblast function, uteroplacental and fetal hemodynamics, and placental histology.

Trophoblast Function

Increased TXA synthase and its receptors were found in trophoblast from preeclamptic placental tissue, and in cell cultures, aspirin reduced the production of TXA2 metabolites by cytotrophoblast [13]. Aspirin also increased production of Interleukin (IL)-3, which supports trophoblast invasion through its ability to increase leukotriene production. However, in human first-trimester extravillous cytotrophoblast HTR-8 cell lines, aspirin did not have a significant effect on production of the cytokines or chemokines IL-8, IL-6, GRO-α or IL-1β, or on production of proangiogenic (VEGF or PlGF) or antiangiogenic factors (sFlt-1 or sEng) [14]. Treatment with aspirin did not induce any changes in the basal migratory capacity of trophoblast cells or in the migratory capacity of trophoblast suppressed by antiphospholipid antibodies [14].

It has been proposed that aspirin may alter trophoblast biology by regulating oxidative-reductive signals associated with placental apoptosis [15]. Oxidative stress induces placental apoptosis and apoptosis has been proposed as an underlying mechanism for placental ischemia in preeclampsia. In BeWo cells, sera from IVF failure increased trophoblast apoptosis, whereas aspirin reversed these effects [15]. However, this effect of aspirin on apoptosis is inconsistent among studies.

Uteroplacental and Fetal Doppler Studies

High levels of impedance in uteroplacental blood flow reflect suboptimal placental function, and advanced stages of uteroplacental insufficiency lead to abnormal fetal Doppler. Aspirin has not shown a beneficial effect on uteroplacental or fetal Doppler in observational, controlled or randomized studies [16–18].

An RCT with 538 healthy nulliparous women receiving aspirin or placebo from 24 weeks showed that monthly umbilical artery Doppler systolic to diastolic (SD) ratio and resistance index (RI) were no different between the two groups, nor was there any correlation with pregnancy outcomes [16]. Grab et al. randomized 43 high-risk women to aspirin or placebo from 20 weeks gestation and performed fortnightly Doppler assessments from 18 weeks until delivery for uterine and umbilical artery PI; fetal middle cerebral artery, aorta and ductus arteriosus PI; and velocities and atrioventricular regurgitation [18]. There was no significant difference in any of the Doppler parameters assessed between the aspirin and control groups.

It has been argued that, to have an impact on placentation, any intervention given for prevention of preeclampsia should be commenced early in gestation. Haapsamo et al. randomized 37 women undergoing IVF/ICSI to aspirin or placebo, commenced before conception [19]. Longitudinal Doppler evaluation in the first and second trimesters showed that at 18 weeks, the uterine artery Doppler PI was lower in those taking aspirin compared to the placebo. Umbilical artery Doppler parameters did not differ significantly between the groups. There were three cases of preeclampsia in the aspirin group and two in the placebo group but all women who developed preeclampsia had normal uterine artery Doppler PI at 18 weeks. This highlights the limitation of correlating changes in uterine artery Doppler impedance with subsequent development of preeclampsia.

Placental Histology

Abnormal uteroplacental perfusion and platelet aggregation are associated with readily identifiable placental lesions, including decidual thrombosis, excessive perivillous fibrin deposition, villous ischemic damage, infarct and abruption [20].

Cusick et al. assessed the impact of aspirin from the first trimester on the placentas of 13 women who had experienced preeclampsia, fetal death or preterm birth and abnormal placental pathology in a previous pregnancy [20]. They found that despite an improvement in clinical outcomes in the aspirin-treated pregnancy, histological evidence of uterine vascular pathology persisted in the majority of women (62%). These findings were also confirmed in a similar study by Tarim et al. [21]. They found no significant difference in the incidence of pathologic placental lesions between the 27 high-risk women taking aspirin from early pregnancy, compared to 29 high-risk women not taking aspirin. This study did not find a significant difference in pregnancy outcomes between the two groups.

Effectiveness of Aspirin for Preventing Preeclampsia and its Complications

Data on the effectiveness of aspirin for prevention of preeclampsia and its complications are now available for more than 37,000 women from 59 RCTs [6]. Although individual large studies do not show significant benefits with aspirin, numerous meta-analyses have consistently shown that aspirin reduces the risk of preeclampsia, albeit the effects are more modest than initially anticipated. The Cochrane review on antiplatelets showed that aspirin is associated with relative risk (RR) reductions for pre-eclampsia by 17%

(95% Confidence Interval (CI) 11–23%), preterm birth by 8% (3–12%), fetal or neonatal death by 14% (2–24%) and a small-for-gestational-age baby by 10% (2–17%) [6].

Uncertainty remained about whether aspirin would have greater benefits if given to specific groups of women, or at particular gestations or in higher doses. To resolve these issues, the PARIS Collaborative Group performed an individual participant data (IPD) meta-analysis from aspirin trials [22]. Raw data were obtained for 90% of women randomized to antiplatelet trials at that time (31 trials, 32,217 women), and analyzed based on numerous participant- and trial-level factors. The IPD review confirmed a 10% statistically significant reduction in the risk of preeclampsia and of a composite serious adverse outcome (death of mother or baby, small-for-gestational-age baby, preterm birth or preeclampsia) with aspirin.

The IPD review did not find any evidence that any one of the prespecified subgroups benefited more or less from the use of antiplatelets, based either on risk factors for preeclampsia or gestation at randomization before or after 20 weeks, or for a dose of 75 mg or less compared to more than 75 mg, for the outcome of preeclampsia.

Although the benefits of aspirin are modest, in the presence of good safety data and low cost, aspirin is now widely recommended for the prevention of preeclampsia and its complications by international guidelines. A low dose of 75 mg aspirin is recommended in all guidelines, although some have considered a higher dose of up to 162 mg. Guidelines vary on when to start aspirin, ranging from late first trimester, before or from 12 weeks, to prior to 16 or 20 weeks.

Adverse Effects of Aspirin

The reported incidence of side effects of low-dose aspirin in the general population include indigestion, nausea, and vomiting in up to 17% of cases, gastrointestinal bleeding in 2.5% of cases, and intracranial hemorrhage in 0.4% of cases [23]. However, the population included a high proportion of elderly patients.

There is now robust evidence from RCTs that low-dose aspirin is safe to use in pregnancy. Despite concerns about potential risk of bleeding with aspirin, there was no increase in the risk of antepartum or postpartum hemorrhage or placental abruption [6, 22].

Aspirin did not increase the risk of intraventricular hemorrhage in the fetus or neonatal bleeding [6]. Daily administration of low-dose aspirin even in the third trimester did not lead to significant constriction or premature closure of the ductus arteriosus [18].

Two randomized trials that followed up babies for up to 18 months after birth did not find any differences in the development of babies whose mothers took aspirin compared to those whose did not [6].

Most aspirin studies have recruited women after 12 weeks gestation. There is reassurance that aspirin does not increase the risk of birth defects when taken from 12 weeks [6]. A review of studies on aspirin therapy *during* the first trimester showed that there is no increase overall in birth defects with aspirin use (odds ratio (OR) 1.33; 95% CI, 0.94–1.89; 8 studies). A number of case-control retrospective studies at higher risk of bias suggested an increased risk of gastroschisis (OR, 2.37; 95% CI, 1.44–3.88; 5 studies) and cleft lip/palate abnormalities (OR, 2.87; 95%CI, 2.04–4.02; 2 studies) with aspirin use. However, these findings have not been substantiated in larger prospective cohort studies or randomized trials on aspirin use in early pregnancy [24].

Unresolved Clinical Dilemmas

Identifying Women at Risk of Preeclampsia for Aspirin Therapy

Traditionally, women at increased risk of preeclampsia have been identified for aspirin therapy based on maternal characteristics such as age and body mass index, and their obstetric, medical and family history [25].

More recently, a number of biophysical and biochemical markers involved in placentation or associated with placental disease have been used to identify high-risk women. In women with preeclampsia, compared with unaffected controls, at 11–13 weeks gestation, the uterine artery PI, mean arterial pressure (MAP), maternal serum or plasma levels of sEng, inhibin-A, activin-A, pentraxin-3 (PTX3) and P-selectin are all increased, whereas serum pregnancy-associated plasma protein-A (PAPP-A), PlGF and placental protein-13 (PP13) are decreased [26]. A model for predicting preeclampsia showed that in screening for preeclampsia by maternal factors alone, at a fixed false-positive rate (FPR) of 5%, the estimated detection rates were 33% for early-onset preeclampsia and 25% for late preeclampsia. The respective detection rates in screening by a combination of maternal factors and biomarkers were 91% and 61% [26].

ASPRE, a recently published large multicentre RCT that screened for high-risk women based on maternal factors and serum PAPP-A, PlGF, MAP and uterine artery PI, for randomization to aspirin 150 mg or placebo in the first trimester found that aspirin reduces the relative risk of preterm pre-eclampsia by 62% but does not reduce term pre-eclampsia [27]. Screening in this way detected 77% of cases of preterm pre-eclampsia and 38 % of term pre-eclampsia at a FPR of of 10%. While this is an improvement on detection rates using only maternal history and characteristics (39% for preterm pre-eclampsia at a FPR of 10%) it remains debatable whether investing in such a combined screening approach is pragmatic, cost-effective or worthwhile in current clinical practice.

Optimal Gestation for Starting Aspirin Therapy

Controversy remains about whether commencing aspirin treatment earlier in pregnancy is associated with greater benefit. The IPD meta-analysis reported no difference in outcomes based on whether randomization was before or after 20 weeks gestation [22]. A more recent meta-analysis of aggregate data has suggested that commencing aspirin prior to 16 weeks is associated with greater benefits for reducing preeclampsia and its complications than commencing after 16 weeks [28]. However, due to the problems of placing women in the correct gestational age category when using aggregate data, this analysis was restricted to 1,479 women recruited before 16 weeks, compared to the IPD dataset which has data for over 9,000 women recruited before 16 weeks. The aggregate data analysis also showed a marked imbalance in the control group between the proportion of women who developed preeclampsia and were randomized before 16 weeks rather than after 16 weeks (17.9% and 8.4% respectively).

An IPD subgroup meta-analysis has recently been published that found no significant difference in the effects of antiplatelet therapy for women randomized before 16 weeks' compared with those randomized after 16 weeks for any of the prespecified outcomes of preeclampsia, death of baby, preterm birth prior to 34 weeks, and having a small-for-gestational-age baby [29]. Therefore, while aspirin may be started before 16 weeks, findings suggest that women who are first seen in clinic after 16 weeks should also be offered aspirin.

Optimizing Dose of Aspirin Therapy

The phenomenon of aspirin resistance or reduced response to aspirin is well established in cardiovascular medicine. It has been defined biochemically as a failure to inhibit platelet function, or clinically as an increased risk of cardiovascular events despite aspirin therapy at recommended doses. Reasons proposed for reduced response to aspirin include enhanced platelet turnover, genetics, drug interactions and noncompliance. A study in patients on two antiplatelet agents after coronary stenting demonstrated that the prevalence of aspirin resistance was significantly reduced by increasing the dose of aspirin [30].

Whether aspirin resistance is also seen in pregnant women at risk of preeclampsia is not clear, but it could provide an explanation for why some women develop preeclampsia despite taking aspirin. Rey et al. assessed a strategy of platelet function testing using a platelet function analyzer (PFA-100), and individualizing the dose of aspirin in women at risk of preeclampsia, with higher dose given for inadequate response to aspirin [31]. The incidence of preeclampsia was lower in women who were tested for aspirin resistance while on aspirin, compared to those who were not tested. Among the group who were tested, the incidence of preeclampsia was higher in those who needed an increase in their aspirin dose compared to those who did not (26% vs. 9%). The authors felt that the modification in dose may have been made too late in gestation to make a difference to outcome. Wojtowicz et al. also reported that women with biochemical aspirin resistance based on u11-dTXB2 concentration levels (urinary metabolite of thromboxane A2) had worse clinical outcomes, including preeclampsia, small-for-gestational-age infants and fetal distress [32].

Tests that assess aspirin resistance measure the degree to which aspirin suppresses platelet activation by measuring thromboxane metabolites, expression of platelet activation markers and the ability of platelets to aggregate. Point-of-care platelet-function tests have become available that are easier to use, and work is currently ongoing to develop platelet function reference ranges for healthy and high-risk pregnant women for such tests (personal communication). Assessing high-risk pregnant women for aspirin resistance may open avenues for more targeted and personalized aspirin therapy in the future.

Conclusions

Aspirin is now widely used for prevention of preeclampsia and its complications. It has modest but consistent benefits, and is safe. There is robust evidence that it alters the TXA2: PGI2 ratio in favor of vasodilatation and inhibition of platelet aggregation in maternal systemic circulation. Evidence for a direct effect of aspirin on placental development is lacking from studies assessing trophoblast function, uteroplacental Doppler hemodynamics and placental histology. Further research is ongoing to assess whether a more personalized approach to aspirin therapy using biomarkers and treating aspirin resistance could be more effective in reducing preeclampsia and its complications.

Key Points

- Evidence from RCTs shows that aspirin is associated with modest but consistent benefits in reducing the risk of preeclampsia and its complications. The exact mechanism through which aspirin improves pregnancy outcome is unclear.

- Aspirin inactivates the cyclooxygenase (COX) enzymes and thereby inhibits the synthesis of cyclic prostanoids. These include thromboxane A2 (TXA2), which is produced by platelets and causes platelet aggregation and vasoconstriction; and prostacyclin (PGI2), which is produced by vascular endothelial cells and induces vasodilatation and inhibition of platelet aggregation.
- Low-dose aspirin preferentially inhibits platelet COX over endothelial COX, and this differential effect has the advantage of enhancing the antithrombotic effects of aspirin by preserving endothelial PGI2 production.
- Controlled studies consistently show that low-dose aspirin selectively inhibits TXA2, and alters the TXA2:PGI2 ratio in favor of vasodilatation and inhibition of platelet aggregation in maternal systemic circulation; this also correlates with improved pregnancy outcomes.
- There is no clear evidence for a direct effect of aspirin on placental development from studies assessing trophoblast function, uteroplacental Doppler hemodynamics and placental histology.
- Research is ongoing to assess whether a more personalized approach to aspirin therapy by treating aspirin resistance with higher doses could be more effective in reducing preeclampsia and its complications.

References

1. Awtry EH, Loscalzo J. Aspirin. *Circulation* 2000;**101**:1206–18.

2. Patrono C, Collar B, Dalen J et al. Platelet-active drugs: the relationships among dose, effectiveness, and side effects. *Chest* 1998;**114**:470S–488S.

3. Farivar RS, Brecher P. Salicylate is a transcriptional inhibitor of the inducible nitric oxide synthase in cultured cardiac fibroblasts. *J Biol Chem* 1996;**271**:31585–92.

4. Bradlow BA, Chetty N. Dosage frequency for suppression of platelet function by low dose aspirin therapy. *Thromb Res* 1982;**27**:99–110.

5. Patrignani P, Filabozzi P, Patrono C. Selective cumulative inhibition of platelet thromboxane production by low-dose aspirin in healthy subjects. *J Clin Invest* 1982;**69**:1366 –72.

6. Duley L, Meher S, Hunter K, Askie L. Antiplatelet agents for preventing preeclampsia and its complications. *Cochrane Database Syst Rev* 2018 (in press).

7. Roberts JM, Hubel CA. The two stage model of preeclampsia: variations on the theme. *Placenta* 2009;**30** Suppl A:S32–7.

8. Young BC, Levine RJ, Karumanchi SA. Pathogenesis of preeclampsia. *Annu Rev Pathol* 2010;**5**:173–92.

9. Pijnenborg R, Bland JM, Robertson WB, et al. Uteroplacental arterial changes related to interstitial trophoblast migration in early human pregnancy. *Placenta* 1983;**4**: 397–413.

10. Viinikka L, Hartikainen-Sorri AL, Lumme R, et al. Low dose aspirin in hypertensive pregnant women: effect on pregnancy outcome and prostacyclin thromboxane balance in mother and newborn. *Br J Obstet Gynaecol* 1993;**100**: 809–15.

11. Schiff E, Peleg E, Goldenberg M, et al. The use of aspirin to prevent pregnancy induced hypertension and lower the ratio of thromboxane A2 to prostacyclin in relatively high risk pregnancies. *New Engl J Med* 1989;**321**: 351–6.

12. Benigni A, Gregorini G, Frusca T, et al. Effect of low-dose aspirin on fetal and maternal generation of thromboxane by platelets in women at risk for pregnancy induced hypertension. *New Engl J Med* 1989;**321**:357–62.

13. Johnson RD, Polakoski K, Everson WV, et al. Aspirin induces increased expression

of both prostaglandin H synthase-1 and prostaglandin H synthase-2 in cultured human placental trophoblast. *Am J Obstet Gynecol* 1997;**177**(1):78–85.

14. Han CS, Mulla MJ, Brosens JJ, et al. Aspirin and heparin effect on basal and antiphospholipid antibody modulation of trophoblast function. *Obstet Gynecol* 2011;**118**(5):1021–8.

15. Bose P, Black S, Kadyrov M, et al. Heparin and aspirin attenuate placental apoptosis in vitro: implications for early pregnancy failure. *Am J Obstet Gynecol* 2005;**192**(1):23–30.

16. Owen J, Maher JE, Hauth JC, et al. The effect of low-dose aspirin on umbilical artery Doppler measurements. *Am J Obstet Gynecol* 1993;**169**(4):907–11.

17. Bar J, Hod M, Pardo J, et al. Effect on fetal circulation of low-dose aspirin for prevention and treatment of pre-eclampsia and intrauterine growth restriction: Doppler flow study. *Ultrasound Obstet Gynecol* 1997;**9**(4):262–5.

18. Grab D, Paulus WE, Erdmann M, et al. Effects of low-dose aspirin on uterine and fetal blood flow during pregnancy: results of a randomized, placebo-controlled, double-blind trial. *Ultrasound Obstet Gynecol.* 2000;**15**(1):19–27.

19. Haapsamo M, Martikainen H, Räsänen J. Low-dose aspirin reduces uteroplacental vascular impedance in early and mid gestation in IVF and ICSI patients: a randomized, placebo-controlled double-blind study. *Ultrasound Obstet Gynecol* 2008;**32**(5):687–93

20. Cusick W, Salafia CM, Ernst L, et al. Low-dose aspirin therapy and placental pathology in women with poor prior pregnancy outcomes. *Am J Reprod Immunol* 1995;**34**(3):141–7.

21. Tarim E, Bal N, Kilicdag E, et al. Effects of aspirin on placenta and perinatal outcomes in patients with poor obstetric history. *Arch Gynecol Obstet* 2006;**274**:209–14.

22. Askie LM, Duley L, Henderson-Smart DJ, et al. Antiplatelet agents for prevention of pre-eclampsia: a meta-analysis of individual patient data. *Lancet* 2007;**369**:1791–8.

23. Baron JA, Senn S, Voelker M, et al. Gastrointestinal adverse effects of short-term aspirin use: a meta-analysis of published randomized controlled trials. *Drugs R D* 2013;**13**:9–16.

24. Kozer E, Nifkar S, Costei A, et al. Aspirin consumption during the first trimester of pregnancy and congenital abnormalities: a meta-analysis. *Am J Obstet Gynaecol* 2002;**187**:1623–30.

25. Duckitt K, Harrington D. Risk factors for pre-eclampsia at antenatal booking: systematic review of controlled studies. *BMJ* 2005;**330**(7491):565.

26. Akolekar R, Syngelaki A, Poon L, et al. Competing risks model in early screening for preeclampsia by biophysical and biochemical markers. *Fetal Diagnosis and Therapy* 2013;**33**(1):8–15.

27. Rolnik DL, Wright D, Poon LC, O'Gorman N, Syngelaki A, de Paco Matallana C, Akolekar R, Cicero S, Janga D, Singh M, Molina FS, Persico N, Jani JC, Plasencia W, Papaioannou G, Tenenbaum-Gavish K, Meiri H, Gizurarson S, Maclagan K, Nicolaides KH. Aspirin versus Placebo in Pregnancies at High Risk for Preterm Preeclampsia. *N Engl J Med* 2017 Aug 17;**377**(7):613–22.

28. Roberge, S, Nicolaides, K, Demers, S, et al. Prevention of perinatal death and adverse perinatal outcome using low-dose aspirin: a meta-analysis. *Ultrasound Obstet Gynecol* 2013;**41**(5):491–9.

29. Meher S, Duley L, Hunter K et al. Antiplatelet therapy before or after 16 weeks' gestation for preventing preeclampsia: an individual participant data meta-analysis. *Am J Obstet Gynecol* 2017;**216**(2):121–8.

30. Neubauer H, Kaiser AF, Endres HG, et al. Tailored antiplatelet therapy can overcome clopidogrel and aspirin resistance–the BOchum CLopidogrel and Aspirin Plan (BOCLA-Plan) to improve antiplatelet therapy. *BMC Med* 2011;**9**:3.

31. Rey E, Rivard G-E. Is testing for aspirin response worthwhile in high-risk pregnancy? *Eur J Obstet, Gynecol Reprode Biol* 2011;**157**(1):38–42.

32. Wojtowicz A, Undas A, Huras H, et al. Aspirin resistance may be associated with adverse pregnancy outcomes. *Neuro Endocrinol Lett* 2011;**32**(3):334–9.

Vascular Endothelial Growth Factor Gene Therapy in the Management of Cardiovascular Problems in Pregnancy

Yuval Ginsberg and Anna David

Summary

Impaired angiogenesis of the uteroplacental circulation is considered to be one of the leading causes of common obstetric complications such as preeclampsia and fetal growth restriction (FGR). Currently, our therapeutic possibilities to improve compromised uteroplacental angiogenesis and to increase the blood flow to the uterus are limited. As research continues to reveal the pathophysiological processes involved in the development of FGR, novel treatments become apparent. Vascular endothelial growth factor (VEGF) is a vascular endothelial cell-specific mitogen which has a pivotal role in uteroplacental vascular development in pregnancy. The proangiogenic role of VEGF has attracted clinical interest for its potential to improve the blood supply to ischemic or damaged tissues. Although not yet fully integrated into the obstetrical field, preclinical studies have demonstrated the ability of VEGF gene therapy, administered to the maternal uterine arteries, to improve fetal growth in an animal model of FGR. In this chapter we will describe the importance of angiogenesis for normal development of the pregnancy. We will review the current use of VEGF and discuss the novel possibility to use maternal VEGF gene therapy for pregnancies complicated with FGR.

Introduction

The development of a well-perfused placental vascular bed is vital for fetal growth and normal placental function. Vascular endothelial growth factor (VEGF) is a key regulator of blood vessel development and blood flow in a wide range of vascular beds, including the coronary, pulmonary and cerebrovascular circulations. In pregnancy it is present from conception and implantation of the conceptus. Abnormal VEGF biology is implicated in the great obstetric syndromes such as preeclampsia and fetal growth restriction (FGR), which are essentially disorders of the cardiovascular system.

VEGF concentration can be manipulated locally or systemically using gene therapy to express the protein and cause a therapeutic effect. Until recently, this "therapeutic angiogenesis" was only explored in traditional cardiovascular beds such as the cerebrovascular systems. Emerging data from animal studies suggests that manipulating VEGF expression locally in the uteroplacental circulation may be of benefit in placental insufficiency and FGR.

This chapter will discuss the link between VEGF and adverse pregnancy outcomes, such as preeclampsia and FGR. It will consider the practicalities of how VEGF gene therapy could be used to treat pregnancies complicated by defective angiogenesis and insufficient placental vascularization. Finally, it will review the current evidence regarding VEGF gene therapy.

Vasculogenesis and Angiogenesis – Normal Physiology

Normal fetal growth is a complex process requiring adequate vascularization in order to supply the fetus with oxygen and nutrients. The establishment and development of a fully functional fetoplacental unit occur through three different vascular processes – vasculogenesis, pseudovasculogenesis and angiogenesis [1]. While vasculogenesis is related to de novo formation of blood vessels from angioblast precursor cells and is responsible for the creation of the primary vascular plexus in the embryo and the placenta, angiogenesis involves neovascularization that arises from existing vessels to form, through cell differentiation, cord formation and tubulogenesis, an adult circulatory system. Both angiogenesis and vasculogenesis are essential for normal placentation and fetal growth. Additionally, in order to increase the blood flow and to enable adequate perfusion of the placental intervillous space, remodeling of the maternal blood vessels is required. During the mid- to late first trimester, in a process termed pseudovasculogenesis [1], cytotrophoblast cells invade the uterine spiral artery walls, destroying the media and transforming the vessels from narrow, high-resistance to flow into wide vessels with low resistance. As described by Konje et al. [2], although this physiological remodeling enables the increase of blood flow through the uterine arteries (uterine artery volume blood flow (UAVBF)), in pregnancies complicated by FGR the total quantified volume is significantly reduced (Figure 17.1), which may imply for uteroplacental insufficiency.

Vascular Endothelial Growth Factor and Its Importance in the Development of a Normal Placental Vascular Bed

The formation of a vascular system involves a complex interaction of various regulatory factors including oxygen, basic fibroblast growth factor (bFGF), epidermal growth factor (EGF), angiopoietins-1 and -2 (Ang-1 and Ang-2) and the VEGF family. The VEGF family is

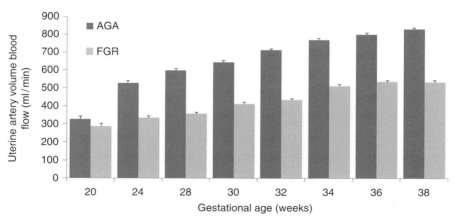

Figure 17.1 Uterine artery volume blood flow (UAVBF) measured in women with normal pregnancy and those with placental insufficiency. UAVBF was measured by color power angiography in 32 women with abnormal uterine artery Doppler velocimetry at 20 and 24 weeks of gestation and with risk factors for FGR and 25 women with normal uterine artery Doppler velocimetry and no risk factors for FGR (AGA group) between 20 and 38 weeks of gestation (Data was taken from Konje et al[2]).

the most studied family of growth factors known to regulate the processes of vasculogenesis and angiogenesis. Since its discovery in guinea pigs, hamsters, and mice by Senger et al. in 1983 [36], VEGF has emerged as the single-most important regulator of blood vessel formation. The VEGF family consists of seven structurally related proteins designated VEGF-A to VEGF-F, and Placental Growth Factor (PlGF), which shares 53% homology with VEGF [3–4]. VEGF-A, also commonly referred to as simply 'VEGF', consists of five splice variants, which are derived from eight exons, the first four of which are present in all of the splice variants. These variants differ in the presence or absence of exons 6 and 7. The larger VEGF molecule contains 189 amino acids (VEGF 189) and comprises all the C-terminal exons (5, 6, 7 and 8). VEGF 165 contains exons 5, 6 and 8. VEGF 121 lacks both exons 6 and 7, whereas VEGF 145 lacks only exon 7. The biological functions of the VEGFs are mediated by a family of cognate protein tyrosine kinase receptors (VEGFRs) [3–4]. VEGF-A binds to VEGFR2 (also called KDR/Flk-1) and VEGFR1 (Flt-1). Flt-1 and KDR have been identified on endothelial cell receptors and are found to share a 44% amino acid homology. VEGF-C and VEGF-D bind VEGFR3 (Flt4) regulating lymphangiogenesis. PlGF and VEGF-B bind only to VEGFR1, and VEGF-E binds only to VEGFR2. In addition, certain VEGF family isoforms bind to non-tyrosine kinase receptors called neuropilins (NRPs) [5].

VEGF During Normal Pregnancy

VEGFs are detectable from the very early stages of pregnancy, with mRNA detectable in the unfertilized oocyte and VEGF protein detected from the 3-cell embryo stage. Supplementation of VEGF-A to early stage embryos improves blastocyst formation, pre-implantation development and embryo outgrowth in vitro [6–7], which implies the importance of VEGF for implantation and early development processes.

VEGFs are also critically required for uteroplacental vascular formation and development. The initial period of vasculogenesis is followed by a phase of branching angiogenesis (the formation of new vessels by sprouting) during which the hemangioblastic cords develop into a richly branched capillary bed [8]. In vitro experiments on the chorioallantoic membrane of the chick have shown that the binding of VEGF-A to Flt-1 and to KDR stimulate branching angiogenesis. Targeted inactivation of a single VEGF allele [9] or disruption of genes encoding for VEGF receptors leads to embryonic death due to abnormal blood vessel formation during embryogenesis.

VEGF and Adverse Pregnancy Outcome

The shift in the normal balance of angiogenic and antiangiogenic factors toward an antiangiogenic state and elevated maternal plasma concentration of antiangiogenic factors has been described in patients with FGR, small-for-gestational-age (SGA) babies, pre-eclampsia and spontaneous preterm birth (PTB) [9–10]. Preeclamptic women and pregnancies affected by FGR were shown to have lower levels of free VEGF and PlGF as well as higher levels of both sFLT-1 and sVEGFR-1 compared with uncomplicated pregnancies. The severity of these conditions may even be determined by the magnitude of the angiogenic imbalance, its timing and the maternal susceptibility. Correcting this angiogenic imbalance and improving the blood supply to the placental-fetal circulation might be a potential strategy for treating these severe obstetric complications.

Current Medical Use of VEGF and Anti-VEGF

Since abnormal angiogenesis is a common pathological pathway, angiogenesis itself might be manipulated for clinical applications using VEGF or its inhibitors. In cases of excessive angiogenesis, as in cancer or chorioretinal vascular diseases, angiogenic inhibitors can be used to attenuate angiogenesis. Angiogenesis is a critical step in cancer progression. Since tumors are unable to grow without a proper blood supply (in the form of a rich network of vessels that provides a conduit for tumor dissemination and metastasis), VEGF is important to cancer pathology. Currently, antiangiogenic therapy is used with proven benefit for multiple types of cancer: renal-cell carcinoma, hepatocellular carcinoma, gastric cancer, gliomas and more [11].

Similarly, chorioretinal vascular diseases, such as age-related macular degeneration [AMD], diabetic retinopathy, retinal vein occlusions and retinopathy of prematurity, are caused by either neovascularization or macular edema, which are both an imbalance of VEGF. Currently, intravitreal injections of anti-VEGF are the preferred treatment of exudative AMD and are gaining popularity as treatment for age-related macular degeneration macular edema caused by diabetic retinopathy [12].

Therapeutic Angiogenesis in Cardiovascular Disease

Drugs which accelerate angiogenesis and improve the pre-existing microvascular network were promoted as a novel treatment for complications of ischemic heart disease or diseases stemming from deficient angiogenesis, such as peripheral artery disease or wound healing. Vectors have been used to deliver VEGF to cells via gene therapy, causing expression of transgenic VEGF protein.

Peripheral artery disease caused by impaired function of the endothelium and inhibition of neovascularization results in critical limb ischemia, tissue damage, ulceration and pain. Preclinical and first-in-man studies using VEGF were promising [13] to reduce the ischemia and to increase the blood flow to the affected limbs by promoting neovascularization and expanding the collateral circulation. The data obtained from large clinical trials, however, is controversial, possibly due to variations in patient selection criteria and assessment methods. Endothelial cell damage and tissue fibrosis in the diseased vessels may also limit angiogenesis, and combined approaches may be required [14].

In ischemic heart disease, therapeutic angiogenesis aims to induce the growth of coronary artery collateral vessels in order to enhance blood flow to the chronically ischemic myocardium and to support the repair and regeneration of muscle tissue. Promising results in large animals and early clinical trials [15] led to the development of randomized controlled trials (RCTs) [16] in which recombinant proteins, plasmid DNA or adenoviral vectors expressing the angiogenic factors were used for treatment of chronic MI patient. The potential of this new treatment paradigm has not been realized yet in late-stage clinical trials, mainly due to difficulties identifying the optimum target within the heart and understanding the required clinical endpoints [17].

VEGF Gene Therapy for Fetal Growth Restriction

As yet, there is no treatment that increases uterine artery perfusion and fetal growth in utero, although promising therapeutics are under investigation [18]. The only current management for severe early-onset FGR is to deliver the fetus before death or irreversible organ damage occurs, but the need for early delivery adds additional risks due to prematurity. Neonatal survival studies suggest that even a modest increase in birthweight and gestational age at the time of delivery are associated with significant improvement in mortality and morbidity rates [19]. A promising new therapy for FGR that may delay the need for extreme preterm birth is the manipulation of VEGF expression. In order to avoid the potential systemic complications of VEGF and given that the protein has a short half-life (t1/2 approximately 90 minutes) it is probably optimal to express VEGF locally in the maternal uterine arteries, bilaterally.

Choice of Vector

As pregnancy is of a finite duration, the ideal vector to deliver gene therapy for the treatment of FGR should produce a short-term rise in VEGF expression in maternal tissues, at the maternal side of the placenta, or possibly within the placenta itself, for the length of gestation remaining, of approximately 3 months. Adenoviral vectors (Ad) efficiently transduce a wide range of cells, producing short-term protein expression, and are the most commonly used vectors in clinical trials of gene therapy, particularly those of therapeutic angiogenesis. There are concerns that longer-term expression of VEGF, as might be achieved using adeno-associated viral vectors and integrating vectors such as lentivirus or retrovirus, might result in vascular tumors. A summary of viral vectors for prenatal therapy is provided here [20].

Maternal VEGF Gene Therapy for FGR in Preclinical Studies

The impact of Ad.VEGF on uterine blood flow (UBF) was first examined at midgestation in uncompromised sheep pregnancies using the VEGF-A_{165} isoform. UBF was quantified at baseline and at 4–7 days following direct uterine artery (UtA) injection of Ad.VEGF-A_{165} at laparotomy. The artery was digitally occluded during vector injection and afterwards for up to 5 minutes total time to maximize transfection of the downstream endothelium [21]. By 4–7 days, volume blood flow in the UtA was increased threefold when compared to a contralateral UtA injection of a nonvasoactive control adenoviral vector endcoding bacterial ß-galactosidase (Ad.LacZ; Figure 17.2).

Ad.VEGF-A_{165} transduced vessels demonstrated an enhanced contractile response to phenylephrine and increased relaxation response to bradykinin when examined in an organ bath, as well as upregulation of endothelial nitric oxide synthase (eNOS) and VEGFR-2 [22]. Further experiments using the preprocessed short-form of Ad.VEGF-D (Ad.VEGF-D$^{\Delta N \Delta C}$) demonstrated similar effects on vasoreactivity, upregulation of phosphorylated eNOS and enhanced UtA endothelial cell proliferation [22].

In a second study, and over a longer time period, the effects of Ad.VEGF-A_{165} on UBF were examined using indwelling ultrasonic flow probes. At 28 days post-injection, vessels treated with Ad.VEGF-A_{165} exhibited a 36.5% increase in UBF compared to just 20.1% in vessels treated with Ad.LacZ [23], which represents a virtual doubling of the normal gestational increase in UBF. A similar trend was observed long-term after injection of Ad.VEGF-D$^{\Delta N \Delta C}$ [22]. In both studies, reduced phenylephrine-induced vasoconstriction continued to be observed but vasorelaxation and VEGFR-2 expression were no longer differed between Ad.VEGF and Ad.LacZ groups. Nevertheless, at 30–45 days following treatment there was evidence of neovascularization within the perivascular adventitia despite a complete lack of ongoing transgenic VEGF expression, which implies that the vasoactive

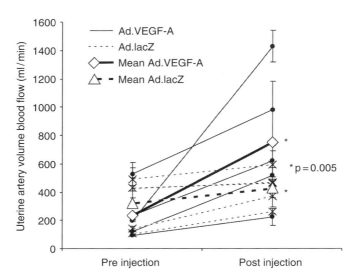

Figure 17.2 Changes in uterine artery volume blood flow as measured by Doppler ultrasound, 4–7 days after injection of Ad.VEGF-A$_{165}$ or Ad.LacZ (a nonvasoactive control vector) in 5 normal midgestation pregnant sheep (David AL et al Gene Ther. 2008 Oct;15(19):1344–50)

effects of Ad.VEGF persist beyond the period of transgene expression, probably via mechanisms of angiogenesis.

Using a well-established ovine model of FGR – the overnourished adolescent ewe – it was determined whether Ad.VEGF-mediated changes in UBF might impact fetal growth. High nutritional intake in adolescent dams promotes maternal tissue growth at the expense of the pregnancy, leading to marked FGR (= fetal weight >2SD below the mean birth weight of genetically matched contemporaneous controls fed an optimum diet) in approximately half of cases [24], and the model replicates many of the key features of uteroplacental FGR in the human.

Serial ultrasonographic measurements of the fetal abdominal circumference (AC), which is the most accurate single marker of fetal growth in humans and sheep [25-26] between mid- and late gestation, were used to monitor fetal growth.

Following bilateral UtA injections of Ad.VEGF-A$_{165}$ in midgestation, AC measurements were significantly increased by ≈20% when examined at three and four weeks following treatment compared to animals with equivalent baseline measurements receiving control treatments (Ad.LacZ or saline only) [27]. There was evidence of an attenuated brain sparing effect (catch up of abdominal to head growth). In pregnancies sacrificed at 0.9 gestation (term = 145 days), significantly fewer fetuses demonstrated marked FGR (fetal weight >2SD below control mean) in Ad.VEGF-A$_{165}$ compared with Ad.LacZ/saline groups (5/18 versus 17/10, respectively, p=0.033, Figure 17.3b). Similar findings were demonstrated in a second cohort, culminating in spontaneous birth, with no evidence of adverse events during postnatal development [28].

Ad.VEGF-A$_{165}$-treated lambs continued to grow faster in absolute terms throughout the first 12 weeks of life in the absence of any change in fractional growth velocity or markers of adiposity. In both studies there was evidence of increased placental function (g fetus/lamb

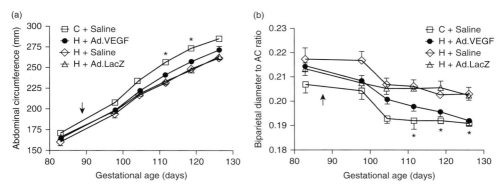

Figure 17.3 Serial ultrasound measurements of: (a) fetal abdominal circumference (AC); and (b) biparietal diameter to AC ratio, following midpregnancy uterine artery injection of Ad.VEGFA$_{165}$, Ad.LacZ or Saline in 57 singleton-bearing overnourished adolescent ewes. Control dams were fed ad lib and did not undergo surgery. AC was significantly higher and biparietal diameter to AC ratio significantly lower in control sheep at days 16, 23, 30 and 37 post-injection, * $p<0.05$. At time points A, B and C there were significant differences between measurements from Ad.VEGF-A$_{165}$ treated fetuses and those receiving Ad.LacZ and Saline. AC, abdominal circumference; Ad, adenovirus; LacZ, b-galactosidase; VEGF, vascular endothelial growth factor (Carr DJ and David AL et al Hum Gene Ther. 2014 Apr;25(4):375–84)

per g placenta), and in late gestation there was increased VEGFR-1 and VEGFR-2 mRNA expression localized to the maternal placental compartment (caruncle) [28].

Complementary experiments were performed in another model of FGR induced by periconceptual nutrient deprivation of Dunkin Hartley guinea pigs [29]. Placentation in this species more closely mimics the human, being hemochorial in nature, and shares a similar process of trophoblast cell invasion and proliferation [30]. Administration of Ad.VEGF-A165 in midgestation FGR guinea pig pregnancy results in an increased pup weight at term with no evidence of gene transfer to the fetus or adverse events [31].

Delivery Method

In the preclinical studies of Ad.VEGF, local delivery to the uterine arteries has been achieved either at laparotomy by direct injection combined with proximal occlusion of the vessel or by application of a thermolabile Pluronic gel to the outside of the vessel wall. This is a technique developed for transduction of vascular beds [32] which achieves high levels of local gene transfer to the guinea pig uterine vasculature when compared to other direct injection methods [33]. In clinical practice direct uterine artery injection could be achieved using a balloon catheter, introduced into each uterine artery in turn via x-ray guided interventional radiology. This technique has been used for over 30 years to treat fibroids and to manage postpartum hemorrhage. It is now being used increasingly during pregnancy, with catheters and deflated balloons placed into the uterine arteries before Cesarean section when severe hemorrhage is anticipated due to, for example, placenta previa [34].

Ethics and Safety of Gene Therapy in Pregnancy

The most important aspect regarding the ethics of a medical intervention is the balance of risks and benefits. The risks of maternal gene therapy are not well characterized, and the efficacy in pregnant women remains to be determined. The ethical and social acceptability of maternal gene therapy for FGR has been explored in a qualitative study with stakeholder groups and women with experience of the condition, using semistructured interviews carried out in four European countries: Germany, Spain, Sweden and the UK [35]. Overall, stakeholders and women/couples viewed the proposed trial in positive terms, and maternal gene therapy to treat severe early-onset FGR appears to be ethically and socially acceptable.

Conclusion

Impaired angiogenesis is the underlying etiology of common severe obstetric complications, such as FGR and preeclampsia. Currently, there are no novel treatments to improve compromised angiogenesis or to improve the blood flow to the uterus as pregnancy progresses. As research continues to uncover the pathophysiological processes involved in the development of FGR, new therapeutic possibilities become apparent. VEGF gene therapy, although not yet fully integrated into the clinic, is a novel solution.

Key Points

- Impaired angiogenesis is the underlying etiology of common severe obstetric complications, such as FGR and preeclampsia.
- Currently, there are no treatment options to improve compromised angiogenesis or to improve the blood flow to the uterus as pregnancy progresses.
- Preclinical studies have demonstrated the ability of VEGF gene therapy, administered to the maternal uterine arteries, to improve fetal growth in an animal model of FGR.

References

1. Charnock-Jones DS, Kaufmann P, Mayhew TM. Aspects of human fetoplacental vasculogenesis and angiogenesis. I. Molecular regulation. Placenta 2004;25:103–13.

2. Konje JC, Howarth ES, Kaufmann P, Taylor DJ. Longitudinal quantification of uterine artery blood volume flow changes during gestation in pregnancies complicated by intrauterine growth restriction. BJOG. 2003;110(3):301–5.

3. Ferrara N, Gerber HP, Le Couter J. The biology of VEGF and its receptors. Nat Med 2003;9:669–76.

4. Holmes DI, Zachary I. The vascular endothelial growth factor (VEGF) family: angiogenic factors in health and disease. Genome Biol. 2005;6:209.

5. Zachary I. Neuropilins: role in signalling, angiogenesis and disease. Chem Immunol Allergy. 2014;99: 37–70.

6. Binder NK, Evans J, Gardner DK, Salamonsen LA, Hannan NJ. Endometrial signals improve embryo outcome: functional role of vascular endothelial growth factor isoforms on embryo development and implantation in mice. Hum Reprod. 2014;29(10):2278–86.

7. Carmeliet P, Ferreira V, Breier G, et al. Abnormal blood vessel development and lethality in embryos lacking a single VEGF allele. Nature 1996;380:435–9.

8. Kaufmann P, Mayhew TM, Charnock-Jones DS. Aspects of human fetoplacental vasculogenesis and angiogenesis. II. Changes during normal pregnancy. Placenta. 2004;25(2–3):114–26.

9. Andraweera PH, Dekker GA, Roberts CT. The vascular endothelial growth factor family in adverse pregnancy outcomes. *Hum Reprod Update*. 2012;**18**(4):436–57.

10. Romero, R, Nien JK, Espinoza J, et al. A longitudinal study of angiogenic (placental growth factor) and anti-angiogenic (soluble endoglin and soluble vascular endothelial growth factor receptor-1) factors in normal pregnancy and patients destined to develop preeclampsia and deliver a small for gestational age neonate. *J. Matern. Fetal Neonatal Med*. 2008;**21**:9–23.

11. Jain RK. Antiangiogenesis strategies revisited: from starving tumors to alleviating hypoxia. *Cancer Cell*. 2014;**26**(5):605–22.

12. Martin DF, Maguire MG. Treatment choice for diabetic macular edema. *N Engl J Med*. 2015 Mar 26;**372**(13):1260–1.

13. Baumgartner I, Pieczek A, Manor O, et al. Constitutive expression of phVEGF165 after intramuscular gene transfer promotes collateral vessel development in patients with critical limb ischemia. *Circulation*. 1998;**97**(12):1114–23.

14. Sanada F, Taniyama Y, Kanbara Y, et al. Gene therapy in peripheral artery disease. *Expert Opin Biol Ther* 2015;**15**(3):381–90.

15. Banai S, Shweiki D, Pinson A, et al. Upregulation of vascular endothelial growth factor expression induced by myocardial ischaemia: implications for coronary angiogenesis. *Cardiovasc Res* 1994;**28**:1176–9.

16. Henry TD, Annex BH, McKendall GR, et al. VIVA Investigators The VIVA trial: vascular endothelial growth factor in ischemia for vascular angiogenesis. *Circulation* 2003;**107**:1359–65

17. Rubanyi GM. Identifying and overcoming obstacles in angiogenic gene therapy for myocardial ischemia. *J Cardiovasc Pharmacol* 2014;**64** (2):109–19.

18. Spencer RN, Carr DJ, David AL. Treatment of poor placentation and the prevention of associated adverse outcomes – what does the future hold? *Prenat Diagn*, 2014;**34**:677–84.

19. Baschat AA, Cosmi E, Bilardo CM, et al. Predictors of neonatal outcome in early-onset placental dysfunction. *Obstet Gynecol*. 2007;**109**(2 Pt 1):253–61.

20. Spencer R, Carr DJ, David A. Gene therapy for obstetric conditions. *Fetal Matern Med Rev*, 2015;**25**(3–4):147–77.

21. David AL, Torondel B, Zachary I, et al. Local delivery of VEGF adenovirus to the uterine artery increases vasorelaxation and uterine blood flow in the pregnant sheep. *Gene Ther* 2008;**15**:1344–50.

22. Mehta V, Abi-Nader KN, Shangaris P, et al. Local over-expression of VEGF-D$^{\Delta N\Delta C}$ in the uterine arteries of pregnant sheep results in long-term changes in uterine artery contractility and angiogenesis. *PLoS One*, 2014;**99**.(6): e100021

23. Mehta V, Abi-Nader K, Peebles D, et al. Long-term increase in uterine blood flow is achieved by local overexpression of VEGF-A(165) in the uterine arteries of pregnant sheep. *Gene Ther* 2011; September: 86–96.

24. Wallace JM, Luther JS, Milne JS, et al. Nutritional modulation of adolescent pregnancy outcome – a review. *Placenta*. 2006; **27** Suppl A: S61–8.

25. Carr DJ, Aitken RP, Milne JS, David AL, Wallace JM. Ultrasonographic assessment of growth and estimation of birthweight in late gestation fetal sheep. *Ultrasound Med Biol*. 2011; **37**(10):1588–95.

26. Smith GC, Smith MF, McNay MB, Fleming JE. The relation between fetal abdominal circumference and birthweight: findings in 3512 pregnancies. *BJOG*. 1997; **104**(2):186–90.

27. Carr DJ, Wallace JM, Aitken RP, et al. Uteroplacental adenovirus vascular endothelial growth factor gene therapy increases fetal growth velocity in growth-restricted sheep pregnancies. *Hum. Gene Ther* 2014;**25**:375–84.

28. Carr DJ, Wallace JM, Aitken R, et al. Peri- and postnatal effects of prenatal adenoviral VEGF gene therapy in growth-restricted sheep. *Biol. Reprod* 2016;**9**: 142.

29. Swanson AM, Mehta V, Ofir K, et al. The use of ultrasound to assess fetal growth in a guinea pig model of fetal growth restriction. *Lab. Anim.* Apr 26. pii: 0023677216637506

30. Carter AM. Animal models of human placentation–a review. *Placenta.* 2007;**28** Suppl A:S41–7.

31. Swanson A, Rossi C, Ofir K, et al. Maternal uterine artery gene therapy with Ad. VEGF-A165 increases weight at term in a guinea pig model of fetal growth restriction. *Hum Gene Ther* 2015;**26**:A14.

32. Feldman LJ, Pastore CJ, Aubailly N., et al. Improved efficiency of arterial gene transfer by use of poloxamer 407 as a vehicle for adenoviral vectors. *Gene Ther* 1997;**4**(3):189–98.

33. Pelage JP, Dref O, Le Mateo J, et al. Life-threatening primary postpartum hemorrhage: treatment with emergency selective arterial embolization. *Radiology* 1998;**208**: 359–62.

34. Angstmann T, Gard G, Harrington T, Ward E, Thomson A, Giles W. Surgical management of placenta accreta: a cohort series and suggested approach. *Am J Obstet Gynecol* 2010;**202**(1):38.e1–9.

35. Sheppard MK, David AL, Spencer R, Ashcroft R. Consortium E, Ethics and ethical evaluation of a proposed clinical trial with maternal uterine artery vascular endothelial growth factor gene therapy to treat severe early onset fetal growth restriction in pregnant. *Hum. Gene Ther* 2014;**25**:A98.

36. Senger DR, Asch BB, Smith BD, Perruzzi CA, Dvorak HF. A secreted phosphoprotein marker for neoplastic transformation of both epithelial and fibroblastic cells. *Nature.* 1983 Apr 21;**302** (5910):714–5.

Chapter 18

Nitric Oxide Donors in Preeclampsia

Thomas Everett, Taminrit Johal and Christoph Lees

Summary

Despite the fact that the mechanisms underlying the disease process are more and more understood, preeclampsia remains a significant cause of maternal and neonatal morbidity and mortality worldwide. The mainstay of current therapies is targeted at treatment of hypertension and seizure control rather than aiming to normalize the underlying endothelial function. While targeting the root cause of preeclampsia should be the ultimate goal for therapy and prevention, however, these processes remain elusive and poorly understood. Until such time as this is feasible, NO donors, or alteration of the NO pathways, either by precursor supplementation (e.g. L-arginine) or through augmentation of downstream effects (e.g. sildenafil), are logical candidates for the treatment of preeclampsia.

This chapter summarizes the current evidence underlining the relevance of exploring NO donors in prevention and treatment of preeclampsia.

Background

Endothelial dysfunction is evident in preeclampsia [1]. The underlying pathological processes of preeclampsia are hypothesized to occur in two stages [2]. Abnormal placentation is suggested to be the initiating event resulting in reduced placental perfusion, in turn leading to increased oxidative stress, which, in combination with a maternal predisposition, results in endothelial dysfunction; this, in turn, is thought to play a major role in the maternal manifestations of preeclampsia, including hypertension, platelet activation, proteinuria and edema. While endothelial dysfunction in preeclampsia results from changes in a number of signaling pathways and homeostatic mechanisms, which remain to be fully elucidated, impaired nitric oxide bioavailability underlies the resultant pathophysiology. NO, originally identified as the endothelium-derived relaxing factor, is the predominant vasodilatory substance produced by the endothelium in response to mechanical and chemical stimuli. It is an autocrine and paracrine signaling molecule that is synthesized from L-arginine by a family of calcium–calmodulin-dependent enzymes called nitric oxide synthetases (NOS), the most important one of which, in this context, is endothelial NOS(eNOS). NO causes relaxation of vascular smooth muscle cells by activating soluble guanylate cyclase (sGC), which in turn causes an increase in intracellular cyclical guanosine-3',5' monophosphate (cGMP) and activation of cGMP-dependent protein kinases.

Asymmetric dimethylarginine (ADMA) is an endogenous eNOS inhibitor. Levels of ADMA are higher in women at high risk of preeclampsia as determined by abnormal uterine artery Doppler waveforms [3]. And, in those women who go on to develop preeclampsia, there is an inverse correlation of ADMA to flow-mediated dilatation

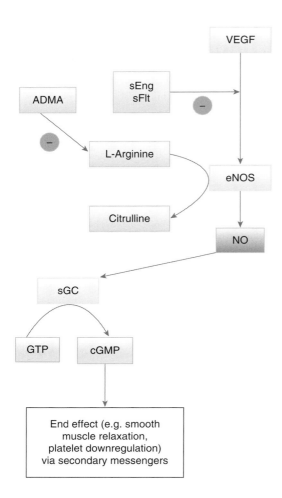

Figure 18.1 Schematic diagram of the effect of NO and soluble factors related to preeclampsia. (A black and white version of this figure will appear in some formats. For the color version, please refer to the plate section.)

(FMD), suggesting that increased ADMA may reduce NO bioavailability and thus contribute to the development of preeclampsia. Increased concentrations of ADMA have also been found in women who go on to develop preeclampsia later in pregnancy [4].

Circulating soluble factors are to be implicated in the endothelial dysfunction of preeclampsia. It is established that circulating levels of VEGF and PlGF are decreased in women with preeclampsia and, indeed, decreased levels are seen prior to the clinical onset of disease [5–7]. Similarly, increased levels of sFlt-1, a soluble receptor for VEGF and PlGF, are found prior to and during the acute phase of preeclampsia. More recently, sEng, a soluble placenta-derived form of a co-receptor for TGFβ-1 and TGFβ-3, has been shown to be raised in and contribute to the pathogenesis of preeclampsia [8].

VEGF and PlGF are closely related angiogenic peptides. On endothelial cells, they act primarily through the VEGF receptors-1 and 2, resulting in phosphorylation and a signal transduction cascade, which ultimately upregulates eNOS expression and NO production [9–11]. The increased circulating levels of sFlt-1 bind, thus neutralizing the free circulating

VEGF and PlGF and in doing so reduce stimulation of NO production in the endothelial cells, contributing to the hypertension and proteinuria of preeclampsia [12, 13]. TGFβ-1 increases eNOS expression in human endothelial cells [14], and endoglin acts as part of the receptor complex to potentiate the effect of TGFβ-1 and increase eNOS expression in endothelial cells [15]. sEng impairs the binding of TGFβ-1 to its receptors and thus reduces the downstream signaling and activation of eNOS [8]. Further support for the effects of sFlt-1 and sEng on endothelial dysfunction is in the inverse relationship between nitric oxide formation and levels of these factors in preeclampsia [16]. It is also suggested the effects of sFlt-1 and sEng on endothelial dysfunction may be synergistic in severe preeclampsia.

Nitric Oxide Donors

Many of the maternal features of preeclampsia, particularly hypertension and disruption of platelet function, are largely manifestations of endothelial dysfunction and disruption of NO bioavailability. While not treating the primary cause, which is rooted in the maternal-placental function and is yet to be fully understood, supplementation with exogenous NO donors is an apparently logical solution to the treatment of the resulting systemic manifestations. The use of NO donors in cardiovascular diseases is well established, and evidence for their role in the prevention and treatment of preeclampsia is emerging. The classes of NO donors that have been studied in the context of preeclampsia include organic nitrates and S-nitrosothiols.

Organic Nitrates

Organic nitrates have been used as vascular smooth muscle relaxants for over a hundred years. The organic nitrates that have been studied in the context of preeclampsia include glyceryl trinitrate (GTN) or nitroglycerine and isosorbide dinitrate (ISDN).

Glyceryl trinitrate

GTN is a widely used organic nitrate in clinical practice, particularly for the treatment of angina pectoris. It releases NO from its terminal nitrate group after enzyme-mediated bioactivation. Although the identity of the activating enzyme remains elusive, recent evidence has proposed mitochondrial aldehyde dehydrogenase (mtADH) as a likely candidate [17].

The use of GTN in women at risk for preeclampsia was first reported in 1994. A study of intravenous GTN infusion in 15 women with abnormal uterine artery Doppler at 24–26 weeks gestation showed a dose-dependent reduction in uterine artery resistance without any effect on the maternal cardiovascular parameters or the fetal circulation [18]. Further studies of intravenous GTN infusion in preeclampsia, however, have shown a significant reduction in the maternal blood pressure [19–21], and umbilical artery resistance [19] without any significant adverse effects [21, 22] after.

Transdermal GTN patches have been the focus of various studies, for both the prevention and management of preeclampsia and related disorders [22, 23]. A randomized placebo-controlled trial of low-dose transdermal GTN patches in women with abnormal uterine artery Doppler at 24–26 weeks, showed that although there was no change in the incidence of preeclampsia, growth restriction or preterm delivery, GTN increased the likelihood of a complication-free pregnancy with a significant reduction in hazard ratio in the GTN treated arm. There was no effect on maternal cardiovascular parameters, or uterine and fetal Dopplers [22]. Studies of both transdermal [24, 25] and sublingual GTN [26] in women affected by preeclampsia consistently showed a significant reduction of both blood pressure and uterine artery resistance indices without adversely affecting fetal Doppler parameters.

The evidence for the clinical use of GTN for the prevention or treatment of preeclampsia is, therefore, limited by the small numbers of women in the studies, which were not powered to identify alterations in maternal or fetal outcomes. These studies have, nonetheless, highlighted the potential use of GTN as a therapeutic agent in preeclampsia. However, whether it offers any competitive advantage over the existing treatment options in preeclampsia remains to be established.

The major disadvantage of organic nitrates in general, and GTN in particular, is the development of tolerance upon continuous dosing, necessitating the requirement of regular "nitrate free" intervals. There are many theories regarding the molecular basis of tolerance, including increased oxidative stress and generation of superoxide anions, uncoupling of NOS leading to worsening of the underlying endothelial dysfunction, and plasma volume expansion due to fluid retention [27]. Continuous exposure to GTN may also reduce the activity of mtADH [17]. Paradoxically, the increase in oxidative stress and potentiation of endothelial dysfunction may also worsen the underlying disease process [28].

The safety profile of these drugs is well established in the nonpregnant population. The side effects observed with their use are not usually serious and include headache, flushing and dizziness, but can be severe enough to affect compliance, causing discontinuation of their use [29].

Isosorbide Dinitrate

Isosorbide dintirate (ISDN) undergoes bioactivation by a similar mechanism to GTN, but has a longer half-life. A few small studies have demonstrated a reduction in maternal blood pressure [30–32] and resistance in the uterine arteries with the use of both transdermal and sublingual ISDN in women with preeclampsia [33, 34]. However, it has the same disadvantages as GTN, including tolerance, worsening of the underlying endothelial dysfunction and lack of platelet effects at vasodilatory doses.

Other Organic Nitrates

Pentaerythrlytetranitrate (PETN) is a long-acting organic nitrate, which, as with other organic nitrates, improves uteroplacental perfusion. A single randomized placebo-controlled double-blinded study of PETN in pregnancies at risk of preeclampsia is necessary. Although, the risk of IUGR, perinatal death and preterm birth was reduced, there was no reduction in the incidence of preeclampsia in the treatment arm [35].

Sodium nitroprusside is a very potent nitrovasodilator used as an antihypertensive in nonpregnant patients for the treatment of hypertensive emergencies. It can cause profound hypotension, hence requiring very cautious dose titration. It also causes significantly greater risk of causing cerebral hypoperfusion [36]. Although it remains within the guidelines of some European countries, such as the Netherlands, its use has been removed from other guidelines [37] (and it should only be used under exceptional circumstances in carefully controlled intensive care settings). Theoretically, a potential adverse effect of sodium nitroprusside is cyanide toxicity. The data for its use in pregnant patients is limited, with animal studies suggesting the risk of fetal toxicity.

S-nitrosothiols

S-nitrosothiols are a class of compounds that have an NO group attached to the thiol (RSH) moiety by a single chemical bond. S-nitrosothiols release the NO moiety by a variety of mechanisms, including exposure to light, heat and transition metals, in addition to enzymatic bioactivation. As a result of this wide array of mechanisms of activation, S-nitrosothiols are not susceptible to tolerance [38]. The NO moiety can be effectively transferred to endogenous thiols, which act as biological NO reservoirs. This protects NO from being rapidly metabolized to nitrites under conditions of oxidative stress [38]. This permits a longer duration of action of S-nitrosothiols than can be expected from the short half-life of NO. S-nitrosothiols can also transfer the NO moiety across plasma membranes by transnitrosation catalyzed by protein disulfide isomerases [28]. The S-nitrosothiol that has been investigated in women with preeclampsia is S-nitrosoglutathione (GSNO).

GSNO is an endogenous S-nitrosothiol that is found ubiquitously in tissues, in concentrations as high as 250nM [39]. GSNO is not currently in clinical use, but has been the focus of research for its therapeutic role in a variety of conditions, including preeclampsia, cardiovascular and cerebrovascular disorders and cystic fibrosis. The effects of GSNO are tissue specific. A significant reduction in platelet aggregation in response to ADP [40, 41], a

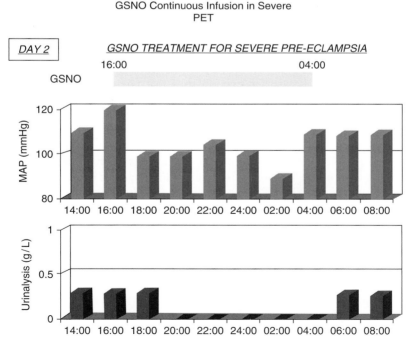

Figure 18.2 Reduction of BP and proteinuria is seen during GSNO infusion in women with early-onset preeclampsia. (A black and white version of this figure will appear in some formats. For the color version, please refer to the plate section.)

reduction in platelet-surface P-selectin and glycoprotein IIbIIIa expression have been shown at doses that have only a minimal cardiovascular effect [42, 43]. This has highlighted its therapeutic potential in conditions associated with platelet over-activation, which include preeclampsia.

The first reported use of GSNO in preeclampsia was in 1994, in a woman with postpartum HELLP syndrome and associated severe thrombocytopenia [44]. A rapid improvement in the patient's clinical condition and improvement in platelet count was seen with GSNO infusion. A further study of GSNO infusion in ten women with severe preeclampsia showed a significant dose-dependent reduction in blood pressure, uterine artery resistance and platelet activation. Despite a fall in maternal blood pressure, no significant effect on the fetal circulation was found [45]. The use of GSNO in women with early-onset preeclampsia has also been the focus of a recent dose ranging study [46]. This demonstrated that intravenous GSNO administration in these women resulted in a significant reduction in augmentation index (which is commonly raised in preeclampsia [47]) and a reduction in platelet activation at doses that did not cause a significant change in mean arterial pressure. A significant post-infusion reduction was observed in urinary protein:creatinine ratio in relation to the pre-infusion value, and the reduction in sEng level approached significance [48]. These studies, albeit small, indicate that GSNO may have a role in targeting the underlying endothelial dysfunction of preeclampsia. However, evidence for an effect of GSNO on clinical end points such as prolongation of pregnancy or improved perinatal outcomes for mother or fetus is lacking. Further research is required to investigate the safety and efficacy of GSNO in women with preeclampsia, and to elucidate effects on maternal and fetal outcomes.

GSNO is known to modulate cell signaling by post-translational S-nitrosylation and S-glutathionylation of redox-sensitive proteins [49]. As previously mentioned, an alteration in the redox state of various plasma proteins, and the oxidative switch of angiotensinogen to its more active form, has been shown in patients with preeclampsia. S-nitrosylation of angiotensinogen by a S-nitrosothiol (S-nitroso-N-acetyl-penicillamine) resulted in a shift toward its less active reduced form [50]. It can, hence, be inferred that post-translational modification of proteins by GSNO may also target the underlying pathophysiological changes in preeclampsia.

Reduced levels of glutathione have been shown in women with preeclampsia [51–53]. It may be hypothesized that exogenous GSNO can replenish these antioxidant reserves of glutathione.

The therapeutic effects of GSNO, a molecule with a very short half-life, persisted up to 24 hours after cessation of the infusion in two studies investigating the reduction of embolic signals from carotid plaque [54, 55]. It is possible that this phenomenon is attributable to the post-translational modification reactions described above. It remains to be elucidated if the changes in cardiovascular parameters, uteroplacental circulation or platelet function similarly persist in preeclamptic women after GSNO infusion.

GSNO has been found to have a favorable toxicity profile in animal toxicology studies using inhalational GSNO, with no biologically significant adverse effects seen [56].

Nitric Oxide Precursors

L-arginine

L-arginine acts as a precursor of NO and is converted into NO and L-citrulline by NOS, as previously described; it has been the focus of studies aimed at investigating its preventive role in women at high risk for developing preeclampsia. A study of intravenous infusion of L-arginine in pregnant women showed a significant reduction in blood pressure – an effect that was greater in women with preeclampsia [57]. Recently, the focus has been on the effects of L-arginine supplementation on the prevention of preeclampsia in high-risk women. A randomized controlled trial showed that dietary supplementation with a combination of L-arginine and antioxidants was associated with a significant reduction in the incidence of preeclampsia, compared with antioxidants alone and placebo [58]. These results, however, have to be interpreted with caution as the effects of L-arginine alone were not studied and it is difficult to ascertain the relative contributions of L-arginine and antioxidants in reducing the incidence of preeclampsia. In addition, the prevalence of recurrent preeclampsia reported in the study population was very high (nearly 30%), hence raising a question about the generalizability of these results to other obstetric populations and low-risk women. Interestingly, a previous study that investigated the effects of L-arginine supplementation in women with chronic hypertension showed less need for antihypertensive medications and fewer maternal and neonatal complications, but no difference in the incidence of superimposed preeclampsia [59]. Since L-arginine is a widely available food supplement, conclusive evidence about its beneficial effects could provide a feasible means of preventing preeclampsia. Hence, further research is warranted into its role in reducing the incidence of preeclampsia in low-risk populations.

Inhibitors of cGMP Breakdown

PDE Inhibitors

Sildenafil citrate (SC) is a cGMP-specific phosphodiesterase type 5 (PDE5) inhibitor commonly used in the treatment of erectile dysfunction. It potentiates the action of NO downstream by inhibiting the degradation of cGMP. SC was the focus of a randomized placebo-controlled trial in 35 women with preeclampsia, which showed no significant difference in randomization to delivery interval. Although SC was well tolerated and did not increase maternal or fetal morbidity or mortality, treatment with SC did not prolong the pregnancy [60]. Further in vivo studies of SC in rat models of preeclampsia have since shown a significant reduction in sFlt-1 and sEng [61], and an improvement in blood pressure, proteinuria and uteroplacental and fetal perfusion after treatment with SC [62]. However, a recent RCT of SC in early-onset growth-restricted fetuses with abnormal umbilical artery Doppler waveforms found sildenafil did not prolong pregnancy or improve pregnancy outcomes in severe early-onset fetal growth restriction.

Inhibitors of NO Donor Metabolism

GSNO Reductase Inhibitors

GSNO is metabolized in vivo by GSNO reductase (GSNOR), an alcohol dehydrogenase that plays a central role in regulating the levels of endogenous GSNO. Small molecule inhibitors of this enzyme have recently been the focus of research. N6022 is a first-in-class compound that is a very potent, specific and fully reversible inhibitor of GSNOR [63] and has been shown to improve endothelial function in vivo [64]. Animal toxicology studies have demonstrated an acceptable safety profile. N6022 is currently the focus of an early phase trial in humans for the treatment of asthma and cystic fibrosis. Hence, it is possible that GSNOR inhibitors hold potential to be studied in the context of preeclampsia, in conjunction with GSNO.

Conclusion

Severe preeclampsia is a rare disease and this, in combination with the poor financial prospects for developing a drug in a high-risk area of medicine, have limited the furthering of drug developments for preeclampsia and, indeed, in obstetrics overall. The current studies on NO donors in pregnancy and preeclampsia have involved small numbers of women. The studies also had extremely limited or no follow-up into the neonatal and early childhood period; improvement of outcomes in this area in particular must be one of the primary outcomes for any drug used to treat preeclampsia. Likewise, improvement in adverse maternal physiological changes, particularly cardiac and renal, need to be carefully elucidated; longer-term improvements in cardiovascular wellbeing will be considerably more difficult to study.

NO donors may hold potential for improving outcomes and reducing the burden of mortality and morbidity in women affected by preeclampsia and in their babies suffering from growth restriction and preterm delivery. Multicenter studies, which are likely to need to be multinational, are required. The financial, ethical, legal and administrative obstacles to this are considerable; however, a treatment for this serious and rare disease is necessitated as a concerted collaborative effort.

Key Points

- From the physiological and pharmacological point of view, NO donors or alterations of the NO pathways are logical candidates for the treatment of preeclampsia.
- The current studies on NO donors in pregnancy and preeclampsia have involved small numbers of women and also had extremely limited follow up into the neonatal and early childhood period.
- Multicenter studies, preferably multinational, are required.

References

1. Poston L. Endothelial dysfunction in pre-eclampsia. *Pharmacol Rep* 2006;**58**:69–74.

2. Roberts JM, Hubel CA. The two stage model of preeclampsia: variations on the theme. *Placenta* 2009;**30**:32–7.

3. Savvidou MD, Hingorani AD, Tsikas D, Frölich JC, Vallance P, Nicolaides KH. Endothelial dysfunction and raised plasma concentrations of asymmetric dimethylarginine in pregnant women who subsequently develop pre-eclampsia. *Lancet* 2003;**361**:1511–7.

4. López-Alarcón M, Montalvo-Velarde I, Vital-Reyes VS, Hinojosa-Cruz JC, Leaños-Miranda A, Martínez-Basila A. Serial determinations of asymmetric dimethylarginine and homocysteine during pregnancy to predict pre-eclampsia: a longitudinal study. *BJOG* 2015;**122**:1586–92.

5. Koga K, Osuga Y, Yoshino O, Hirota Y. Elevated serum soluble vascular endothelial growth factor receptor 1 (sVEGFR-1) levels in women with preeclampsia. *J Clin Endocrinol Metab* 2003;**88**:2348–51.

6. Krauss T, Pauer H-U, Augustin HG. Prospective analysis of placenta growth factor (PlGF) concentrations in the plasma

of women with normal pregnancy and pregnancies complicated by preeclampsia. *Hypertens Pregnancy* 2004;**23**:101–11.

7. Romero R, Nien JK, Espinoza J, et al. A longitudinal study of angiogenic (placental growth factor) and anti-angiogenic (soluble endoglin and soluble vascular endothelial growth factor receptor-1) factors in normal pregnancy and patients destined to develop preeclampsia and deliver a small for gestational age neonate. *J Matern Fetal Neonatal Med* 2008;**21**:9–23.

8. Venkatesha S, Toporsian M, Lam C, et al. Soluble endoglin contributes to the pathogenesis of preeclampsia. *Nat Med* 2006;**12**:642–9.

9. Hood JD, Meininger CJ, Ziche M, Granger HJ. VEGF upregulates ecNOS message, protein, and NO production in human endothelial cells. *Am J Physiol* 1998;**274**: H1054–8.

10. Kroll J, Waltenberger J. VEGF-A induces expression of eNOS and iNOS in endothelial cells via VEGF receptor-2 (KDR). *Biochem Biophys Res Commun* 1998;**252**:743–6.

11. Ahmad S, Hewett PW, Wang P, et al. Direct evidence for endothelial vascular endothelial growth factor receptor-1 function in nitric oxide-mediated angiogenesis. *Circ Res.* 2006;**99**:715–22.

12. Maynard SE. Excess placental soluble fms-like tyrosine kinase 1 (sFlt1) may contribute to endothelial dysfunction, hypertension, and proteinuria in preeclampsia. *J Clin Invest.* 2003;**111**:649–58.

13. Levine RJ, Maynard SE, Qian C, et al. Circulating angiogenic factors and the risk of preeclampsia. *N Engl J Med* 2004;**350**:672–83.

14. Inoue N, Venema RC, Sayegh HS, Ohara Y, Murphy TJ, Harrison DG. Molecular regulation of the bovine endothelial cell nitric oxide synthase by transforming growth factor-beta. *Arterioscler Thromb Vascular Biol.* 1995;**15**:1255–61.

15. Santibanez JF, Letamendia A, Perez-Barriocanal F, et al. Endoglin increases eNOS expression by modulating Smad2 protein levels and Smad2-dependent TGF-beta signaling. *J Cell Physiol* 2007;**210**:456–68.

16. Sandrim VC, Palei ACT, Metzger IF, Gomes VA, Cavalli RC, Tanus-Santos JE. Nitric oxide formation is inversely related to serum levels of antiangiogenic factors soluble fms-like tyrosine kinase-1 and soluble endogline in preeclampsia. *Hypertension* 2008;**52**:402–7.

17. Chen Z, Zhang J, Stamler JS. Identification of the enzymatic mechanism of nitroglycerin bioactivation. *Proc Natl Acad Sci USa* 2002;**99**:8306–11.

18. Ramsay B, de Belder A, Campbell S, Moncada S, Martin JF. A nitric oxide donor improves uterine artery diastolic blood flow in normal early pregnancy and in women at high risk of pre-eclampsia. *Eur J Clin Invest* 1994;**24**:76–8.

19. Grunewald C, Kublickas M, Carlström K, Lunell NO, Nisell H. Effects of nitroglycerin on the uterine and umbilical circulation in severe preeclampsia. *Obstet Gynecol.* 1995;**86**:600–4.

20. Cetin A, Yurtcu N, Guvenal T, Imir AG, Duran B, Cetin M. The effect of glyceryl trinitrate on hypertension in women with severe preeclampsia, HELLP syndrome, and eclampsia. *Hypertens Pregnancy* 2004;**23**:37–46.

21. Manzur-Verástegui S, Mandeville PB, Gordillo-Moscoso A, Hernández-Sierra JF, Rodríguez-Martínez M. Efficacy of nitroglycerine infusion versus sublingual nifedipine in severe pre-eclampsia: a randomized, triple-blind, controlled trial. *Clin Exp Pharmacol Physiol* 2008;**35**:580–5.

22. Lees C, Valensise H, Black R, et al. The efficacy and fetal-maternal cardiovascular effects of transdermal glyceryl trinitrate in the prophylaxis of pre-eclampsia and its complications: a randomized double-blind placebo-controlled trial. *Ultrasound Obstet Gynecol* 2002;**12**:334–8.

23. Picciolo C, Roncaglia N, Neri I. Nitric oxide in the prevention of pre-eclampsia. *Prenat Neonatal Med* 2000;**5**:212–5.

24. Cacciatore B, Halmesmäki E, Kaaja R, Teramo K, Ylikorkala O. Effects of

transdermal nitroglycerin on impedance to flow in the uterine, umbilical, and fetal middle cerebral arteries in pregnancies complicated by preeclampsia and intrauterine growth retardation. *Am J Obstet Gynecol* 1998;**179**:140–5.

25. Trapani A, Gonçalves LF, Pires MM de S. Transdermal nitroglycerin in patients with severe pre-eclampsia with placental insufficiency: effect on uterine, umbilical and fetal middle cerebral artery resistance indices. *Ultrasound Obstet Gynecol* 2011;**38**:389–94.

26. Luzi G, Caserta G, Iammarino G, Clerici G, Di Renzo GC. Nitric oxide donors in pregnancy: fetomaternal hemodynamic effects induced in mild pre-eclampsia and threatened preterm labor. *Ultrasound Obstet Gynecol* 1999;**14**:101–9.

27. Gori T, Parker JD. Nitrate Tolerance. A Unifying Hypothesis. *Circulation* 2002;**106**:2510–3.

28. Miller MR, Megson IL. Recent developments in nitric oxide donor drugs. *Br J Pharmacol.* 2009;**151**:305–21.

29. Davis DG, Brown PM. Re: glyceryl trinitrate (GTN) patches are unsuitable in hypertensive pregnancy. *Aust N Z J Obstet Gynaecol* 2001;**41**:474.

30. Thaler I, Amit A, Kamil D, Itskovitz-Eldor J. The effect of isosorbide dinitrate on placental blood flow and maternal blood pressure in women with pregnancy induced hypertension. *Am J Hypertens.* 1999;**12**:341–7.

31. Martínez-Abundis E, González-Ortiz M, Hernández-Salazar F, Huerta-J-Lucas MT. Sublingual isosorbide dinitrate in the acute control of hypertension in patients with severe preeclampsia. *Gynecol Obstet Invest* 2000;**50**:39–42.

32. Nakatsuka M, Takata M, Tada K, et al. A long-term transdermal nitric oxide donor improves uteroplacental circulation in women with preeclampsia. *J Ultrasound Med* 2002;**21**:831–6.

33. Thaler I, Amit A, Jakobi P, Itskovitz-Eldor J. The effect of isosorbide dinitrate on uterine artery and umbilical artery flow velocity waveforms at mid-pregnancy. *Obstet Gynecol.* 1996;**88**:838–43.

34. Makino Y, Izumi H, Makino I, Shirakawa K. The effect of nitric oxide on uterine and umbilical artery flow velocity waveform in pre-eclampsia. *Eur J Obstet Gynecol Reprod Biol* 1997;**73**:139–43.

35. Groten T, Lehmann T, Fitzgerald J, et al. Reduction of preeclampsia related complications with with the NO-donor penterythriltetranitrat (PETN) in risk pregnancies – a prospective randomized double-blind placebo pilot study. *Pregnancy Hypertens.* 2012; Jul;**2**(3):181.

36. Immink RV, van den Born B-JH, van Montfrans GA, Kim Y-S, Hollmann MW, van Lieshout JJ. Cerebral hemodynamics during treatment with sodium nitroprusside versus labetalol in malignant hypertension. *Hypertension* 2008;**52**:236–40.

37. National Institute for Health and Care Excellence (2010) *Hypertension in Pregnancy.* CG107. London: National Institute for Health and Care Excellence.

38. Sayed N, Kim DD, Fioramonti X, Iwahashi T, Duran WN, Beuve A. Nitroglycerin-induced S-nitrosylation and desensitization of soluble guanylyl cyclase contribute to nitrate tolerance. *Circ Res* 2008;**103**:606–14.

39. Bryan NS, Rassaf T, Maloney RE, et al. Cellular targets and mechanisms of nitros(yl)ation: an insight into their nature and kinetics in vivo. *Proc Natl Acad Sci USa* 2004;**101**:4308–13.

40. de Belder AJ, MacAllister R, Radomski MW, Moncada S, Vallance PJ. Effects of S-nitroso-glutathione in the human forearm circulation: evidence for selective inhibition of platelet activation. *Cardiovasc Res* 1994;**28**:691–4.

41. Ramsay B, Radomski M, de Belder A, Martin JF, Lopez-Jaramillo P. Systemic effects of S-nitroso-glutathione in the human following intravenous infusion. *Br J Clin Pharmacol* 1995;**40**:101–2.

42. Langford EJ, Brown AS, Wainwright RJ, et al. Inhibition of platelet activity by

S-nitrosoglutathione during coronary angioplasty. *Lancet* 1994;**344**:1458–60.

43. Langford E, Wainwright R, Martin J. Platelet activation in acute myocardial infarction and unstable angina is inhibited by nitric oxide donors. *Arterioscler Thromb Vasc Biol* 1996;**16**:51–55.

44. de Belder A, Lees C, Martin J, Moncada S, Campbell S. Treatment of HELLP syndrome with nitric oxide donor. *Lancet* 1995;**345**:124–5.

45. Lees C, Langford E, Brown AS, et al. The effects of S-nitrosoglutathione on platelet activation, hypertension, and uterine and fetal Doppler in severe preeclampsia. *Obstet Gynecol* 1996;**88**:14–9.

46. Everett TR, Wilkinson IB, Mahendru AA, et al. S-Nitrosoglutathione improves haemodynamics in early-onset pre-eclampsia. *Br J Clin Pharmacol* 2014;**78**:660–9.

47. Hausvater A, Giannone T, Sandoval Y-HG, et al. The association between preeclampsia and arterial stiffness. *J Hypertens.* 2012;**30**:17–33.

48. Martínez-Ruiz A, Lamas S. Signalling by NO-induced protein S-nitrosylation and S-glutathionylation: convergences and divergences. *Cardiovasc Res* 2007;**75**:220–8.

49. Kaposzta Z, Clifton A, Molloy J, Martin JF, Markus HS. S-nitrosoglutathione reduces asymptomatic embolization after carotid angioplasty. *Circulation* 2002;**106**:3057–62.

50. Zhou A, Carrell RW, Murphy MP, et al. A redox switch in angiotensinogen modulates angiotensin release. *Nature* 2010;**468**:108–11.

51. Rani N, Dhingra R, Arya DS, Kalaivani M, Bhatla N, Kumar R. Role of oxidative stress markers and antioxidants in the placenta of preeclamptic patients. *J Obstet Gynaecol Res* 2010;**36**:1189–94.

52. Knapen MF, Mulder TP, Van Rooij IA, Peters WH, Steegers EA. Low whole blood glutathione levels in pregnancies complicated by preeclampsia or the hemolysis, elevated liver enzymes, low platelets syndrome. *Obstet Gynecol* 1998;**92**:1012–5.

53. Raijmakers MT, Zusterzeel PL, Steegers EA, Hectors MP, Demacker PN, Peters WH. Plasma thiol status in preeclampsia. *Obstet Gynecol* 2000;**95**:180–4.

54. Kaposzta Z, Martin JF, Markus HS. Switching off embolization from symptomatic carotid plaque using S-nitrosoglutathione. *Circulation* 2002;**105**:1480–4.

55. Colagiovanni DB, Borkhataria D, Looker D, et al. Preclinical 28-day inhalation toxicity assessment of s-nitrosoglutathione in beagle dogs and Wistar rats. *Int J Toxicol* 2011;**30**:466–77.

56. Facchinetti F, Neri I, Piccinini F, et al. Effect of L-arginine load on platelet aggregation: a comparison between normotensive and preeclamptic pregnant women. *Acta Obstet Gynecol Scand* 1999;**78**:515–9.

57. Vadillo-Ortega F, Perichart-Perera O, Espino S, et al. Effect of supplementation during pregnancy with L-arginine and antioxidant vitamins in medical food on pre-eclampsia in high risk population: randomised controlled trial. *BMJ* 2011;**342**:d2901.

58. Neri I, Monari F, Sgarbi L, Berardi A, Masellis G, Facchinetti F. L-arginine supplementation in women with chronic hypertension: impact on blood pressure and maternal and neonatal complications. *J Matern Fetal Neonatal Med* 2010;**23**:1456–60.

59. Samangaya RA, Mires G, Shennan A, et al. A randomised, double-blinded, placebo-controlled study of the phosphodiesterase type 5 inhibitor sildenafil for the treatment of preeclampsia. *Hypertens Pregnancy* 2009;**28**:369–82.

60. Ramesar SV, Mackraj I, Gathiram P, Moodley J. Sildenafil citrate decreases sFlt-1 and sEng in pregnant l-NAME treated Sprague-Dawley rats. *Eur J Obstet Gynecol Reprod Biol* 2011;**157**:136–40.

61. Herraiz S, Pellicer B, Serra V, et al. Sildenafil citrate improves perinatal outcome in fetuses from pre-eclamptic rats. *BJOG* 2012;**119**:1394–402.

62. Stanley JL, Andersson IJ, Poudel R, et al. Sildenafil citrate rescues fetal growth in the

catechol-O-methyl transferase knockout mouse model. *Hypertension* 2012;**59**:1021–8.

63. Nassar AH, Masrouha KZ, Itani H, Nader KA, Usta IM. Effects of sildenafil in Nω-nitro-L-arginine methyl ester-induced intrauterine growth restriction in a rat model. *Amer J Perinatol* 2012;**29**:429–34.

64. Sharp A, Cornforth C, Jackson R, et al. Maternal sildenafil for severe fetal growth restriction (STRIDER): a multicentre, randomised, placebo-controlled, double-blind trial. *Lancet Child Adolesc Health* 2018;**2**:93–102.

65. Colagiovanni DB, Drolet DW, Langlois-Forget E, Piché M-P, Looker D, Rosenthal GJ. A nonclinical safety and pharmacokinetic evaluation of N6022: a first-in-class S-nitrosoglutathione reductase inhibitor for the treatment of asthma. *Regul Toxicol Pharmacol* 2012;**62**:115–24.

Chapter 19

Vasodilatation and Fluid Expansion

Herbert Valensise, Damiano Lo Presti and Marc Spaanderman

Summary

Pregnancies complicated by IUGR and/or hypertension are associated with a reduced expansion of the maternal intravascular space, a lack of increase in cardiac output in the very early phase of pregnancy and a decreased preload as compared to normal pregnancies. For hypertensive mothers of severely growth-restricted fetuses, the combined therapy of plasma volume expansion (PVE) and vasodilators, such as NO donors, might be beneficial in improving maternal hemodynamics and prolonging pregnancy.

This chapter summarizes the current evidence supporting the rationale for further research into this area.

Introduction

Cardiovascular physiological adaptations occur during pregnancy, becoming apparent even during the first 8 weeks of pregnancy [1]. This altered hemodynamic function is permitted by several factors, which allows adequate fetus demand of nutrients and oxygen. Moreover, these changes persist in the puerperium and tend to show again, in a more remarkable way, in successive pregnancies [2]. The main changes include a higher cardiac output [3] due to an increase in terms of plasma volume, especially between weeks 10 and 20, which involves a higher preload volume, and heart rate. Furthermore, a decrease of systemic vascular resistance occurs with subsequent reduced values of mean arterial pressure. This parameter begins to decrease in the first trimester and reaches its maximum level in the middle of the second trimester [4]. Regarding the vascular resistance, they appear to undergo the effect of an increased production of several vasodilator factors by the maternal endothelium.

Preeclampsia and the Impaired Placentation Theory

Preeclampsia is a multifactorial pregnancy-related disorder defined as the onset of hypertension (systolic blood pressure ≥ 140 and/or diastolic blood pressure ≥ 90 mmHg) and proteinuria (>300 mg/24 h) after 20 weeks of gestation in a previously normotensive woman. It occurs in about 2–8% of pregnancies [5, 6] and could represent, especially in severe forms, a leading cause of maternal and perinatal morbidity and mortality.

Preeclampsia can manifest in different clinical forms, being extremely variable in onset time, progression and involvement of several compartments, leading to eclampsia (seizures), hemorrhagic stroke, hemolysis, elevated liver enzymes and low platelets (HELLP) syndrome, diffuse intravascular coagulation (DIC), oliguria and renal failure, pulmonary edema, placental infarction, abruption placentae, fetal growth restriction and preterm birth.

Clinically, it is observed as:

- Increased cardiac ejection
- Increased systemic resistance
- Unstable and increased arterial pressure with the loss of normal reduction at rest

Maternal plasma volume appears to be reduced with a wrong distribution of fluid with an increase of sediment in the interstitial space, edema and decrease of vascular compartment (hypovolemia). Another relevant factor is hypoalbuminemia, which causes a low osmotic-colloid pressure and a subsequent worsening of edema. A complication of fluid retention is ascites and the risk of formation of pulmonary or laryngeal edema [7]. Furthermore, the normal gestational hypercoagulability status is markedly augmented in preeclampsia and could lead to an imbalance condition such as DIC, first highlighted through a reduction of platelets.

Even though the origin of preeclampsia remains uncertain, the presence of the placenta is a necessary and sufficient condition to provoke the disease [8]. The theory of the association with the systemic endothelial dysfunction is widely accepted. Along with theories describing immunological maladaptive tolerance between maternal, paternal and fetal tissue, maternal maladaptation to cardiovascular or inflammatory changes of normal pregnancy and genetic factors including inherited predisposing genes and epigenetic influences, currently the main cause of preeclampsia is thought to be impaired placentation [9]. This condition is commonly considered as deriving from an inadequate trophoblastic invasion of uterine vessels, which leads to a failure of physiological loss of remodeling and relaxation of spiral arteries with a lack of proper blood supply. As a consequence, it develops an increased uterine vessels resistance and a subsequent reduced blood perfusion with placental hypoxia and ischemic events, determining an abnormal function of endothelial cells, possibly as result of oxidative stress [10]. Therefore, a generalized vasoconstriction is produced with a reflected increase of total vascular resistance, along with alterations in angiogenic factor signaling, platelet activation and thrombosis, and decreased plasma volume, with subsequently reduced blood supply to multiple organs [11]. In conclusion, placental hypoxia and endothelial dysfunction may lead to preeclampsia through an exacerbated systemic inflammatory reaction [12].

Placental impairments in endovascular trophoblastic invasion and the subsequent estimation of resistance to uteroplacental blood flow are assessed through the measurement of uterine artery blood flow velocity. Impedance to uterine artery blood flow is decreased after the end of placental formation. On the contrary, alterations of this process show an abnormal high-resistance persistence [13–15]. In addition, the presence of a notching in the Doppler waveform is indicated as another sign of increased risk for preeclampsia and fetal growth restriction [16], even though having a low predicted value except for early-onset severe disease [17].

The definitive treatment for preeclampsia is delivery, particularly in severe forms with multi-organ alterations and placental insufficiency. In these cases, the risk of prematurity is the main point of focus, together with the resolution of maternal disease.

The Role of Endothelium Dysfunction

The instauration of a hypoxic environment within the placenta stimulates oxidative stress and the release of placental factors such as soluble fms-like tyrosine kinase 1 (sFlt-1), soluble endoglin, agonistic autoantibodies to the angiotensin type 1 receptor (AT1-AA) and inflammatory cytokines [18]. These factors, along with the presence of additional maternal risk factors for preeclampsia, contribute to a generalized systemic vascular endothelial dysfunction and result in increased systemic vascular resistance and hypertension [19].

Vascular endothelium has several hemostatic functions, many of which are mediated by nitric oxide (NO).

Therapies Targeting the Vasodilation

Restoring the balance of vascular tone to favor systemic vasodilation might be considered as the new target to treat preeclampsia, linking the concept of systemic endothelial dysfunction as the intrinsic cause of signs and symptoms. Potential therapies may include those that target the nitric oxide pathway. Other new targets may consider hydrogen sulfide, in order to increase its levels, or reduce the vasoconstrictor effect of elements such as endothelin-1 (ET-1).

Nitric Oxide

Nitric oxide (NO) belongs to the vasodilator family and is released by endothelial cells determining important changes in modifying maternal vascular resistance through a physiological vasodilatation, decreased responsiveness to vasopressors and therefore increasing blood flow; it is also an inhibitor of platelet aggregation and adhesion [20]. Moreover, it determines inhibition of vascular smooth muscle cell proliferation [21] and inhibition of inflammatory cell activation [22], and also can modulate protein function through S-nitrosylation, which may be of biological importance. It is an autocrine- and paracrine-signaling molecule that is synthesized from L-arginine by a family of calcium–calmodulin-dependent enzymes called nitric oxide synthases (NOS). Nitric oxide causes relaxation of vascular smooth muscle cells regulating the placental vascular tone and development [23, 24] by activating soluble guanylatecyclase (sGC), which determine an increase in intracellular cyclic guanosine $3'$, $5'$-monophosphate (cGMP) and activation of cGMP-dependent protein kinases. During pregnancy it appears to play a relevant role in normal placental development; its production occurs in the uteroplacental tissues and endothelial cells, in order to reduce the vascular resistance of the fetoplacental and uterine circulations [25]. Impairment in its production is associated with diseases such as atherosclerosis, hypertension, cerebral and coronal vasospasm and ischemic-reperfusion injury.

Preeclampsia and Nitric Oxide Therapeutic Strategies

Reduced availability of nitric oxide may have a role in the pathophysiology of preeclampsia and therefore drugs, which aim at increasing this element, or nitric oxide donors and precursors may be considered as therapeutic agents that prevent or treat preeclampsia. It is controversial whether the real availability or its production is indeed reduced, or whether this is due to increased degradation of nitric oxide. Increased degradation of nitric oxide may result from oxidative stress, which occurs in preeclampsia [26, 27]. The production may be reduced if there is a deficiency of its precursor, L-arginine, or an increase in NOS enzyme inhibitor activity. Davidge and Seligman have found evidence of decreased nitric oxide production in the serum and urine of women with preeclampsia [28, 29]. There is evidence that NOS activity within platelets is reduced [30, 31], and that the normal inhibitor of NOS enzyme, asymmetric dimethylarginine, is increased in women with preeclampsia [32].

Some studies have demonstrated decreased L-arginine concentrations [33] and reduced NOS activity [34] in the placenta of women with preeclampsia. All these considerations have led to the conclusion that nitric oxide may have a role in prevention and treatment of preeclampsia.

As the abnormal placentation with the subsequent endothelial dysfunction are the crucial elements by which preeclampsia develops, therapies which increase NO bioavailability are seen as potential tools in the prevention and treatment of preeclampsia and several methods might be considered, including:

- administration of NO precursors (L-arginine or L-citrulline)
- use of NO donors (such as glyceryl trinitrate (GTN))
- inhibition of the production of asymmetric dimethylarginine (ADMA) interferes with L-arginine in the production of NO
- the clearance of NO downstream messengers (sildenafil citrate)
- a reduced production of reactive oxygen species – such as superoxide anions – which will react with NO

L-Arginine and L-Citrulline

The real precursor of NO is L-arginine [27], which is converted into NO and L-citrulline by NOS. Its endothelial relaxing effect in patients with cardiovascular risk factors have been demonstrated [35]. A 40% reduction of the risk of preeclampsia in women at increased risk for family history has been shown in a randomized trial of L-arginine in combination with antioxidant vitamins [36]. This study also showed a reduction in preeclampsia with antioxidant vitamins alone, which is not consistent with meta-analysis of other clinical trials [37]. The use of nitric oxide precursor L-arginine in one small trial was associated with a reduction in the risk of preeclampsia [38]. It is commercially available, and may be given orally as tablets, or solution, or by intravenous injections. Known side effects include diarrhea.

L-citrulline is the precursor of L-arginine. A recent study investigated the effect of L-citrulline treatment in a cohort of obese pregnant women. Treatment, which commenced at week 16 of gestation and lasted for 3 weeks, was associated with significant beneficial effects such as a reduction in blood pressure, improved endothelial function (as measured via flow-mediated dilation), and improved uterine artery Doppler indices [39]. This study certainly supports further investigation of L-citrulline as a potential new treatment.

Sildenafil Citrate

Sildenafil citrate is a phosphodiesterase-5 inhibitor potentiating and prolonging the action of NO downstream by inhibiting the degradation of cGMP. Currently sildenafil is used predominantly for male erectile dysfunction, and also in the treatment of pulmonary hypertension, including its successful use in pregnancy as part of a treatment regimen for Eisenmenger's syndrome [40, 41].

Several animal studies support the efficacy of sildenafil as a treatment for preeclampsia, confirming it is well tolerated. Evidence from clinical trials is currently too limited to provide conclusions about the benefit in preeclampsia, but suggests that use may be associated with improved fetal growth. Sildenafil has been shown to improve endothelial dysfunction in myometrial vessels of women who have pregnancies complicated by intrauterine growth restriction, and increased dilation of chorionic plate arteries obtained from women with healthy pregnancies [42, 43], improving uterine artery blood flow [44]. A pilot study of women with severely growth-restricted pregnancies found a significant increase in abdominal circumference growth with sildenafil treatment (25 mg three times daily), compared with nontreated controls [45].

Nitric Oxide Donors

As already mentioned, endothelial dysfunction and NO bioavailability impairment play a role in the maternal manifestations of preeclampsia, thus supplementation with exogenous NO donors would be an apparently logical solution.

Nitric oxide (NO) donors such as glyceryl trinitrate (GTN) are attractive treatment strategies as they have been shown to improve uterine [46–48] and umbilical blood flow [46, 49], and appear to protect the syncytiotrophoblast from apoptosis, lipid peroxidation, and superoxide formation following hypoxia-reperfusion insults [50].

In many cases, uterine arteries are found to be increased in preeclampsia, compromising blood flow to the placenta. Some studies have demonstrated that administration of nitric oxide donors is associated with a reduction in uterine artery resistance in women with preeclampsia [51–52].

Nitric oxide donors include glyceryl trinitrate (or nitroglycerin), isosorbide mononitrate, isosorbide dinitrate, S-nitroglutathione and sodium nitroprusside.

Many means of administration are available, such as oral or sublingual tablets, aerosol spray under the tongue, skin patches and intravenous injection. Transdermal administration appears to be the most feasible as a long-term treatment option.

The most common side effects include:

- headache
- flushing
- postural hypotension
- local irritation with patches.

Headache is the most common side effect, observed in about 80% of patients [46, 53, 54]. However, headaches are well controlled with common analgesics, and disappeared or decreased with adaptation to the medication. There are no known risks associated with the use of nitric oxide donors in pregnancy. A potential risk associated with all vasodilators is hypotension with subsequent reduction in the blood supply to the fetus and placenta. Treatment with GTN has been associated with falls in maternal arterial pressure and/or a rise in maternal heart rate in most studies of pregnancy [46, 47, 49, 55].

Transdermal GTN patches have been the focus of various studies, for both prevention and management of preeclampsia and related disorders [54, 56]. A randomized, placebo-controlled trial of low-dose transdermal GTN patches in women with abnormal uterine artery Doppler velocimetry at 24–26 weeks showed that although there was no change in the incidence of preeclampsia, growth restriction or preterm delivery, GTN increased the likelihood of a complication-free pregnancy, with a significant reduction in hazard ratio in the GTN treated group. Another study has demonstrated that transdermal nitroglycerin improved Doppler velocimetry parameters of the uterine arteries and umbilical artery without modifying fetal cerebral blood flow. The pulsatility index (PI) and the resistivity index (RI) of the middle cerebral artery remained unaltered following GTN administration, indicating that the fetal cerebral arterial vascular tonus is not dependent on external nitric oxide supply [46].

Sublingual administration has a short duration so would potentially require half-hourly dosing [55]. Tolerance can develop quickly, with reduced therapeutic effect, but is minimized by carefully timed, intermittent administration. Other observed disadvantages include lack of platelet effects at vasodilatory doses; moreover, continuous exposure to GTN may reduce the activity of mitochondrial aldehyde dehydrogenase [57]. Paradoxically, the increase in oxidative stress and potentiation of endothelial dysfunction may also worsen the underlying disease process [58].

Isosorbide dintirate has similar action to GTN, but a longer half-life, and shares the same disadvantages, including tolerance.

Some trials were conducted to compare the effect of nitric oxide donors or precursors versus placebo or no intervention. Four trials compared nitric oxide donors (glycerol trinitrate) or precursors (L-Arginine) with controls (either placebo or no nitric oxide donor or precursor). Overall, there are insufficient data for reliable conclusions about the effects on preeclampsia (four trials, 170 women; relative risk (RR) 0.83, 95% confidence interval (CI) 0.49 to 1.41), perinatal death (three trials, 114 women; RR 0.25, 95% CI 0.03 to 2.34), preterm birth (three trials, 154 women; RR 0.48, 95% CI 0.21 to 1.07) or having a small-for-gestational-age baby (two trials, 108 women; RR 0.78, 95% CI 0.36 to 1.70) [11].

Glyceryl trinitrate was associated with an increased relative risk of headache compared to placebo (two trials, 56 women; RR 6.85, 95% CI 1.42 to 33.04). Both glyceryl trinitrate and a placebo were given as skin patches, and there was no clear difference between the groups in the risk of skin rashes (two trials, 56 women; RR 0.68, 95% CI 0.22 to 2.07). Women allocated glyceryl trinitrate were more likely to stop treatment than those allocated a placebo (two trials, 56 women; RR 4.02, 95% CI 1.15 to 14.09). This was due to headaches for women allocated glyceryl trinitrate in one small trial [59]. In the other trial [54], equal numbers of women in the two groups stopped treatment due to skin rashes.

The increase in the relative risk of headaches, and stopping treatment, was due to an extreme result in one small study [59] (7/7 versus 0/9 for both outcomes). There were no clear differences between the two groups for any other outcome. There was no statistically significant heterogeneity between the trials [11].

Furthermore, one trial (36 women) compared nitric oxide donors with nifedipine. The confidence intervals for all outcomes reported were wide, and crossed the line of no effect. There are insufficient data for any reliable conclusions about the differential effects of these agents [11].

Nitric Oxide Donors and Plasma Volume Expansion

Pregnancies complicated by intrauterine growth restriction (IUGR) are associated with a reduced expansion of the maternal intravascular space, a lack of increase in cardiac output in the very early phase of pregnancy [60–61], and a decreased preload compared with normal pregnancies. These findings suggest that the combined therapy of PVE and NO donors in hypertensive mothers of severely growth-restricted fetuses might be beneficial in improving maternal hemodynamics and prolonging pregnancy. Valensise et al. conducted a case-control study in order to evaluate the effect of PVE and NO donors in addition to antihypertensive therapy for gestational hypertensive pregnancies complicated by IUGR with absent end-diastolic flow (AEDF) in the umbilical artery (UA) [62]. Improvement in maternal cardiac function was apparently linked to the action of the pharmacological treatment on the maternal circulation, with an increase in maternal heart rate, stroke volume and cardiac output, and a fall in peripheral vascular resistance. Apart from the potential benefit of afterload decrease, NO donors cause a dilatation of the capacitance vessels (i.e. the venous bed), which increases venous pooling and decreases the preload, which is already defective in mothers of IUGR fetuses. Mothers of growth-restricted fetuses show reduced preload, stroke volume and cardiac output. Fluid management (with PVE) induces an increase in preload. Its efficacy in enhancing maternal circulation is linked to a concomitant increase in stroke volume. The latter might be obtained by administering nitrates (NO donors), which reduce the afterload (peripheral resistances). It would be reasonable to suggest that PVE might induce an increase in preload, synergistically acting with the reduction of total vascular resistance (TVR) due to NO donors, and thus improving stroke volume and cardiac output. The consequence of the preload increase (obtained by PVE) and the afterload decrease (obtained by NO donor administration) was the enhancement of left atrial and ventricular emptying, with an increase in stroke volume. The positive synergistic effects of the combined administration of NO donors and PVE on the maternal circulation were also evident in the uterine region, with a reduction, although not significant, of the uterine artery resistance index. This is plausible since this region is part of the total maternal peripheral circulation and contributes to the determination of TVR [63, 64]. Improvement in maternal cardiovascular function was found to influence positively fetal hemodynamics. In fact, in this study it is described as an improvement in terms of reappearance of end-diastolic flow in the UA and therefore a prolongation of pregnancy with a delayed time of delivery [62]. In conclusion, the combined therapeutic approach of NO donor administration and PVE in hypertensive mothers of growth-restricted fetuses apparently improves both maternal and fetoplacental hemodynamics, thus prolonging gestation. Moreover there is some evidence that nitrates and fluid therapy added to standard antihypertensive treatment improve maternal hemodinamics and fetal growth more than standard antihypertensive treatment alone [65].

Hydrogen Sulfide

Hydrogen sulfide (H_2S) has the same structural and functional properties as NO and is produced by endothelial and vascular smooth muscle cells. It shows a vasorelaxation effect [66, 67], including vasodilation of the fetoplacental vasculature [68], and also proangiogenic effects [69]. This endothelium is a site of expression of two types of enzyme, cystathionine-glyase (CSE) and cystathionine-b-synthase (CBS), which are designated to produce H_2S [70]. Holwerda et al. demonstrated the effects of H_2S donors in adenovirus-mediated sFlt-1 overexpression in (nonpregnant) rats in terms of reduction of hypertension, proteinuria and a reduction in glomerular endotheliosis with treatment [71].

Endothelin Receptor Antagonists

Endothelin (ET) receptor antagonists are used in the treatment of numerous cardiovascular diseases, including systemic and pulmonary hypertension, congestive heart failure, myocardial infarction, vascular restenosis and atherosclerosis, renal failure, cancer and cerebrovascular disease. Endothelin-1 has a vasoconstrictor effect and seems to be activated by inflammatory and antiangiogenic factors. Its levels are demonstrated to be increased in women with preeclampsia [72–75]. Therefore, its effect might be modulated as a target to prevent the progression of disease [76]. Some benefits are reported for preeclampsia treatment and the role of endothelin receptor antagonist (BQ123), which lead to attenuated hypertension [77]. Blockade of endothelin type A receptors in animal models of preeclampsia resulted in attenuation of hypertension as well as a small increase in pup weight. Interestingly, no change in arterial pressure was seen in nonpregnant animals [78].

Conclusion

The rationale for using a combination of PVE and vasodilators in the management of pregnancies complicated with maternal hypertension and fetal growth restriction remains mainly a theoretical issue. Since experimental data and few clinical studies show promising results, much more research is required to evaluate the relevance of this interesting approach.

Key Points

- As compared to uncomplicated pregnancies, those complicated by IUGR and/or hypertension are associated with a reduced expansion of the maternal intravascular space, a lack of increase in cardiac output in the very early phase of pregnancy and a decreased preload.
- For hypertensive mothers of severely growth-restricted fetuses, the combined therapy of PVE and vasodilators, such as NO donors, might be beneficial in improving maternal hemodynamics and prolonging pregnancy. More research is needed to evaluate the relevance of this approach.

References

1. Hibbard JU, Shroff SG, Cunningham FG. Cardiovascular alterations in normal and preeclamptic pregnancies. In Taylor RN, Roberts JM, Cunningham FG (eds): *Chesley's Hypertensive Disorders in Pregnancy*, 4th edn. Amsterdam, Academic Press, 2014.

2. Clapp JF, Capeless E. Cardiovascular function before, during, and after the first and subsequent pregnancies. *Am J Cardiol* 1997;**80**(11):1469–73.

3. Duvekot JJ, Cheriex EC, Pieters FA, et al: Early pregnancy changes in hemodynamics and volume homeostasis are consecutive adjustments triggered by a primary fall in systemic vascular tone. *Am J Obstet Gynecol* 1993;**169**:1382.

4. MacGillivray I, Rose GA, Rowe B. Blood pressure survey in pregnancy. *Clin Sci.* 1969;**37**(2):395–407.

5. World Health Organization International Collaborative Study of Hypertensive Disorders in Pregnancy. Geographic variation in the incidence of hypertension in pregnancy. *Am J Obstet Gynecol.* 1988;**158**: 80–3.

6. Sibai B, Dekker G, Kupferminc M. Pre-eclampsia. *Lancet* 2005;**365**:785–99.

7. Cedergren M. Effects of gestational weight gain and body mass index on obstetric outcome in Sweden. *Int. J. Gynaecol Obstet* 2006; **93**:269–74.

8. Redman CW, Sargent IL. Latest advances in understanding preeclampsia. *Science* 2005;**308**:1592–4.

9. Khong TY, De Wolf F, Robertson WB, Brosens I. Inadequate maternal vascular response to placentation in pregnancies complicated by pre-eclampsia and by small-for-gestational age infants. *Br J Obstet Gynaecol* 1986;**93**:1049–59.

10. Widmer M, Villar J, Benigni A, Conde-Agudelo A, Karumanchi SA, Lindheimer M. Mapping the theories of preeclampsia and the role of angiogenic factors: a systematic review. *Obstet Gynecol.* 2007 Jan;**109**(1):168–80.

11. Meher S, Duley L. Prevention of Pre-eclampsia Cochrane Review Authors. Interventions for preventing preeclampsia and its consequences: generic protocol. *Cochrane Database of Systematic Reviews* 2005; 2. [doi: 10.1002/ 14651858. CD005301]

12. Redman CW, Sacks GP, Sargent IL. Preeclampsia: an excessive maternal inflammatory response to pregnancy. *Am J Obstet Gynecol* 1999;**180**: 499–506.

13. Everett TR, Mahendru AA, McEniery CM, Wilkinson IB, Lees CC. Raised uterine artery impedance is associated with increased maternal arterial stiffness in the late second trimester. *Placenta.* 2012;**33** (7):572–7. doi: 10.1016/j. placenta.2012.04.001. Epub 2012 Apr 24.

14. Ghidini A, Locatelli A. Monitoring of fetal well-being: role of uterine artery Doppler. *Semin Perinatol.* 2008;**32**(4):258–62. doi: 10.1053/j.semperi.2008.04.019.

15. Napolitano R, Thilaganathan B. Mean, lowest, and highest pulsatility index of the uterine artery and adverse pregnancy outcome in twin pregnancies. *Am J Obstet Gynecol.* 2012;**206**(6):e8–9; author reply e9. doi: 10.1016/j.ajog.2012.02.030. Epub 2012 Mar 6.

16. Groom KM, North RA, Stone PR, et al. SCOPE Consortium. Patterns of change in uterine artery Doppler studies between 20 and 24 weeks of gestation and pregnancy outcomes. *Obstet Gynecol.* 2009;**113**(2, Pt 1):332–8. doi: 10.1097/ AOG.0b013e318195b223.

17. Myatt L, Clifton RG, Roberts JM, et al. First-trimester prediction of preeclampsia in nulliparous women at low risk. *Obstet Gynecol.* 2012;**119**(6):1234–42. doi: 10.1097/AOG.0b013e3182571669.

18. George EM, Granger JP. Mechanisms and potential therapies for preeclampsia. *Curr Hypertens Rep* 2011;**13**:269–75.

19. Goulopoulou S, Davidge ST. Molecular mechanisms of maternal vascular dysfunction in preeclampsia. *Trends Mol Med* 2015;**21**:88–97.

20. Moncada S, Higgs A. The L-arginine-nitric oxide pathway. *N Engl J Med.* 1993;**329** (27):2002–12.

21. Jeremy JY, Rowe D, Emsley AM, Newby AC. Nitric oxide and the proliferation of vascular smooth muscle cells. *Cardiovasc Res* 1999; **43**:580–94.

22. Gaboury JP, Niu XF, Kubes P. Nitric oxide inhibits numerous features of mast cell-induced inflammation. *Circulation* 1996; **93**:318–26.

23. Krause BJ, Hanson MA, Casanello P. Role of nitric oxide in placental vascular development and function. *Placenta.* 2011; **32**(11): 797–805. doi: 10.1016/j. placenta.2011.06.025.

24. Kulandavelu S, Whiteley KJ, Bainbridge SA, et al. Endothelial NO synthase augments fetoplacental blood flow, placental vascularization, and fetal growth in mice. *Hypertension.* 2013;**61**(1):259–66. doi: 10.1161/ HYPERTENSIONAHA.112.201996. Epub 2012 Nov 12.

25. Learmont JG, Poston L. Nitric oxide is involved in flow-induced dilation of isolated human small fetoplacental arteries. *Am J Obstet Gynecol* 1996; **174**: 1056–60.

26. Hubel CA, Kagan VE, Kisin ER, McLaughlin MK, Roberts JM. Increased ascorbate radical formation and ascorbate depletion in plasma from women with preeclampsia: implications for oxidative stress. *Free Radic Biol Med* 1997;**23**:597–609.

27. Lowe DT. Nitric oxide dysfunction in the pathophysiology of preeclampsia. *Nitric Oxide* 2000;**4**(4):441–58.

28. Davidge ST, Stranko CP, Roberts JM. Urine but not plasma nitric oxide metabolites are decreased in women with preeclampsia. *Am J Obstet Gynecol* 1996;**174**(3):1008–13.

29. Seligman SP, Buyon JP, Clancy RM, Young BK, Abramson SB. The role of nitric oxide

in the pathogenesis of preeclampsia. *American Journal of Obstetrics and Gynecology* 1994;**171**:944–8.

30. Delacretaz E, DeQuay N, Waeber B, et al. Differential nitric oxide synthase activity in human platelets during normal pregnancy and preeclampsia. *Clin Sci* 1995;**88**:607–10.

31. Neri I, Piccinini F, Marietta M, Facchinetti F, Volpe A. Platelet responsiveness to L-arginine in hypertensive disorders of pregnancy. *Hypertension in Pregnancy* 2000;**19**(3):323–30.

32. Fickling SA, Williams D, Vallance P, Nussey SS, Whitley GStJ. Plasma concentrations of endogenous inhibitor of nitric oxide synthesis in normal pregnancy and preeclampsia. *Lancet* 1993;**342**:242–3.

33. Noris M, Todeschini M, Cassis P, et al. L-arginine depletion in preeclampsia orients nitric oxide synthase toward oxidant species. *Hypertension* 2004;**43**(3):614–22.

34. Morris NH, Sooranna SR, Learmont JG, et al. Nitric oxide synthase activities in placental tissue from normotensive, preeclamptic, and growth retarded fetuses. *Br J Obstet Gynaecol* 1995;**102**:711–4.

35. Wu G, Meininger CJ. Arginine nutrition and cardiovascular function. *J Nutr* 2000;**130**(11):2626–9

36. Vadillo-Ortega F, Perichart-Perera O, Espino S, et al. Effect of supplementation during pregnancy with L-arginine and antioxidant vitamins in medical food on pre-eclampsia in high risk population: Randomised controlled trial. *BMJ* 2011;**342**:d2901

37. Rumbold A, Duley L, Crowther CA, Haslam RR. Antioxidants for preventing pre-eclampsia. *Cochrane Database Syst Rev* 2008;1. CD004227. doi: 10.1002/14651858. CD004227.pub3.

38. Meher S, Duley L. Nitric oxide for preventing pre-eclampsia and its complications. *Cochrane Database Syst Rev.* 2007;**18**(2):CD006490.

39. Powers R, Weissgerber TL, McGonigal S, et al. [7-OR]: L-citrulline administration increases the arginine/ ADMA ratio, decreases blood pressure and improves vascular function in obese pregnant women. *Pregnancy Hypertens* 2015;**5**(1):4

40. Molelekwa V, Akhter P, McKenna P, et al. Eisenmenger's syndrome in a 27 week pregnancy-management with bosentan and sildenafil. *Ir Med J* 2005;**98**(3):87–8

41. Lacassie HJ, Germain AM, Valdes G, et al. Management of eisenmenger syndrome in pregnancy with sildenafil and L-arginine. *Obstet Gynecol* 2004;**103**(5, Pt 2):1118–20.

42. Wareing M, Myers JE, O'Hara M, Baker PN. Sildenafil citrate (Viagra) enhances vasodilatation in fetal growth restriction. *J Clin Endocrinol Metab* 2005;**90**:2550–5.

43. Maharaj CH, O'Toole D, Lynch T, et al. Effects and mechanisms of action of sildenafil citrate in human chorionic arteries. *Reprod Biol Endocrinol* 2009;**7**:34

44. Malinova M. Sildenafil – for treatment of preeclampsia and intrauterine growth restriction. *Akush Ginekol (Sofiia)*. 2014;**53**(1):40–3.

45. Von Dadelszen P, Dwinnell S, Magee LA, et al. Sildenafil citrate therapy for severe early-onset intrauterine growth restriction. *BJOG* 2011;**118**(5):624–8.

46. Trapani A Jr, Gonçalves LF, Pires MM. Transdermal nitroglycerin in patients with severe preeclampsia with placental insufficiency: Effect on uterine, umbilical and fetal middle cerebral artery resistance indices. *Ultrasound Obstet Gynecol* 2011;**38**(4):389–94.

47. Cacciatore B, Halmesmäki E, Kaaja R, et al. Effects of transdermal nitroglycerin on impedance to flow in the uterine, umbilical, and fetal middle cerebral arteries in pregnancies complicated by preeclampsia and intrauterine growth retardation. *Am J Obstet Gynecol* 1998;**179**(1):140–5.

48. Ramsay B, De Belder A, Campbell S, et al. A nitric oxide donor improves uterine artery diastolic blood flow in normal early pregnancy and in women at high risk of pre-eclampsia. *Eur J Clin Invest* 1994;**24**(1):76–8.

49. Grunewald C, Kublickas M, Carlström K, et al. Effects of nitroglycerin on the uterine and umbilical circulation in severe

preeclampsia. *Obstet Gynecol* 1995;**86**(4 Pt 1):600–4.

50. Belkacemi L, Bainbridge SA, Dickinson MA, Smith GN. Glyceryl trinitrate inhibits hypoxia/reoxygenation-induced apoptosis in the syncytiotrophoblast of the human placenta: Therapeutic implications for preeclampsia. *Am J Pathol* 2007;**170** (3):909–20.

51. Lees C, Langford E, Brown AS, de Belder A, Pickles A, Martin JF. The effects of S-nitrosoglutathione on platelet activation, hypertension, and uterine and fetal Doppler in severe preeclampsia. *Obstetrics & Gynecology* 1996;**88**:14–19.

52. Thaler I, Amit A, Kamil D, Itskovitz-Eldor J. The effect of isosorbide dinitrate on placental blood flow and maternal blood pressure in women with pregnancy induced hypertension. *Am J Hypertens* 1999;**12**(4 Pt 1):341–7.

53. Cetin A, Yurtcu N, Guvenal T, Imir AG, Duran B, Cetin M. The effect of glyceryl trinitrate on hypertension in women with severe preeclampsia, HELLP syndrome, and eclampsia. *Hypertens Pregnancy* 2004; **23**: 37–46.

54. Lees C, Valensise H, Black R, et al. The efficacy and fetal–maternal cardiovascular effects of transdermal glyceryl trinitrate in the prophylaxis of preeclampsia and its complications: a randomized double-blind placebo-controlled trial. *Ultrasound Obstet Gynecol* 1998; **12**:334–8.

55. Giles W, O'Callaghan S, Boura A, Walters W. Reduction in human fetal umbilical-placental vascular resistance by glyceryl trinitrate. *Lancet* 1992;**340**(8823):856.

56. Picciolo C, Roncaglia N, Neri I, Pasta F, Arreghini A, Facchinetti F. Nitric oxide in the prevention of pre-eclampsia. *Prenat Neonatal Med* 2000; **5**: 212–15.

57. Chen Z, Zhang J, Stamler JS. Identification of the enzymatic mechanism of nitroglycerin bioactivation. *Proc Natl Acad Sci U S A* 2002; **99**: 8306–11.

58. Miller MR, Megson IL. Recent developments in nitric oxide donor drugs. *Br J Pharmacol* 2007; **151**: 305–21.

59. Davis G, Brown M. Glyceryl trinitrate patches are unsuitable in hypertensive pregnancy. *Aust N Z J Obstet Gynaecol* 2001;**41**(4):474.

60. Duvekot JJ, Cheriex EC, Pieters FA, Peeters LH. Severely impaired fetal growth is preceded by maternal hemodynamic maladaptation in very early pregnancy. *Acta Obstet Gynecol Scand* 1995; **74**: 693–7.

61. Duvekot JJ, Cheriex EC, Pieters FA, Menheere PP, Schouten HJ, Peeters LH. Maternal volume homeostasis in early pregnancy in relation to fetal growth restriction. *Obstet Gynecol* 1995;**85**:361–7.

62. Valensise H, Vasapollo B, Novelli GP, et al. Maternal and fetal hemodynamic effects induced by nitric oxide donors and plasma volume expansion in pregnancies with gestational hypertension complicated by intrauterine growth restriction with absent end-diastolic flow in the umbilical artery. *Ultrasound Obstet Gynecol* 2008;**31**:55–64.

63. Valensise H, Novelli GP, Vasapollo B, et al. Maternal cardiac systolic and diastolic function: relationship with uteroplacental resistances. A Doppler and echocardiographic longitudinal study. *Ultrasound Obstet Gynecol* 2000; **15**: 487–97.

64. Curran-Everett D, Morris Jr KG, Moore LG. Regional circulatory contributions to increased systemic vascular conductance of pregnancy. *Am J Physiol* 1991;**261**:H1842–H1847.

65. Valensise H, Vasapollo B, Novelli GP, Altomare F, Arduini D. Nitric oxide donors and fluid therapy increase fetal growth in gestational hypertension. 15th World Congress on Ultrasound in Obstetrics and Gynecology Poster abstracts.

66. Ariyaratnam P, Loubani M, Morice AH. Hydrogen sulphide vasodilates human pulmonary arteries: A possible role in pulmonary hypertension? *Microvasc Res* 2013;**90**:135–7.

67. Zhao W, Zhang J, Lu Y, Wang R. The vasorelaxant effect of H(2)S as a novel endogenous gaseous K(ATP) channel opener. *EMBO J* 2001;**20**(21):6008–16.

68. Cindrova-Davies T. Reduced cystathionine glyase and increased miR-21 expression are associated with increased vascular resistance in growth-restricted pregnancies: Hydrogen sulfide as a placental vasodilator. *Am J Pathol* 2013;**182**(4):1448.

69. Cai W, Wang M, Moore PK, et al. The novel proangiogenic effect of hydrogen sulfide is dependent on Akt phosphorylation. *Cardiovasc Res* 2008;**76**(1):29–40.

70. Holwerda KM. Hydrogen sulfide producing enzymes in pregnancy and preeclampsia. *Placenta* 2012;**33**(6):518–21.

71. Holwerda KM, Burke SD, Faas MM, et al. Hydrogen sulfide attenuates sFlt1-induced hypertension and renal damage by upregulating vascular endothelial growth factor. *J Am Soc Nephrol* 2014;**25**(4):717–25.

72. Sharma D, Singh A, Trivedi SS, Bhattacharjee J. Role of endothelin and inflammatory cytokines in pre-eclampsia – a pilot North Indian study. *Am J Reprod Immunol* 2011;**65**(4):428–32.

73. Taylor RN, Varma M, Teng NN, Roberts JM. Women with preeclampsia have higher plasma endothelin levels than women with normal pregnancies. *J Clin Endocrinol Metab* 1990;**71**(6):1675–7.

74. Dekker GA, Kraayenbrink AA, Zeeman GG, van Kamp GJ. Increased plasma levels of the novel vasoconstrictor peptide endothelin in severe pre-eclampsia. *Eur J Obstet Gynecol Reprod Biol* 1991;**40**(3):215–20.

75. Clark BA, Halvorson L, Sachs B, Epstein FH. Plasma endothelin levels in preeclampsia: Elevation and correlation with uric acid levels and renal impairment. *Am J Obstet Gynecol.* 1992;**166**(3):962–8.

76. George EM, Palei AC, Granger JP. Endothelin as a final common pathway in the pathophysiology of preeclampsia: Therapeutic implications. *Curr Opin Nephrol Hypertens* 2012;**21**(2):157–62.

77. Olson GL, Saade GR, Buhimschi I, et al. The effect of an endothelin antagonist on blood pressure in a rat model of preeclampsia. *Am J Obstet Gynecol* 1999;**181**(3):638–41.

78. Alexander BT, Rinewalt AN, Cockrell KL, et al. Endothelin type a receptor blockade attenuates the hypertension in response to chronic reductions in uterine perfusion pressure. *Hypertension* 2001;**37**(2 Pt 2):485–9.

Chapter 20

Beyond Temporal Classification of Early and Late Preeclampsia

Enrico Ferrazzi, Daniela Di Martino, Tamara Stampalija and Maria Muggiasca

Summary

The numerous exceptions and failures in epidemiology, prediction, diagnosis and treatment of temporal classification of preeclampsia and other hypertensive disorders of pregnancy (HDPs) prompted many scholars to warn that preeclampsia is a syndrome and not a progression of a single disease.

There is growing evidence that when the two partners of the disease – the mother and the fetus (the placenta being just a transient intrauterine organ of the fetus) – are considered with equal worth, we can try to make sense of these puzzling clinical phenotypes of HDP.

Fetal abdominal circumference and uterine arteries Doppler velocimetry can be easily used at the bedside of a pregnant woman affected by high blood pressure to ascertain which woman is suffering the consequences of endothelial dysfunction associated with a small placenta and a growth-restricted fetus (IUGR) as such from the first trimester shallow trophoblastic invasion, or who is suffering primarily from maternogenic endothelial dysfunction with a different placental pathology with normal impedance to uterine flow and an appropriate-for-gestational age (AGA) fetus.

Temporal classification of HDP with an abrupt switch at 34 weeks of gestation does not accommodate these two mainstream physio-pathological conditions determined by the placenta and the mother, nor accommodate different maternal cardiovascular adaptations that are associated with HDP-IUGR fetuses and HDP-AGA fetuses.

Can the Temporal Model of Preeclampsia Fit the Clinical Phenotypes of this Syndrome

At eight thirty a.m., after a preliminary stabilization of a severely symptomatic hypertensive crisis in the emergency department, a Cesarean section was performed on a multiparous woman, 34 years old, with a body mass index (BMI) of 31, who had been oliguric in the last day and a half, at 31+2 weeks of gestation. A female newborn baby of 1760 gr. (approximately 60th percentile of local standards) was delivered in good condition; the Apgar score was 9 at 5 minutes. Uterine arteries Doppler velocimetry had been reported normal at first trimester screening, at 20 weeks of gestation, and at admission. Pregnancy had been reported as uneventful until 28 weeks of gestation, the time of her last visit at the low-risk outpatient clinic.

On the same day, in the same labor and delivery unit, a preeclamptic nulliparous woman, 25 years old with a BMI of 24, at 37+4 weeks of gestation was delivered by Cesarean section for persistent ACOG class 2 cardiotocography (CTG) in latent phase of labor, after she had been induced for "late preeclampsia" and intrauterine growth restriction

(IUGR). A male baby of 1820 gr. (approx. the 3rd centile of local standard) was delivered; the Apgar score was 8 at 5 minutes. She had been admitted directly from the outpatient clinic, on the occasion of her scheduled visit 12 days after the diagnosis of mild IUGR that had been done at 35 weeks of gestation. The diagnosis of IUGR was based on the combination of an abdominal circumference <5th centile for gestation and uterine artery Doppler pulsatility index >95th centile and a normal brachial blood pressure.

This narrative describes two clinical scenarios that frequently occur in any obstetric unit worldwide, and that do not have citizenship in the temporal model so far adopted to classify preeclampsia.

In science, for a model to be applicable, beyond being elegant, it should accommodate as few exceptions as possible and explain with the same principles the whole of the natural phenomena and allow to predict future observations [1]. As described above, that is probably not the case with the temporal model of classification of preeclampsia. Early-onset preeclampsia is supposed to be "more" frequently associated with early shallow trophoblastic invasion [2], detectable by abnormal uterine arteries Doppler velocimetry [3], and consequently associated with IUGR. This clinical phenotype usually occurs with the first pregnancy. Late-onset preeclampsia is more frequently associated with maternal pre-existing risk factors for endothelial and cardiovascular dysfunction that sum up to low-grade inflammation [4] and decidual lesions due to pregnancy and/or pre-existing dyslipidemia [5] until the traditional clinical signs are observed: high blood pressure and proteinuria (though not always).

Notes on Epidemiology of Preeclampsia and Hypertensive Disorders of Pregnancy

A clinical or epidemiological observer living in Western Europe or in the rich states of the USA is very likely to affirm that early-onset preeclampsia is the most severe form, whereas late preeclampsia or gestational hypertension (GH), which are by far more frequent, are the least severe forms of this syndrome. The tenets of an observer sitting somewhere in South America could be quite the opposite. In 2000, Conde-Agudelo [6] reported an epidemiological survey on more than 800,000 women from 700 hospitals in South America: the observed prevalence of preeclampsia was 4.8% and the mean gestational age at delivery was 38 weeks (±3) vs. 39 (±2) in the uneventful pregnancies. Women developing preeclampsia were older, with a higher BMI, higher prevalence of gestational diabetes and previous hypertension – all factors that conjure to design a background of metabolic syndrome (or, according to Baschat, cardiovascular and metabolic individual risk profile [7]). From this and other epidemiological reports from "developing" countries we can understand why preeclampsia associated to these risk factors is one of the main causes of pregnant women's death worldwide, as reported by WHO analysis of causes of maternal death in 2011 [8]. The phenotype of preeclampsia associated to these risk factors is quite different from the form of preeclampsia that we tend to consider as early-onset preeclampsia, as described by Steegers [2].

In countries were pregnancy is not only valued, but assisted by prenatal screening programs, high blood pressure is usually identified prior to the development of severe complications, therapy and rest are prescribed, and near-term delivery is usually induced, minimizing the risk for the mother and the fetus.

In poor countries, or in rich countries without health care programs for mother-to-be and without maternity-leave provision, women are referred late to hospital, only when symptoms arrive (such as headache, severe oliguria or worse seizures). This is why the two clinical observers described as sitting in different countries perceived such a different epidemiology.

Preeclampsia Beyond Maternal Medicine Only, into the Maternal-fetal Medicine (MFM) World

The plentiful exceptions and failures in epidemiology, prediction, diagnosis and treatment of temporal classification of preeclampsia and other HDPs induced many scholars to warn that preeclampsia is a syndrome and not a progression of a single disease of different severity, as supported by some [9], and that to overcome present deadlocks prospective studies should be designed to include all clinical characteristics of the syndrome [10]. This message was sent out, hopefully, to disentangle the syndrome and come up with well-ordered different diseases, although with common tertiary downstream pathways in the mother, as already observed in the nineteenth century: the high blood pressure and foamy urines. A key factor, to distinguish among the clinical phenotypes, was the introduction of the fetus in the evaluation of preeclampsia, as proposed by the CoLab group in their consensus paper [10] and by a group of scholars into clinical guidelines [11]. Eventually, fetal medicine was added to what had been for decades apparently a maternal medicine problem only, and with the fetus the different placental pathologies are taken into consideration and the appropriate diagnostic tools that can be added to the traditional sphygmomanometer and dipstick.

If, for the classification of preeclampsia and other HDPs, we consider also the fetal condition and different placental pathologies that are associated with IUGR fetuses, or appropriate-for-gestational-age fetuses (AGAf), then it might be possible to redesign a model that accommodates the physio-pathology and not "simply" the calendar date at clinical onset of hypertension and proteinuria. If the mother-to-be is properly investigated in the first trimester for her risk profile (placental or cardiovascular-metabolic, or both) then the epidemiological description will no longer be confused by a different local case-mix of different clinical phenotypes and the objectives of predictive tests and prevention programs could be tailored on completely different interventions.

Prediction of Preeclampsia in the "MFM World"

A seminal paper by Oliveira et al. [12] proved that predictive algorithms applied to different populations underperform compared to the original prospective studies (Table 20.1). In this study, a prospective cohort of 3,422 women had been recruited in the Baltimore metropolitan area, where obesity is up to 36% [32]. The mean BMI was around 30, which means that 75% of women were overweight, obese or severely obese. The risk factors for metabolic syndrome (cardiovascular and diabetogenic) embedded in this population were not comparable with those of populations on which the original models were developed. In fact, for example, the model by Scazzochio was developed in the metropolitan area of Barcelona, where the mean BMI of recruited woman was 24 (Table 20.1). These observations had been the background for additional research on predictive models by the same group [7]. Adjusted proportional distribution of individual

Table 20.1 Observed and reported sensitivity of different models developed on European populations when applied to populations affected by obesity epidemics [12]. To further prove the role of obesity on prevalence of HDP-AGAf fetuses in women affected by metabolic syndrome, the only model which proved to work was the one developed by Odibo [31] in Louisiana, with a female obesity epidemic affecting 37% of the population.

Reference	Sensitivity (%) at fixed 10% FPR	
	Reported	Observed
Early preeclampsia		
Parra-Cordero	47	29
Scazzocchio	81	43
Poon	89	53
Poon	95	52
Odibo	68	80
Caradeux	63	30
Late preeclampsia		
Parra-Cordero	29	18
Scazzocchio	40	31

variables that increase the risk for preeclampsia were calculated based on seven major published predictive studies. At the top of the individual risk factors, apparently by contradiction, were the BMI (cardiovascular and metabolic risk factors due to maternal low-grade inflammation) and the uterine arteries Doppler velocimetry (early abnormal placental vascular development).

If this information is included in a model in which the temporal domain is ousted, it could be eventually be acknowledged that small placentas deriving from shallow trophoblastic invasion which are the cause of IUGR and that are detectable by uterine arteries Doppler velocimetry in the first trimester do not end at 33+6 weeks of gestation. Similarly, obesity and its metabolic impact on endothelium and placental dysfunction do not ignite their inflammatory role only at and beyond 34+0 weeks of gestation. Indeed, these findings were used by Baschat to address the problem of individual risk factors, and five risk profiles were proposed: "personal, placental, cardiovascular, metabolic and prothrombotic." One might challenge the appropriateness of the basket of "personal risk factors" or "prothrombotic risk factors" that had been studied for decades now, with controversial association with preeclampsia and IUGR. Yet, the idea that there exists a placental risk factor and a maternal metabolic syndrome risk factor (cardiovascular and metabolic are part of the metabolic syndrome and probably do not need further partition) perfectly suits a model based on preeclampsia associated with shallow trophoblastic invasion and IUGR, and preeclampsia substantially associated with maternal risk factors acutely blown up by placental oxidative stress due to placenta villi overcrowding [4] and decidual lesions associated with maternal low-grade inflammation and dyslipidemia [5] with AGA fetuses. We could make these brief remarks even more critical if we consider the fact that the same predictive tests that are significantly associated with early preeclampsia are also good predictors of IUGR without clinical maternal hypertension [13].

Predicting Early Preeclampsia or IUGR Preeclampsia?

In our recent prospective study, in an unselected cohort of 4,290 women examined in the first trimester, the model based on uterine arteries Doppler velocimetry performed better in predicting IUGR-preeclampsia (area under the receiver operating curve [AUC] 0,84) than early preeclampsia (AUC 0,71, p<0.0001) in the gestational period from 25 to 40 weeks (Figure n 1) [14]. The better prediction of uterine arteries Doppler velocimetry of women that will develop IUGR-preeclampsia from 25 weeks of gestation to term was observed in spite of the fact that the most "severe" cases occurred, as expected, prior to 34 weeks of gestation. However, additional cases of IUGR-preeclampsia were identified that occurred beyond 34 weeks of gestation. In fact, according to the temporal classification, the "early" group (<34 weeks of gestation) included a mixture of cases with IUGR-preeclampsia and AGAf-preeclampsia. The latter had a normal uterine arteries Doppler velocimetry in the first trimester, thereby lowering the predictive values of the model based on temporal classification.

In a subset of this cohort, additional items of maternal history and central aortic pressure were collected and included in the predictive model. The BMI (23 vs. 21; p<0.05), the family history of hypertension (60% vs. 40%; p<0.05) and the mean aortic and brachial pressure (81 mmHg, and 85 mmHg, vs. 72 mmHg and 77 mmHg, respectively; p<0.01) were significantly higher in women who later developed AGAf-preeclampsia than in uncomplicated pregnancies. There were no significant differences of these first trimester parameters between IUGR-preeclampsia and uncomplicated pregnancies.

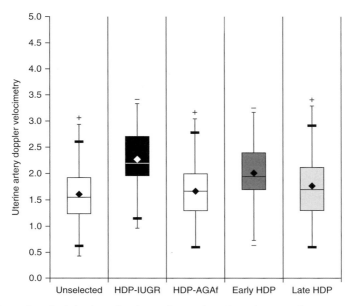

Figure 20.1 Uterine Doppler Pulsatility Index observed in unselected populations and in women affected by HDP. Observed values in cases were analyzed and compared with unaffected women according the temporal and physic-pathological classification. The only significant difference (p<0.01) was observed between unselected cases and HDP-IUGR [14].

Clinical Diagnosis of Different Phenotypes of Hypertensive Disorders of Pregnancy

There is growing evidence that when the two partners of the disease, the mother and the fetus (the placenta being just a transient intrauterine organ of the fetus), are considered with equal worth, then we can try to make sense of a puzzling condition, as vividly summarized in the introduction of the seminal paper by Redman and co-workers [4]:

> pre-eclampsia is associated with poor placentation and incomplete remodelling of the uteroplacental spiral arteries. However … poor placentation may occur with IUGR without features of pre-eclampsia or with partial features such as PIH … However FGR is not a consistent feature of pre-eclampsia being confined largely to the early onset syndrome. In pre-eclampsia, at or beyond term, neonates are not growth restricted and may even be large for date.

These key remarks underline a possible different way to interrogate preeclampsia. First of all, the name itself might be challenged. Eclampsia has become so rare that in medical parlance the prefix "pre" has lost its original meaning as a warning to identify a disease that precedes eclampsia ("pre" from the latin "prae": before in time). Proteinuria is no longer either a prognostic factor or a unique diagnostic criterion, hence it might be more appropriate to use the definition of Hypertensive Disorder of Pregnancy and, when appropriate, to articulate the main functions and organ damages associated with the hypertensive disorder that so far remain the only common denominator.

The Placenta

Preeclampsia – or more broadly, HDP – is determined by the placenta, whatever be its lesions and its downstream effects. Once the placenta is removed and its microparticles later disappear from the maternal circulation, preeclampsia ebbs away, although sometimes there might be residual permanent organ damage.

Placenta pathology is of great help in the partition of HDP. The most widely known placental lesion derives from an abnormal shallow trophoblastic invasion, poor and patchy changes of the spiral arteries, a small placenta with fewer and poorly branched terminal villi [3], and syncithio trophoblast oxidative (STB) stress. More recently, pathological description of placental lesions proved, opposite to this, an increased terminal villi branching with a relative reduction and under-perfusion of the intervillous space [15–17] resulting in a similar STB stress. The former placental lesion is associated with IUGR fetuses, and the latter with AGA fetuses.

In agreement with the two patterns of placental lesions, during an interim analysis of placental lesions classified according to Redline into maternal vascular supply lesions (the extrinsic placental lesions) and fetal vascular supply lesions, we observed in 15 cases of HDP-IUGR and in 10 cases of HDP-AGAf a highly significant association of the former group with maternal vascular supply lesions, and of the latter group with fetal vascular supply lesions, namely villi immaturity and excessive branching restricting intervillous perfusion (Figure 20.2).

Doppler Velocimetry of Uterine Arteries

Doppler velocimetry of the uterine arteries is now widely accepted as a useful proxy of placental vascular damage and abnormal release of vasoreactive mediators, caused by early shallow trophoblastic invasion [3]. Its bedside use has proved valuable to identify a possible

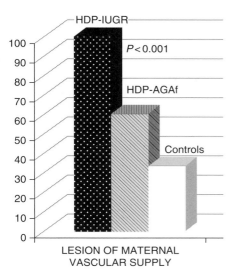

Figure 20.2 Placental lesions associated with HDP-IUGR and with HDO-AGAf. Maternal vascular supply according to Redline classification [16] includes, among others: superficial implantation/decidual arteriopathy, undergrowth/distal villous hypoplasia, increased syncytial knots, agglutination, intervillous fibrin and villous infarction.

dual etiology, at least as regards late HDPs [18]. Indeed, uterine blood flow volume measurements might add interesting information to the simple waveform analysis [19]. In our previous studies, we proved that pregnant women with an abnormal uterine arterial waveform at midgestation, that delivered at term of AGA newborns, had an absolute blood flow volume of uterine arteries at 30 weeks of gestation (105 ml/min/kg; i.q.r.: 82–135) that was halfway between that of pregnancies with an abnormal uterine Doppler velocimetry, delivered of IUGR fetuses (81ml/min/kg; i.q.r. 67–134) and those delivered of AGA fetuses with a normal uterine arterial waveform at midgestation (193ml/min/kg; i.q.r.144–260). These findings add experimental evidence that abnormal findings on uterine arteries Doppler velocimetry are a good proxy of abnormal uterine arteries blood flow volume, even in those cases considered to be false positives of the test. Figure 20.3 shows the absolute values observed in these three groups.

The Fetus

The fetus is ideally the best target for the definition of IUGR or appropriate-for-gestational-age fetal growth. Obviously there is a difference between the criteria to define a small-for-gestational-age newborn (all newborns delivered prematurely) and an IUGR fetus. A seminal paper by Marconi and Battaglia clearly highlighted this difference [21]. Figure 20.4 shows how a significant share of fetuses with a strict diagnosis of IUGR were then classified as AGA according to local newborn weight standards.

However, a common universal criterion to "close" the diagnosis of IUGR is still missing. It is very likely that the abdominal circumference according to local standard or universal reference standard [20] when below the 5th percentile associated with a complementary finding such as an abnormal uterine Doppler velocimetry might satisfy the diagnosis of a growth-restricted fetus; even more prudent is a criterion of an abdominal circumference below the 10th percentile with an abnormal umbilical Doppler velocimetry.

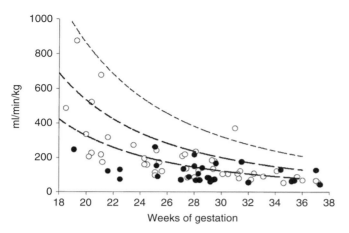

Figure 20.3 Uterine blood flow volume (ml7min/kg) in control pregnant women (dotted lines: 10th, 50th and 90th centile), in cases with abnormal Uterine Doppler Velocimetry delivered of IUGR newborns (full circles), and delivered of AGA newborns (empty circles) [19].

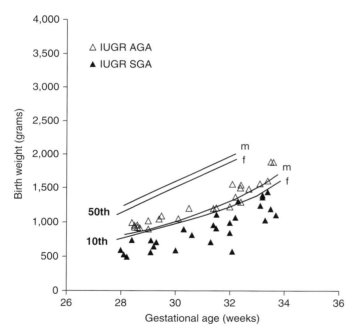

Figure 20.4 Newborn weight plotted versus the 50th and 10th centile for females and males newborns according to local standards. All newborns (triangles) had been diagnosed to be IUGR according to abnormal Umbilical artery pulsatility index and abdominal circumference below the 5th centile. Empty triangles = IUGR fetuses diagnosed as AGA newborns according to newborn weight standards. Full triangles IUGR = fetuses diagnosed as SGA newborns [21].

The Mother

Since the late 2010s [22] to recent studies [23], data has shown that "early" and "late" preeclampsia had different maternal cardiovascular maladaptations to pregnancy. In a nutshell, the idea was that early preeclampsia is associated with low cardiac output and high total vascular peripheral resistance. In a brilliant recent overview of maternal cardiovascular adaptation, Melchiorre, Sharma and Tilanghanathan [24] described the preclinical phase of preeclampsia as follows:

In the preclinical phase of preeclampsia, vascular reactivity, hemodynamic indices, and left ventricular (LV) properties are subtly impaired, especially in those women destined to develop preterm preeclampsia (Level 2 evidence). At midgestation, there is a shift toward a low cardiac index associated with a high total vascular resistance index, increased mean arterial pressure, contracted intravascular volume, and reduced venous reserve capacity (Level 2). In contrast, the hemodynamic profile of women destined to develop late-onset preeclampsia is not well delineated, with some authors reporting a normal cardiac index and increased total vascular resistance index at midgestation, and others reporting a high cardiac output/ low TVR status.

The confusing factor we point to in studies on so-called "late-onset preeclampsia" is that these include a large percentage of less severe HDP-IUGR cases that blur the picture of cardiovascular adaptation, since it is obvious that the occurrence of HDP associated with IUGR (and its typical placental disease, and possibly different maternal adaptation) do not end abruptly at 34 weeks of gestation.

The other debated hypothesis regards the different criteria adopted to test cardiac performance: cardiac output or cardiac index – cardiac output normalized for BMI or body surface. This second approach assumes that uterus placenta and fetus can be equalized to fat tissue. This is obviously not the case, since the fat tissue, visceral and subcutaneous, absorbs a negligible percentage of cardiac output – the opposite of the fetoplacental unit that drains up to 20% of cardiac output. These observations might be further confused by the prevalence of obesity and metabolic syndrome in the population examined. For instance, the HUNT studies from Norway observed that "These results suggest that the positive association of preeclampsia and gestational hypertension with post-pregnancy cardiovascular risk factors may be due largely to shared prepregnancy risk factors rather than reflecting a direct influence of the hypertensive disorder in pregnancy" [25]. A survey performed in a population affected by obesity epidemics concluded the opposite [26].

In our studies on the cardiovascular adaptation of the mother we analyzed the findings by taking into account the two different classifications: the temporal classification, and the one based on clinical phenotypes (the association of HDP with IUGR or with AGA fetuses diagnosed according to fetal biometry and uterine arteries Doppler velocimetry). When the behavior of maternal cardiovascular indices are observed according to these two classifications, in a population not affected by obesity epidemics, then the difference between women affected by HDP-IUGR and HDP-AGAf becomes quite clear, as shown in Figure 20.5. These findings are in agreement with recent findings on the abnormal diastolic function and different behavior of the venous compartment [27] in different phenotypes of HDP. Even a more sophisticated approach, such as the analysis of the autonomic control of the heart-rate variability by the means of the Phase Rectified Signal averaging (PRSA)[28], showed a significant difference between mothers affected by HDP-IUGR and controls, but not between mothers with HDP-AGA and controls (Figure 20.6).

Bedside Criteria to Differentiate HDP-IUGR and HDP-AGAf

The two ultrasound criteria briefly described above – fetal abdominal circumference and uterine arteries Doppler velocimetry – can be easily used at the bedside of a pregnant woman affected by high blood pressure to ascertain which woman is suffering the consequences of endothelial abnormal reactivity associated with a small placenta, such as from the first trimester shallow trophoblastic invasion, or who is suffering from endothelial

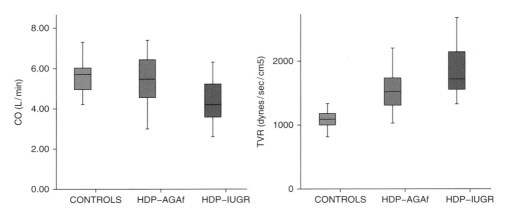

Figure 20.5 E/a diastolic ratio and cardiac output in women affected by HDP classified according to the physio-pathologic phenotypes (p<0.05). (A black and white version of this figure will appear in some formats. For the color version, please refer to the plate section.)

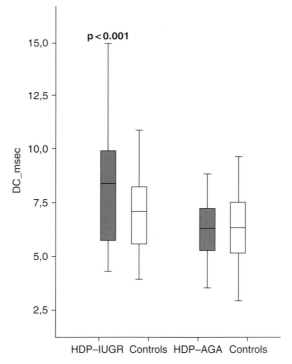

Figure 20.6 PRSA analysis of deceleration capacity of maternal heart rate in women affected by HDP–IUGR and HDP–AGAf from 26–37 weeks of gestation compared with matched controls. A significant difference in the index of autonomic heart rate variability was observed only in women affected by HDP–IUGR vs. their matched controls [28].

dysfunction with a normal grown placenta with normal impedance to uterine flow and an AGA fetus. It is very likely that these two conditions require different surveillance of the fetus, and different therapies and supportive interventions for the mothers-to-be, as we will speculate in the next paragraph.

In a large retrospective study on HDPs [29], we tested the hypothesis that these two criteria alone, when coherently associated in the same pregnant patient or when both absent, could differentiate the two different physio-pathological conditions as regards placental nutritional/vascular function. Figure 20.7 shows how the criteria adopted to classify women affected by HDP with AGA fetuses yielded a mean birthweight centile with a growth curve close to that of local reference neonates. This proved that newborns from mothers with AGAf are not just a group of "less small" fetuses, as one could have also expected from the criteria of selection of the abdominal circumference above the 5th centile. In addition to this, we observed that regardless of the temporal cut-off, women with preeclampsia and GH delivered AGA and IUGR fetuses, before and after 34 weeks of gestation.

Conclusions

A careful reconstruction of possible physio-pathological pathways of different clinical phenotypes of preeclampsia could allow modeling of tailored predicting strategies, better prevention interventions, and overcome the present deadlock in therapy of preeclampsia or even HDP.

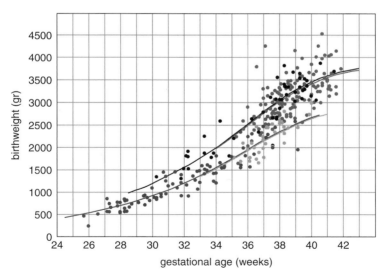

Figure 20.7 Birthweight as a function of gestational age at delivery in HDP-AGAf and HDP-IUGR groups with early (34 weeks of gestation) or late (≥34 weeks of gestation) gestational age at diagnosis [29].
Dark green dots and line: birthweight in HDP-AGAf group <34, and fitted curve.
Light green dots and line: birthweight in HDP-AGAf group ≥ 34, and fitted curve.
Dark red dots and line: birthweight in HDP-IUGR group <34, and fitted curve.
Light red dots and line: birthweight in HDP-IUGR group ≥ 34, and fitted curve.
(A black and white version of this figure will appear in some formats. For the color version, please refer to the plate section.)

We still read from an extraordinary authoritative body (Report of the American National High Blood Pressure Education Program Working Group (NHBPEPWG) on High Blood Pressure in Pregnancy, 2000) that labetalol and hydralazine are equipollent drugs for the treatment of PE, where one has a predominantly peripheral vaso-dilatatory action and the other has a combined blocking effect on alpha-beta adrenergic receptors. HDP-AGAf or a large share of "late PE" is associated with low peripheral vascular resistance, which gives reason to use hydralazine, a peripheral vasodilator. Or why not adopt an alpha-beta blocking drug to treat hypertensive women with a low cardiac output?

If HDP-AGAf with different placental pathology were to become a proven disease by itself, then a more preventive and therapeutic strategy could be tailored addressing each one of the risk factors that might lead to its clinical expression, such as cardiovascular risk factors, low-grade inflammation caused by visceral fat, increased abdominal venous pressure, abnormal pro-inflammatory intestinal microbiota associated with obesity, pre-existing endothelial dysfunction, etc.

Similarly, if women affected by HDP-IUGR were assessed all along gestation and not censored at 34 weeks of gestation, preventive and therapeutic interventions more focused on original early vascular placental oxidative stress and immune dysregulation could be studied [30], hopefully in the near future.

When these two different diagnoses are well defined, their overlapping and their relative contribute to single clinical cases can be considered to include all phenotypes of this syndrome.

Key Points

- Experimental, observational and epidemiological data suggest that two different types of preeclampsia, the so-called placental and maternal types, coexist and have different pathophysiologic background mechanisms.
- From the clinical point of view, it makes sense to classify preeclampsia according to type-specific cardiovascular characteristics, rather than the currently used classifications of early and late-onset preeclampsia.
- The relevance of an alternative classification system is to be determined in future research.

References

1. Hawking S, Mlodinow L. The Grand Design. In *What is Reality*. Bantam Books, USA. 2010.

2. Steegers EA, Dadelszen von P, Duvekot JJ, Pijnenborg R. Pre-eclampsia. *The Lancet*. 2010;**376**:631–44.

3. Burton GJ, Woods AW, Jauniaux E, Kingdom JCP. Rheological and physiological consequences of conversion of the maternal spiral arteries for uteroplacental blood flow during human pregnancy. *Placenta*. 2010;**30**:473–82.

4. Redman CW, Sargent IL, Staff AC. IFPA Senior Award Lecture: Making sense of pre-eclampsia. *Placenta*. 2014;**35**: S20–5.

5. Staff AC, Redman CWG. IFPA Award in Placentology Lecture: Preeclampsia, the decidual battleground and future maternal cardiovascular disease. *Placenta*. 2014;**35**: S26–S31.

6. Conde-Agudelo A, Belizán JM. Risk factors for pre-eclampsia in a large cohort of Latin American and Caribbean women. *BJOG*. 2000;**107**:75–83.

7. Baschat AA. First-trimester screening for pre-eclampsia: moving from personalized risk prediction to prevention. *Ultrasound Obstet Gynecol.* 2015;45:119–29.

8. Khan KS, Wojdyla D, Say L, Gulmezoglu AM, Van Look PF. WHO analysis of causes of maternal death: a systematic review. *Lancet.* 2005;367: 1066–74.

9. Akolekar R, Syngelaki A, Poon L, Wright D, Nicolaides KH. Competing risks model in early screening for preeclampsia by biophysical and biochemical markers. *Fetal Diagn Ther.* 2013;33:8–15.

10. Myatt L, Redman CW, Staff AC, Hansson S. Strategy for standardization of preeclampsia research study design. *Hypertension.* 2014;6332(6):1293–301.

11. Magee L, Pels A, Helewa M, Rey E, Dadelszen von P. Diagnosis, evaluation, and management of the hypertensive disorders of pregnancy: *Executive Summary. J Obstet Gynaecol Can.* 2014;307: 416–38.

12. Oliveira N, Magder LS, Blitzer MG, Baschat AA. First-trimester prediction of pre-eclampsia: external validity of algorithms in a prospectively enrolled cohort. *Ultrasound Obstet Gynecol.* 2014;44:279–85.

13. Poon LCY, Syngelaki A, Akolekar R, Lai J, Nicolaides KH. Combined screening for preeclampsia and small for gestational age at 11–13 weeks. *Fetal Diagn Ther.* 2013;33:16–27.

14. Stampalija T, Monasta L, Di Martino DD, Quadrifoglio M, Lo Bello L, D'Ottavio G, Zullino S, Mastroianni C, Casati D, Signorelli V, Rosti E, Cecotti V, Ceccarello M, Ferrazzi E. The association of first trimester uterine arteries Doppler velocimetry with different clinical phenotypes of hypertensive disorders of pregnancy: a longitudinal study. J Matern Fetal Neonatal Med. 2017 Nov 20:1–9.

15. Egbor M, Ansari T, Morris N, Green CJ, Sibbons PD. Pre-eclampsia and fetal growth restriction: How morphometrically different is the placenta? *Placenta.* 2006;27 (6–7):727–34.

16. Redline RW. Placental pathology: a systematic approach with clinical correlations. *Placenta.* 2008;29 Suppl A: S86–91.

17. Mayhew TM, Ohadike C, Baker PN, Crocker IP, Mitchell C, Ong SS. Stereological investigation of placental morphology in pregnancies complicated by pre-eclampsia with and without intrauterine growth restriction. *Placenta.* 2003;24(2–3):219–26.

18. Verlohren S, Melchiorre K, Khalil A, Thilaganathan B. Uterine artery Doppler, birth weight and timing of onset of pre-eclampsia: providing insights into the dual etiology of late-onset pre-eclampsia. *Ultrasound Obstet Gynecol* 2014;44(3): 293–8.

19. Ferrazzi E, Rigano S, Padoan A, Boito S, Pennati G, Galan HL. Uterine artery blood flow volume in pregnant women with an abnormal pulsatility index of the uterine arteries delivering normal or intrauterine growth restricted newborns. *Placenta.* 2011 Jul 1;32(7):487–92.

20. Villar J, Cheick ismail L, Victoria CG, Ohuma EOA, Bertino E, Altman DG, et al. International standards for newborn weight, length, and head circumference by gestational age and sex: the Newborn Cross-Sectional Study of the INTERGROWTH-21st Project. *Lancet.* 2014;384: 857–68.

21. Marconi AM, Ronzoni S, Bozzetti P, Vailati S, Morabito A, Battaglia FC. Comparison of Fetal and Neonatal Growth Curves in Detecting Growth Restriction. *Obstet Gynecol.* 2008;112: 1227–34.

22. Valensise H, Vasapollo B, Gagliardi G, Novelli GP. Early and Late Preeclampsia: Two Different Maternal Hemodynamic States in the Latent Phase of the Disease. *Hypertension.* 2008;52: 873–80.

23. Gyselaers W, Mullens W, Tomsin K, Mesens T, Peeters L. Role of dysfunctional maternal venous hemodynamics in the pathophysiology of pre-eclampsia: a review. *Ultrasound Obstet and Gynecol.* 2011;38:123–9.

24. Melchiorre K, Sharma R, Thilaganathan B. Cardiovascular implications in preeclampsia: an overview. *Circulation.* 2014;**130**:703–14.

25. Romundstad PR, Magnussen EB, Smith GD, Vatten LJ. Hypertension in pregnancy and later cardiovascular risk: common antecedents? *Circulation.* 2010;**122**:579–84.

26. Lisonkova S, Joseph KS. Incidence of preeclampsia: risk factors and outcomes associated with early- versus late-onset disease. *Am J Obstet Gynecol* 2013;**209**:544–e12.

27. Gyselaers W. Hemodynamics of the maternal venous compartment: a new area to explore in obstetric ultrasound imaging. *Ultrasound Obstet Gynecol.* 2008;**32**:716–7.

28. Stampalija T, Casati D, Ferrazzi E. et al. Maternal Cardiac Deceleration Capacity: a novel way to explore maternal autonomic function in pregnancies complicated by hypertensive disorders and intrauterine growth restriction. *Eur J Obstet Gynecol Reprod Biol..* 2016; **206**:6–11.

29. Ferrazzi E, Zullino S, Stampalija T, et al. Bedside diagnosis of two major clinical phenotypes of hypertensive disorders of pregnancy. *Ultrasound Obstet Gynecol.* 2016;**48**(2):224–31.

30. Ferrazzi E, Muggiasca M, Gervasi MT. Low molecular weight heparin: does it represent a clinical opportunity for preventing preeclampsia associated with fetal growth restriction? *J Matern Fetal Neonatal Med.* 2015 Sep;**28**(13):1525–9.

31. Odibo AO, Zhong Y, Goetzinger KR, et al. First-trimester placental protein 13, PAPP-A, uterine artery Doppler and maternal characteristics in the prediction of pre-eclampsia. *Placenta.* 2011;**32**(8):598–602.

32. Institute for Health Metrics and Evaluation, US County Profile: Baltimore County, Maryland. Seattle, WA: IHME, 2015

Chapter 21

Chemotherapy and Cardiovascular Function in Pregnancy

Kristel van Calsteren

Summary

In this chapter the occurrence and mechanisms of chemotherapy-induced cardiotoxicity are discussed, together with the maternal and fetal cardiac problems that are seen when chemotherapy is administered during pregnancy, and cardiac problems that are seen during pregnancy in women that had been treated for cancer before.

Introduction

The problem of cardiovascular problems in pregnancy due to chemotherapy exposure is rather rare. Nevertheless, situations of chemotherapy administration for cancer diagnosed during pregnancy and pregnancies after cancer treatment have occurred in increasing numbers over recent years. Treatment of (childhood) cancer has improved, resulting in more cancer survivors that reach reproductive life and become pregnant. Most frequently seen tumors in children and young women are hematological malignancies, tumors of the central nervous system and breast cancer. Chemotherapy is part of the treatment for all these tumor types. For breast and hematological malignancies the standard chemotherapy schedules contain anthracyclines. Chemotherapy-induced cardiotoxicity is a serious complication that poses a grave threat to life and limits the clinical use of various chemotherapeutic agents, particularly anthracyclines. This cardiotoxicity can present shortly after chemotherapy exposure, but might also become clear only decennia after the cancer treatment.

As extensively discussed in other chapters of this volume, pregnancy is a specific physiologic state associated with significant cardiovascular changes and adaptations resulting in increased cardiac output and workload, and a reduced peripheral vascular resistance. These circulatory adaptations could result in increased sensitivity to cardiovascular side effects of cancer treatments.

Apart from the effect on the maternal heart, chemotherapy exposure during pregnancy can also influence the development of the fetal heart. Cytotoxic treatment is given with the aim of killing tumor cells by interfering with the process of cell division. Since embryological and fetal development is characterized by highly proliferating cells, fetal tissues are more vulnerable to toxic effects of chemotherapy than adult tissues with a low proliferating index.

In this chapter we will discuss the occurrence and mechanisms of chemotherapy-induced cardiotoxicity, even as the cardiac problems that are seen when chemotherapy is administered during pregnancy – for both the mother and the fetus, and cardiac problems that are seen during pregnancy of women that had been treated for cancer before the pregnancy.

Table 21.1 Chemotherapeutic agents associated with cardiotoxicity [1]

Chemotherapeutic agent	Cardiac effect
Anthracycline	Acute (3%): • Left ventricular systolic and/or diastolic dysfunction • Acute heart failure • Arrhythmias • Pericarditis/myocarditis syndrome Chronic (50%): • Subclinical cardiac abnormalities • Congestive Heart Failure
Antimetabolites Capecitabine, Cytarabine, 5-FU Cyclophosphamide	Ischemia (3–68%), pericarditis, thrombophlebitis Heart failure (8–27%), (myo)pericarditis
Antimicrotubule agents Docetaxel Paclitaxel	Heart failure (2–8%), ischemia (0.6–1.5%) Bradycardia (1–31%)
Small molecule tyrosine kinase inhibitors	Heart failure (0.5–1.1%), ischemia (2–3%), hypertension (5–47%), QT prolongation (1–10%)
Monoclonal antibodies Trastuzumab Bevacizumab	Heart failure (2–28%) Heart failure (1.7–3%), ischemia (0.6–1.5%), hypertension (4–35%)

Different chemotherapeutic agents have been associated with cardiotoxic effects. Best known are the anthracyclines, but antimetabolites, antimicrotubule agents and targeted therapy agents are also known to cause cardiac damage (Table 21.1) [1]. The cardiovascular complications that have been described are heart failure, hypertension, arrhythmia, (myo) pericarditis, ischemic lesions and thrombo-embolic complications (Table 21.1) [1].

The mechanisms involved in the induction of cardiac dysfunction are various. Since anthracyclines are widely used and are clearly associated with cardiac side effects, the cardiac effects of this drug group have been examined extensively. We discuss the mechanisms of chemotherapy-induced hypertension shortly.

Anthracycline-induced Cardiotoxicity

Anthracycline exposure has been associated with both acute and chronic cardiotoxicity [2].

Of all patients receiving anthracycline-containing chemotherapy, 3% will develop acute cardiotoxic effects, consisting of left ventricular systolic and/or diastolic dysfunction, arrhythmias, pericarditis/myocarditis syndrome and myocardial necrosis leading to dilated cardiomyopathy and acute heart failure.

The chronic cardiotoxicity which has been described after anthracycline exposure consists of two groups. First, patients with subclinical cardiac abnormalities including reduced left ventricular mass and contractility; thirty years after chemotherapy exposure, this is seen in 50% of the patients. The second group reveals progressive myofibrillar loss and degeneration of the left ventricular cardiomyocytes leading to congestive heart failure.

Thirty years after chemotherapy exposure, this complication is seen in 7.5% of patients receiving more than 250 mg/m^2 anthracyclines.[2] For comparison, the incidence of heart failure in the general population aged between 25 and 45 years is estimated around 0.02 per 1,000.

In 2009, Mulrooney et al. performed a retrospective cohort study including 14,358 five-year survivors of childhood cancer in the USA [2]. Main outcome measures were the incidence of and risk factors for congestive heart failure, myocardial infarction, pericardial disease and valvular abnormalities in survivors of cancer compared with siblings. The data were collected based on a questionnaire that was completed by the patients or their parents. This study showed that survivors of cancer were significantly more likely than siblings to report congestive heart failure (hazard ratio (HR) 5.9, 95% confidence interval 3.4 to 9.6; P<0.001), myocardial infarction (HR 5.0, 95% CI 2.3 to 10.4; P<0.001), pericardial disease (HR 6.3, 95% CI 3.3 to 11.9; P<0.001), or valvular abnormalities (HR 4.8, 95% CI 3.0 to 7.6; P<0.001). Exposure to 250 mg/m^2 or more of anthracyclines increased the relative hazard of congestive heart failure, pericardial disease and valvular abnormalities by two to five times compared with survivors who had not been exposed to anthracyclines. The cumulative incidence of adverse cardiac outcomes in cancer survivors continued to increase up to 30 years after diagnosis [2].

Risk factors for developing cardiac problems after anthracycline exposure are a higher cumulative dose, a higher C_{max}, concomitant radiation therapy involving heart region (vascular injury, endothelial dysfunction), female sex, younger age at diagnosis, longer time of follow up, black ethnicity, Trisomy 21, pre-existing cardiac risk factors (diabetes, obesity, renal failure, congenital heart disease) and additional treatment with amasacrine, trastuzumab, cyclophosphamide, bleomycin, vincristine or different anthracycline derivates [2, 3].

For example, the risk of developing heart failure and asymptomatic decline in systolic function after exposure to trastuzumab is around 4% [4], but increases to up to 25% when trastuzumab is administered concurrently with or shortly after anthracycline treatment [5].

Studies have shown that multiple mechanisms are involved in anthracycline-induced cardiotoxicity, including oxidative damage, changes in calcium metabolism and activation of apoptotic pathways [3, 6]. Cell death results in a decreased number of myocardial cells and an increased loading on surviving muscle cells. Also, the normal cardiac repair mechanisms are affected by anthracycline exposure and there is a depletion of cardiac stem cells. These effects influence the function of the surviving cells and can cause a progressive deterioration in cardiac function.

Chemotherapy-induced Hypertension

The incidence of de novo hypertension induced by Vascular Endothelial Growth Factor (VEGF) inhibitors is 17–80%, by alkylating agents 36% and by DNA methylation inhibitors 8–9%. Moreover, patients treated with chemotherapy also receive co-medication, such as steroids and erythropoietin, that are also associated with induction of hypertension [7]. Underlying mechanisms are shown in Table 21.2.

Pregnancy is a specific physiologic state associated with major hemodynamic adaptations resulting in increased cardiac output and workload, and therefore requires some cardiac reserve capacity. Echocardiographic measurements show an important increase in

Table 21.2 Mechanisms of drug induced hypertension [7]

Chemotherapeutic agent	Blood pressure increasing mechanism
VEGF inhibitors (e.g. bevacizumab)	– Increased vascular tone due to the decrease in nitric oxide production (no smooth muscle relaxation) – Increased peripheral resistance due to VEGF inhibitor induced endothelial damage and dysfunction
Alkylating agents (e.g. cyclophosphamide, ifosfamide)	– Renal endothelial damage leading to delayed hypertension and microalbuminuria – Endothelial dysfunction leading to spasm
Erythropoietin	– Vasopressor action – Rise in blood viscosity and correction of anemia – Changes in production or sensitivity to endogenous vasopressors – Alterations in vascular smooth-muscle ionic milieu – Dysregulation of production or responsiveness to endogenous vasodilatory factors – Arterial remodeling through stimulation of vascular cell growth
Steroids	– Increase in blood pressure through mineralocorticoid receptor activation – Increased sodium and blood volume, hypokalemia with metabolic alkalosis, and suppressed plasma renin and aldosterone levels – Increased vascular sensitivity to circulating vasoactive amines

left ventricular mass index. These circulatory changes require a cardiac reserve capacity before getting pregnant and could result in increased sensitivity to cardiovascular side effects of cancer treatments administered during pregnancy.

When chemotherapy is administered in pregnancy several aspects need to be considered, namely pharmacokinetics of chemotherapeutic agents in pregnant women, and maternal and fetal cardiovascular effects of chemotherapy exposure in pregnancy.

Pharmacokinetics of Chemotherapy in Pregnant Women

Apart from the cardiac adaptations mentioned before, during pregnancy the total body water and plasma volume increases with 50%, glomerular filtration rate increases by 40%, hepatic metabolism changes and the body fat mass increases till 30% [8, 9]. This results in lower drug plasma levels, which is important because (side)effects of chemotherapy are related to the C_{max} and Area Under the Curve (AUC).

A study comparing pharmacokinetics characteristics of chemotherapeutic agents in pregnant and nonpregnant women reveals a lower peak plasma concentration and AUC and an increased distribution volume in pregnancy for all tested agents (doxorubicin, epirubicin, paclitaxel, docetaxel) [10, 11]. This finding would suggest that higher drug dosages should be prescribed to pregnant women than to nonpregnant women. On the other hand, we know that the risk of toxic effects –for both the mother and the fetus – increases with higher C_{max} and cumulative drug dose.

As current data do not show a worse maternal outcome for women treated with chemotherapy during pregnancy at standard dose (based on BSA) [12–14], international guidelines advise to use standard dosed chemotherapy [15, 16].

Maternal Cardiovascular Effects of Chemotherapy Administered During Pregnancy

In women with established cardiac disease, the physiologic changes associated with late pregnancy and labor may cause cardiac decompensation. Even so, the impact of chemotherapy in pregnancy might be higher, seen increased hemodynamic loading in pregnancy.

Nevertheless, in the current literature there is no mention of an increased frequency of heart failure, left ventricular dysfunction or hypertensive complications when chemotherapy is administered during pregnancy [1, 13, 17, 18]. The data are, however, very limited and different monitoring strategies have been used in different centers. Therefore, close cardiac monitoring remains advisable for these patients.

Fetal Cardiovascular Effects of Prenatal Exposure to Chemotherapy

Maternal illness and cancer treatment during pregnancy can affect fetal development. Current data show an increased risk of congenital malformations after exposure to chemotherapy in the first gestational trimester [18]. When chemotherapy is administered in the second and third trimester, there is an increased risk of fetal growth restriction and preterm birth [17]. These complications have been linked to cardiovascular problems later in life, such as hypertension, higher body fat percentages, waist circumferences, plasma uric acid levels, alanine aminotransferase levels and aspartate transaminase levels [19, 20].

Since anthracyclines are known to induce a dose-related cardiotoxicity in children and adults, the fetal heart could be affected. Fetal myocardium differs from adult myocardium because fetal myocytes are smaller, and typically have a single nucleus compared with the multinuclear cells prevalent after birth. The myocytes also contain fewer sarcomeres per mass unit, and different isoforms of contractile proteins are expressed [21, 22]. Also, the sarcoplasmic reticulum is immature, affecting excitation–contraction coupling and calcium metabolism. The myocytes contain lower numbers of mitochondria and the antioxidant pathways are still underdeveloped. All these factors might make the fetal myocardium more vulnerable to damage by chemotherapeutic agents. There might also be an effect on the fetal stem cell population that might influence cardiac repair mechanisms, but no data are currently available.

There are a few case reports showing fetal cardiac damage after prenatal exposure to anthracyclines. Germann et al. reported on two cases of cardiac dysfunction after prenatal anthracycline exposure, with one fetal death in the third gestational trimester and one reversible heart dysfunction [23]. Achtari and Hohlfield described a case of reversible biventricular dysfunction which normalized 3 days after birth [24]. Reynoso and Huerta reported on one fetal death 3 days after idarubicin administration to the mother [25]. Baumgartner described one reversible cardiac dysfunction at 24 weeks [26]. Mhallem Gziri et al. reported on one case of supraventricular tachycardia at 24 weeks [27].

Meyer-Wittkopf, on the other hand, reported on a case where detailed prenatal and pediatric echocardiographic follow-up was performed after doxorubicin administration in pregnancy, revealing normal cardiac findings at all exams [28].

Yet, patient series (n=26[29] and n=81[30]) examining the short and long-term cardiac outcome after prenatal exposure to anthracyclines do not show an impaired heart function on echocardiography in these children [1, 29–31].

Since the cardiotoxic effect is dose related, this reassuring finding can be explained by the limited transplacental transfer of anthracyclines. Preclinical and ex-vivo placenta perfusion studies showed a transfer rate of 3–7% for doxorubicin and epirubicin [32–34].

Cardiac Problems in Pregnancies of Cancer Survivors

An increasing number of female childhood cancer survivors reach reproductive age and, although infertility often occurs after cancer treatment, a significant number of them will become pregnant. As mentioned earlier, pregnancy includes cardiac stress. In the general population the incidence of peripartum heart failure is estimated to be 1 per 3000–4000 live births (0.03%) [35].

Apart from the increased gender-related risk of developing heart failure, female cancer survivors who have been treated with anthracyclines might be more vulnerable to cardiac decompensation at times of increased cardiac stress, as is seen in pregnancy [36–38].

An example is the case reported by Katz et al. in 1997 of a young woman treated for a large B-cell lymphoma with doxorubicin-containing chemotherapy (cumulative dose of 270 mg/m^2) at the age of 18 years. Two months after finalizing the treatment a normal cardiac function with Left Ventricle Ejection Fraction (LVEF) of 58% was reported. At the age of 28 years she had an uncomplicated pregnancy and delivery. Nevertheless, 3 months postpartum she developed congestive heart failure (Ejection Fraction (EF) 20%). She was treated with loop diuretics and an angiotensin-converting enzyme inhibitor, resulting in a relief of symptoms. However, 12 months later the EF was still 25% [39].

The incidence of heart failure during pregnancy in female cancer survivors treated with anthracyclines has been studied by different groups.

Van Dalen et al. reported in 2006 on the outcome of 53 patients (100 pregnancies) with an average follow-up period of 20.3 years. The mean cumulative anthracycline dose was 267 mg/m^2. Pregnancy ended in miscarriage in 13 cases, abortion in 4 cases and in live birth in 83 cases. There were no peripartum cardiomyopathies registered. Clinical heart failure prior to the pregnancy was documented in 2 cases. The first patient had a normalized Left Ventricle (LV) function after anticongestive therapy was stopped. The second patient stopped medication after 3.5 years with a LV shortening fraction of 27% at that time. She had a full-term pregnancy and vaginal delivery without need for medication. However, 2.5 years after the delivery the symptoms returned (LVSF: 17%) and medication was initiated again [36].

The study of Bar et al. (2003) reported on 37 patients with 72 pregnancies, of which there were 63 deliveries, 6 miscarriages and 3 pregnancy terminations (of which 2 were because of maternal cardiac deterioration) [40]. Division of the patients by a FS cut-off value of 30% showed that the 29 women with FS values of >30% at baseline had no change in cardiac function, whereas the 8 women (22%) with FS values of <30% before the first pregnancy had a nonsignificant deterioration in cardiac function (FS 26% to 21% after last delivery; 19% decrease, P =.08). In the women with FS values of <30%, pregnancy outcome was worse than in those with FS >30%. Two women (5%) were admitted to ICU because of cardiac deterioration. One had pulmonary edema immediately after the first delivery and progressed to severe heart failure after the second delivery. She was subsequently placed on the heart transplantation list. The other patient had congestive heart failure, which resolved after 24 hours in the ICU.

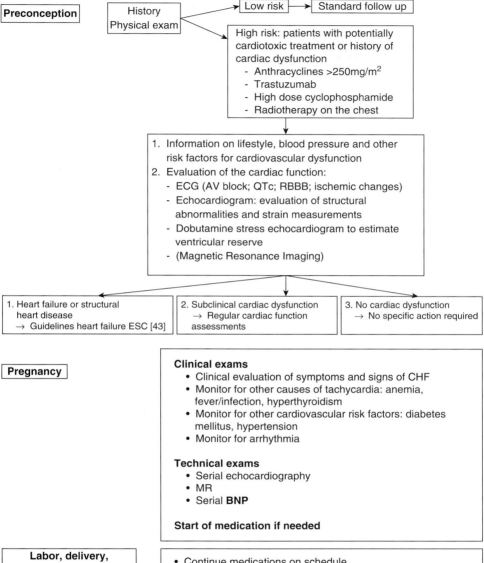

Figure 21.1 Work up for cancer survivors with pregnancy (wish) (adapted from Altena et al. [42])

Recently, Hines et al. performed a retrospective cohort study of female cancer survivors with at least one successful pregnancy [41]. Pregnancy-associated cardiomyopathy was defined as shortening fraction <28% or ejection fraction <50% or treatment for cardiomyopathy during or up to 5 months after completion of pregnancy. Among the 847 female cancer survivors with 1,554 completed pregnancies, only 3 (0.3 %) developed pregnancy-associated cardiomyopathy, and 40 developed nonpregnancy-associated cardiomyopathy either 5 months postpartum (n = 14) or prior to pregnancy (n = 26). Among those with cardiomyopathy prior to pregnancy (n = 26), cardiac function deteriorated during pregnancy in eight patients (three patients with normalization of cardiac function prior to pregnancy, three with persistently abnormal cardiac function, and two for whom resolution of cardiomyopathy was unknown prior to pregnancy). Patients that developed cardiomyopathy received a higher median dose of anthracyclines compared to those that did not (321 versus 164 mg/m^2; p < 0.01).

Based on these studies we can conclude that most female childhood cancer survivors will have no cardiac complications during or after childbirth; however, those with a history of cardiotoxic therapies should be followed carefully during pregnancy and postpartum. Patients with baseline left ventricular dysfunction should be considered at increased risk for worse pregnancy outcome and further deterioration in myocardial function.

Therefore, a standardized work up has been suggested for cancer survivors with pregnancy wish, which is summarized in Figure 21.1 [42, 43].

Key Points

- Some chemotherapeutics – especially anthracyclins – may have acute or chronic cardiotoxic side effects, presenting as heart failure, hypertension, arrhythmia, (myo) pericarditis, ischemic lesions and thrombo-embolic complications.
- Current data do not show a worse maternal or fetal outcome for women treated with chemotherapy during pregnancy at standard dose, which therefore is the current international recommended treatment dose in pregnancy.
- Most female childhood cancer survivors will have no cardiac complications during or after childbirth. Nevertheless, a careful follow-up during pregnancy and postpartum is recommendable for those with a history of cardiotoxic therapies.

References

1. Gziri MM, Amant F, Debieve F, et al. Effects of chemotherapy during pregnancy on the maternal and fetal heart. *Prenat Diagn* 2012;32:614–19.

2. Mulrooney DA, Yeazel MW, Kawashima T, et al. Cardiac outcomes in a cohort of adult survivors of childhood and adolescent cancer: retrospective analysis of the Childhood Cancer Survivor Study cohort. *BMJ* 2009; 339:b4606.

3. Trachtenberg BH, Landy DC, Franco VI, et al. Anthracycline-associated cardiotoxicity in survivors of childhood cancer. *Pediatr Cardiol* 2011;32:342–53.

4. Telli ML, Hunt SA, Carlson RW, Guardino AE. Trastuzumab-related cardiotoxicity: calling into question the concept of reversibility. *J Clin Oncol* 2007;25:3525–33.

5. Chien AJ, Rugo HS. The cardiac safety of trastuzumab in the treatment of breast cancer. *Expert Opin Drug Saf* 2010;9:335–46.

6. Sawyer DB, Peng X, Chen B, et al. Mechanisms of anthracycline cardiac injury: can we identify strategies for cardioprotection? *Prog Cardiovasc Dis* 2010;**53**:105–13.

7. Abi Aad S, Pierce M, Barmaimon G, et al. Hypertension induced by chemotherapeutic and immunosuppresive agents: a new challenge. *Crit Rev Oncol Hematol* 2015;**93**:28–35.

8. Ke AB, Rostami-Hodjegan A, Zhao P, Unadkat JD. Pharmacometrics in pregnancy: An unmet need. *Annu Rev Pharmacol Toxicol* 2014;**54**:53–69.

9. Zhao Y, Hebert MF, Venkataramanan R. Basic obstetric pharmacology. *Semin Perinatol* 2014;**38**:475–86.

10. van Hasselt JG, van Calsteren K, Heyns L, et al. Optimizing anticancer drug treatment in pregnant cancer patients: pharmacokinetic analysis of gestation-induced changes for doxorubicin, epirubicin, docetaxel and paclitaxel. *Ann Oncol* 2014;**25**:2059–65.

11. Van Calsteren K, Verbesselt R, Ottevanger N, et al. Pharmacokinetics of chemotherapeutic agents in pregnancy: a preclinical and clinical study. *Acta Obstet Gynecol Scand* 2010;**89**:1338–45.

12. Stensheim H, Moller B, van Dijk T, Fossa SD. Cause-specific survival for women diagnosed with cancer during pregnancy or lactation: a registry-based cohort study. *J Clin Oncol* 2009;**27**:45–51.

13. Cardonick E, Dougherty R, Grana G, et al. Breast cancer during pregnancy: maternal and fetal outcomes. *Cancer J* 2010;**16**:76–82.

14. Amant F, von Minckwitz G, Han SN, et al. Prognosis of women with primary breast cancer diagnosed during pregnancy: results from an international collaborative study. *J Clin Oncol* 2013;**31**:2532–9.

15. Loibl S, Schmidt A, Gentilini O, et al. Breast cancer diagnosed during pregnancy: adapting recent advances in breast cancer care for pregnant patients. *JAMA Oncol* 2015; **1**(8):1145–53.

16. Amant F, Halaska MJ, Fumagalli M, et al. Gynecologic cancers in pregnancy: guidelines of a second international consensus meeting. *Int J Gynecol Cancer* 2014;**24**:394–403.

17. Van Calsteren K, Heyns L, De Smet F, et al. Cancer during pregnancy: an analysis of 215 patients emphasizing the obstetrical and the neonatal outcomes. *J Clin Oncol* 2010;**28**:683–9.

18. Cardonick E, Iacobucci A. Use of chemotherapy during human pregnancy. *Lancet Oncol* 2004;**5**:283–91.

19. Juonala M, Cheung MM, Sabin MA, et al. Effect of birth weight on life-course blood pressure levels among children born premature: the Cardiovascular Risk in Young Finns Study. *J Hypertens* 2015;**33**: 1542–8.

20. Sipola-Leppanen M, Vaarasmaki M, Tikanmaki M, et al. Cardiometabolic risk factors in young adults who were born preterm. *Am J Epidemiol* 2015;**181**:861–73.

21. Siedner S, Kruger M, Schroeter M, et al. Developmental changes in contractility and sarcomeric proteins from the early embryonic to the adult stage in the mouse heart. *J Physiol* 2003;**548**:493–505.

22. Rudolph AM. Myocardial growth before and after birth: clinical implications. *Acta Paediatr* 2000;**89**:129–33.

23. Germann N, Goffinet F, Goldwasser F. Anthracyclines during pregnancy: embryo-fetal outcome in 160 patients. *Ann Oncol* 2004;**15**:146–50.

24. Achtari C, Hohlfeld P. Cardiotoxic transplacental effect of idarubicin administered during the second trimester of pregnancy. *Am J Obstet Gynecol* 2000;**183**:511–12.

25. Reynoso EE, Huerta F. Acute leukemia and pregnancy–fatal fetal outcome after exposure to idarubicin during the second trimester. *Acta Oncol* 1994;**33**:709–10.

26. Baumgartner AK, Oberhoffer R, Jacobs VR, et al. Reversible foetal cerebral ventriculomegaly and cardiomyopathy under chemotherapy for maternal AML. *Onkologie* 2009;**32**:40–3.

27. Gziri MM, Debieve F, De Catte L, et al. Chemotherapy during pregnancy: effect of anthracyclines on fetal and maternal cardiac function. *Acta Obstet Gynecol Scand* 2012;**91**:1465–8.

28. Meyer-Wittkopf M, Barth H, Emons G, Schmidt S. Fetal cardiac effects of doxorubicin therapy for carcinoma of the breast during pregnancy: case report and review of the literature. *Ultrasound Obstet Gynecol* 2001;**18**:62–6.

29. Amant F, Vandenbroucke T, Verheecke M, et al. Pediatric Outcome after Maternal Cancer Diagnosed during Pregnancy. *N Engl J Med* 2015; **373**(19):1824–34.

30. Aviles A, Neri N, Nambo MJ. Long-term evaluation of cardiac function in children who received anthracyclines during pregnancy. *Ann Oncol* 2006;**17**:286–8.

31. Gziri MM, Hui W, Amant F, et al. Myocardial function in children after fetal chemotherapy exposure. A tissue Doppler and myocardial deformation imaging study. *Eur J Pediatr* 2013;**172**:163–70.

32. Van Calsteren K, Verbesselt R, Beijnen J, et al. Transplacental transfer of anthracyclines, vinblastine, and 4-hydroxy-cyclophosphamide in a baboon model. *Gynecol Oncol* 2010;**119**:594–600.

33. Grohard P, Akbaraly JP, Saux MC, et al. Transplacental passage of doxorubicin. *J Gynecol Obstet Biol Reprod (Paris)* 1989;**18**:595–600.

34. Gaillard B, Leng JJ, Grellet J, et al. Transplacental passage of epirubicin. *J Gynecol Obstet Biol Reprod (Paris)* 1995;**24**:63–8.

35. Pearson GD, Veille JC, Rahimtoola S, et al. Peripartum cardiomyopathy: National Heart, Lung, and Blood Institute and Office of Rare Diseases (National Institutes of Health) workshop recommendations and review. *JAMA* 2000;**283**:1183–8.

36. van Dalen EC, van der Pal HJ, van den Bos C, et al. Clinical heart failure during pregnancy and delivery in a cohort of female childhood cancer survivors treated with anthracyclines. *Eur J Cancer* 2006;**42**: 2549–53.

37. Krischer JP, Epstein S, Cuthbertson DD, et al. Clinical cardiotoxicity following anthracycline treatment for childhood cancer: the Pediatric Oncology Group experience. *J Clin Oncol* 1997;**15**: 1544–52.

38. Silber JH, Jakacki RI, Larsen RL, et al. Increased risk of cardiac dysfunction after anthracyclines in girls. *Med Pediatr Oncol* 1993;**21**:477–9.

39. Katz A, Goldenberg I, Maoz C, et al. Peripartum cardiomyopathy occurring in a patient previously treated with doxorubicin. *Am J Med Sci* 1997;**314**:399–400.

40. Bar J, Davidi O, Goshen Y, et al. Pregnancy outcome in women treated with doxorubicin for childhood cancer. *Am J Obstet Gynecol* 2003;**189**:853–7.

41. Hines MR, Mulrooney DA, Hudson MM, et al. Pregnancy-associated cardiomyopathy in survivors of childhood cancer. *J Cancer Surviv* 2016;**10**(1):113–21.

42. Altena R, Gietema JA, van Veldhuisen DJ, Reyners AK. Pregnancy unbosoms the heart of breast cancer survivors. *Ann Oncol* 2012;**23**:2206–8.

43. European Society of Gynecology (ESG), Association for European Paediatric Cardiology (AEPC), German Society for Gender Medicine (DGesGM), et al. ESC Guidelines on the management of cardiovascular diseases during pregnancy: the Task Force on the Management of Cardiovascular Diseases during Pregnancy of the European Society of Cardiology (ESC). *Eur Heart J* 2011;**32**: 3147–97.

Chapter 22

Maternal Cardiovascular Disease After Pregnancy Complications

Johannes Duvekot

Summary

During pregnancy, most maternal organ systems increase in function or size. This is indeed also the case for cardiovascular function and maternal hemodynamics. Most systems show enormous changes that put a serious strain on these systems. Gestational complications develop when an organ system is unable to meet the increased physiological demands of pregnancy. Pregnancy can be considered as the ultimate stress test for these organ systems. Preeclampsia may be considered as a derangement of the hemodynamic and cardiovascular system during pregnancy. Delivery eventually solves the problem, but this is only a transient relief. During later life the hemodynamic and cardiovascular system again derails when aging takes its toll. Cardiovascular morbidity and mortality is greatly increased after pregnancies afflicted by gestational complications. This is true not only for preeclampsia and other hypertensive disorders in pregnancy, but also for gestational complications such as preterm delivery, gestational diabetes, fetal growth restriction and placental abruption. Excessive weight gain and weight retention postpartum also pose risks for maternal health in later life. Gestational complications have to be acknowledged by health care providers as a risk factor for later cardiovascular disease. The care of women after previous gestational complications has to be focused on prevention and early detection of signs of cardiovascular deterioration. Specific prevention programs are needed for this group of future patients.

Introduction

During uncomplicated pregnancies, total blood volume shows an increase of more than 40%, of which both plasma volume and, to a lesser extent, erythrocyte volume show large increments. There is a distinct relationship with the relative increase in total blood volume and fetal weight. It is not clear whether a decreased or attenuated augmentation of the blood volume is a sign or a cause of inadequate fetal growth. Pregnancy is also characterized by large changes in cardiovascular parameters. These changes arise more or less simultaneously with the changes in volume homeostasis but tend to precede these changes by some weeks. Gestational complications, and especially the hypertensive syndromes, show an aberrant cardiovascular and hemodynamic adaptation to pregnancy. Preeclampsia may be considered as a cardiovascular disease (CVD) since the characteristic generalized endothelial dysfunction, which is pathognomonic for the disease, is also one of the clinical features for CVD. During otherwise uncomplicated pregnancies there are also major changes occurring in the metabolic system, such as increased insulin resistance, upregulation of the inflammatory cascade and dyslipidemia. Metabolic changes that resemble changes that are seen in the metabolic syndrome are even exaggerated during gestational complications. It has long been thought that the effects of these gestational syndromes are reversed when the baby is delivered and (most) values return to normal. However, the detrimental effects of the gestational syndromes in combination with the effect of aging may precipitate those women later in life to develop chronic disease. Probably, the increased abnormal metabolic changes may also add to the later development of CVD. This means that in later life the effect of aging of the cardiovascular system in these women leads to an increased risk of developing cardiovascular morbidity and mortality. The limited reserves of the organ system of those women at risk will be unmasked during pregnancy and form a serious warning. Therefore, pregnancy is the ultimate stress test for an early failure of organ systems in later life. This may also explain why women with pre-existing disease may be struck more frequently by gestational complications [1].

History

Already during the nineteenth century, German scientists reported that previously pre-eclamptic women had chronic impairment of their renal function. In that era preeclampsia was still considered as a renal disease, and that when the disease was maintained long enough, renal damage would ensue [2]. From the beginning of the twentieth century blood pressure measurement came into use, linking preeclampsia and eclampsia to hypertension. [3] Until the beginning of the twentieth century, follow-up studies of formerly (pre)eclamptic patients were indeterminate. In his classical article on the follow-up of 270 women that had an eclamptic insult between 1931 and 1951, Chesley described in 1976 the whereabouts of all but three of these women until 1973–74 [4]. Chesley noticed an increase in mortality during these years that was two to five times higher than in unselected women. Surprisingly, this increased mortality rate was only found in white multiparous women and in black women, irrespective of their parity. According to Chesley, the reason for this difference in outcome is due to the presence or development of essential hypertension in the multiparous women. Chesley also studied the development of hypertension in this series of patients and compared that to the then-current published literature on the subject of subsequent hypertension after eclampsia. He described in this series that after a follow-up of 6 weeks to 44 years, 2.637 women were re-examined, of which 23.8% were shown to have hypertension. To compile these data, 53 studies from the beginning of the twentieth century until 1970 were used. Since this first review on this subject, these longlasting effects of gestational complications have received increasing attention.

Cardiovascular Disease and Pregnancy in General

Number of Pregnancies

Two leading theories of aging, The Antagonistic Pleiotropy Theory [5] and The Disposable Soma Theory [6], suggest a tradeoff between increased fertility and decreased human life span. The Disposable Soma Theory suggests that because of the competing demands of reproduction, less effort is invested in the maintenance of somatic tissues than is necessary for long survival. The Antagonistic Pleiotropy Theory proposes that certain alleles that are favored because of beneficial early effects also have deleterious later effects. This means that resources allocated to fertility and child raising in the early to middle part of life may be at the expense of longevity. Several studies have investigated the relationship between number of children and longevity. The occurrence of CVD after pregnancy may be an indirect measure.

Two large American studies in the nineties of the last century showed that the risk of developing CVD is increased in women after having six or more children. In the Framingham Heart Study, the rate risk ratio to develop coronary heart disease adjusted for age and educational level was calculated as 1.6 (95% CI 1.1–2.2), and a similar ratio of 1.5 (95% CI 1.1–1.9) was calculated in the National Health and Nutrition Examination Survey National Epidemiologic Follow-up Study (NHEFS) [7]. Adjustments for other risk factors, such as BMI, did not change these calculations.

On the other hand, a large Swedish cohort study showed that having no children is also associated with increased risk of developing CVD [8]. In this study 1,332,062 women older than 50 years were followed. Even after accounting for socioeconomic factors and pregnancy-related complications, parity and the occurrence of CVD was associated in a J-shaped curve. The lowest chance of acquiring CVD is after delivering 1–2 children. Thereafter, this risk increases with parity (Figure 22.1).

Although having more children poses only a relatively limited increased risk of developing CVD, life expectancy looks to be markedly influenced by the number of children. With respect to life expectancy, a Dutch cohort study showed that the optimal number of children is two to three (Figure 22.2) [9]. More children or one or no child decreases life expectancy substantially. These findings are in line with the finding in the previous study on CVD and parity. The same findings were described in a British study [10].

This means that not only after complicated pregnancies, but also after uncomplicated pregnancies the incidence of CVD and longevity in the mothers might be influenced by the reproductive process (Figure 22.2).

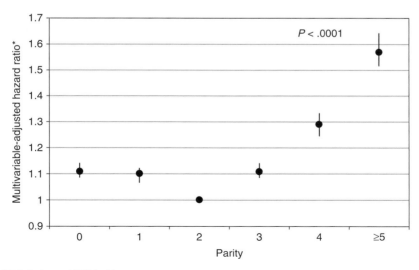

Figure 22.1 Parity and CVD incidence
(Source: Adapted from Parikh et al. [72]).

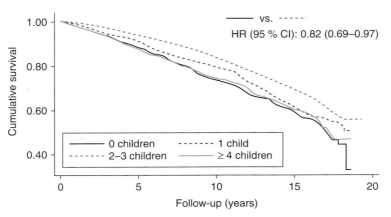

Figure 22.2 Number of children and survival (Source: Adapted from Kuningas et al. [73] (A black and white version of this figure will appear in some formats. For the color version, please refer to the plate section.)

Interpregnancy Interval

Not only pregnancy itself and the number of pregnancies but also the interval between pregnancies probably determines the risk of developing CVD in later life. Short intervals (less than 18 months) between pregnancies in a cohort of women born between 1911 and 1920 were associated with a higher mortality rate [11]. A study from Norway confirmed these findings. This study also showed that mortality seemed to be lower for longer intervals (30–41 months) and longer average birth intervals [12]. One large cohort study from Australia evaluated the risk of developing CVD in association with interpregnancy interval. If the interpregnancy interval between the first birth and the start of the second pregnancy was 18–23 months the risk of subsequent CVD was at its lowest point. Maternal CVD risk follows a J-shaped curve (Figure 22.3) [13]. A shorter interval increases the risk, as does a longer interval also. A possible explanation for this finding is the fact that pregnancy really adds to the risk of developing CVD and that a short interval may be more harmful because the vascular system is not able to recover completely from the first pregnancy and a subsequent pregnancy may aggravate the possible vascular damage even more by hitting the still wea-kened vasculature again. The reason for this may be found in pathways of maternal nutrition and especially folate status. The results for longer intervals are possibly because of the aging of the vascular tree, which makes vasculature also more vulnerable. The fact is that this higher incidence of CVD after longer intervals contradicts with life expectancy overall [11]. More research is needed to elucidate this question more thoroughly.

In line with these findings is that the recurrence rate of pregnancy complications in a next pregnancy is, in a similar fashion, dependant on the pregnancy interval [14]. This finding led to the WHO recommendation to keep an interval of at least 24 months between pregnancies. This advice also seems wise with respect to the future health of the mother (Figure 22.3).

Maternal Age

Finally, teenage pregnancies are linked with higher mortality, where older age pregnancies (above 39 years) are linked with lower mortality [11]. In a British study, a cohort of women born between 1911 and 1940 were followed until their fiftieth birthday for their mortality and health status. A correction was made for socio-demographic characteristics. For women

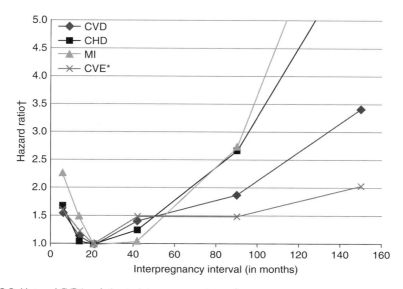

Figure 22.3 Maternal CVD in relation to interpregnancy interval.
(Source: Adapted from Ngo et al. [74])
(A black and white version of this figure will appear in some formats. For the color version, please refer to the plate section.)

with teenage pregnancies the risk of dying by the age of fifty was increased and the odds ratio was 1.15 (95% CI 1.06–1.25) to 1.30 (95% CI 1.11–1.53) for, respectively, the cohorts born in 1911–1920 and in 1931–1940. The role of CVD was not separately investigated in this study.

Pregnancy Complications and Future Cardiovascular Risk

Pregnancy may not be considered as a strict physiologic process. The risk of gestational complications such as hypertensive disorders of pregnancy, fetal growth restriction, gestational diabetes, placental abruption and preterm delivery is more than 20% [15]. With the exception of preterm delivery, all other complications can be summarized as placental syndromes. This makes the placenta the most important factor in influencing the maternal vascular tree, subclinical endothelial dysfunction being the pathophysiologic entity.

Although it seems that pregnancy itself has an effect on cardiovascular health in later life, pregnancy complications seem to add to this risk. Most pregnancy complications have been described as increasing the risk of developing CVD. This is especially true for the group of hypertensive disorders of pregnancy. In 2002, Sattar and Greer published their theory on this phenomenon and drew their famous figure, which illustrates how women that are more susceptible to develop CVD acquire during pregnancy a form of CVD, preeclampsia or another pregnancy complication (Figure 22.4) [16]. The disease disappears and seems to heal after pregnancy, but returns earlier with aging than in women not so susceptible for CVD. Several pregnancy complications have been suggested as increasing risk, preeclampsia and eclampsia being the most important ones. For this reason, the American Heart Association incorporated assessment for a history of preeclampsia, gestational diabetes

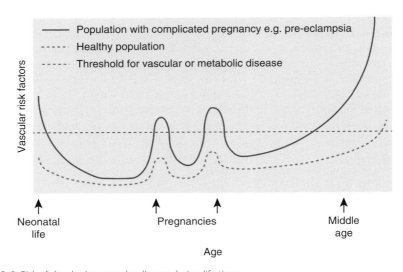

Figure 22.4 Risk of developing vascular disease during life time.
(Source: Adapted from Sattar et al. [75])
(A black and white version of this figure will appear in some formats. For the color version, please refer to the plate section.)

and pregnancy-induced hypertension into its CVD effectiveness-based guidelines [17] (Figure 22.4).

Although pre-existent cardiovascular risk factors predispose strongly to develop pregnancy complications, it is often not known whether these pre-existing factors were already present in those women that develop CVD after complicated pregnancies. Pre-existing hypertension predisposes women to develop preeclampsia greatly (OR 7.3, 95% CI 3.1–17.2). Increased pre-existent cholesterol levels (>5.6 mmol/L) show also an increased risk (OR 2.1, 95% CI 1.2–3.8). Pre-existent hypertension is also associated with an increased CVD death hazard ratio of 3.5 (95% CI 2.4–5.1) 50 years after uncomplicated pregnancy [18]. In combination with preterm delivery this association increases to 7.1 (95% CI 3.5–14.6). A literature-based study, evaluating all studies on CVD risk after preeclampsia, concluded that pre-existing cardiovascular risk factors do not fully explain the risk of CVD after preeclampsia. From this study it was concluded that the difference between observed and estimated odds ratios may be explained by an additional risk by the disease of preeclampsia itself [19].

Hypertensive Disorders of Pregnancy

The incidence of preeclampsia shows an increasing trend in the latest years. Rates have increased by 25% during the last two decades in the United States [20]. This development poses preeclampsia more and more as a serious threat to female health in later life through the increased chance of developing CVD in later life.

Hypertension

It has long been known that women with pregnancies complicated by hypertensive disorders more frequently develop hypertension in later life. Although blood pressure in most cases of preeclampsia initially normalizes after delivery, the risk of developing hypertension in later life is increased in comparison to women after uncomplicated pregnancies. In several studies investigating this relationship, the risks of developing hypertension are reported with ranges from 1.50 to 20.00. More recent studies with larger numbers demonstrate relative risks for hypertension of between 2.35 and 3.70, which looks to be a more reasonable figure [21]. An older and leading meta-analysis written by Bellamy et al. previously showed a relative risk of 3.70 (95% CI 2.70–5.05) [22].

A pitfall of these studies is the recovery phase after complicated pregnancies. It is important to note that hypertension after preeclamptic pregnancies may take a long time to recover and to disappear. A study of 205 preeclamptic women showed that it may take up to two years postpartum before hypertension has disappeared. After three months 39% still had hypertension, decreasing to 18% two years postpartum [23]. This means that 50% of cases of hypertension still disappear between three months and two years postpartum. Studies describing remaining hypertension after pregnancies complicated by hypertensive disorders should attend to this relatively long period in which hypertension may still disappear.

Severity of the hypertensive disease during pregnancy plays also a role. Normalization time after gestational hypertension was significantly shorter than after preeclampsia (6 ± 5.5 days versus 16 ± 9.5 days) [24]. Unfortunately, in this study women that still had hypertension 50 days postpartum were excluded. Aside from the severity, normalization of blood pressure after preeclampsia may also be dependent on the period of onset of the disease during pregnancy. The earlier the onset, the longer normalization lasts.

One of the effects of (chronic) hypertension is left ventricular hypertrophy. Ventricular hypertrophy can be more often found in women that had pregnancies complicated by hypertensive disorders [25]. In this study women were evaluated at the age of 56 years. Adjusted for the several usual risk factors for developing left ventricular hypertrophy, the odds ratio for developing left ventricular hypertrophy was 1.42 (95% CI 1.01–1.99) for previously preeclamptic women as compared to women with uncomplicated pregnancies. After additional adjustment for the duration of hypertension after pregnancy this significance disappeared. The latter suggests that following hypertensive disorders in pregnancy, women should receive timely treatment for their (remaining) hypertension in an effort to reduce the effects of longstanding hypertension. Diastolic function is also slightly impaired, as can be deduced from the larger left atrial diameter and the different left ventricular filling patterns. Systolic function was still found to be normal in this study.

The development of hypertension after preeclamptic pregnancies in previously normotensive women is possibly heralded by the persistence of gestational structural changes of the heart, and especially left ventricular hypertrophy, that is still present several months or years postpartum [26,27]. In cases where gestational hypertension had disappeared, left ventricular hypertrophy and an increased left atrial dimension was predictive for development of hypertension in later life. Especially in women with early-onset preeclampsia, these abnormalities were present in more than 50% of all cases. Two years postpartum, 50% of the women with echocardiographic abnormalities presented with essential hypertension versus only 3.5% when no abnormalities had previously been seen.

Ischemic Heart Disease

The risk of future ischemic heart disease after a preeclamptic pregnancy lies between 1.65 and 3.61 (Figure 22.5) with an average relative risk of 2.16 (95% CI 1.86–2.52), as demonstrated by the forest plot from Bellamy's study (Figure 22.5) [22].

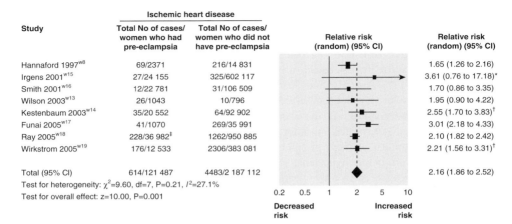

Figure 22.5 Forest plot of studies investigating the relation between preeclampsia and the development of ischemic heart disease.
(Source: Adapted from Bellamy et al. [76])

The large meta-analysis of Bellamy also gives a subdivision for the development of ischemic disease after different phenotypes of preeclampsia (Figure 22.6) [22]. So-called mild preeclampsia leads to an increased risk of developing ischemic disease of 1.92 (95% CI 1.65–2.24), whereas the risk after severe preeclampsia is 2.86 (95% CI 2.25–3.65). Early preeclampsia with an onset before 34 weeks of gestation shows the largest risk (7.71: 95% CI 4.40–13.52).

Another discussion is whether prolongation of preeclamptic pregnancies for longer periods aggravates the endothelial damage and has an influence on future CVD. No studies have looked at this aspect, but it seems likely that a longer disease period might influence the later effects of the disease (Figure 22.6).

These risks are in line with other risk factors for CVD. Lifetime hazard ratios for smoking and other lifestyle factors are shown in Table 22.1.

Later studies even showed differences in future risk for CVD after only gestational hypertension [28]. These risks range from 1.5 to 2.8. The occurrence of hypertension, but to a lesser extent ischemic heart disease and stroke, is more frequent among women that had gestational hypertension during their pregnancies [29]. Since the different studies on this subject evaluate different outcomes only two studies really evaluated the occurrence of ischemic heart disease [30, 31]. Risk ratios in these two studies, both from Scandinavia, were almost identical (1.6, 95% CI 1.4–2.0) for ischemic heart disease. In studies evaluating the long-term effects of gestational hypertension, the major problem is always whether there had been pre-existent hypertension before pregnancy.

Cerebrovascular Disease

Cerebrovascular risk, an often forgotten form of CVD, varies between 1.39 and 3.59 after preeclamptic pregnancies [21]. Of all cardiovascular events, stroke occurs predominantly during and within two years after preeclamptic pregnancies, closely followed by myocardial infarction. A large study from Taiwan found an overall risk for CVD of more than 7.0 but a higher risk for stroke of 14.5 (Hazard Ratio, 95% CI 1.3–165.1) than for myocardial

Table 22.1 Risk ratios for the main causes of CVD

Risk factor	Risk ratio for CVD	95% CI	Reference
Preterm delivery	1.8	1.3–2.5	28
IUGR	1.9	1.5–2.4	28
Preeclampsia	2.2	1.86–2.52	22
Obesity	2.26	1.90–2.68	70
Smoking	2.86	2.36–3.48	70
Hypertension	2.95	2.57–3.39	70
Diabetes	4.26	3.51–5.18	70
Early preeclampsia	7.71	4.40–13.52	22
Familiar hypercholesterolemia	8.54	5.29–13.80	71

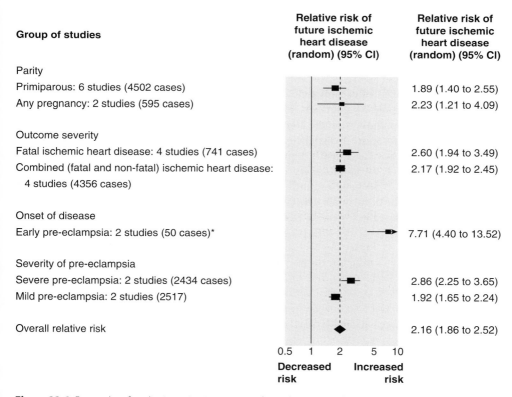

Figure 22.6 Forest plot of studies investigating severity of preeclampsia in relation to the development of ischemic heart disease.
(Source: Adapted from Bellamy et al. [77])

infarction (13.0, 95% CI 4.6–6.3) [32]. In this population-based cohort study patients were followed for up to three years, and more than 70% of cardiovascular events were stroke cases.

Mortality

As already observed by Chesley in the 1960s and 1970s, studies have shown that maternal mortality is increased after complicated pregnancies, and especially after pregnancies complicated by preeclampsia (Figure 22.7). Maternal mortality following preeclamptic pregnancies is somewhat increased, and overall risks of mortality vary between 1.20 and 3.00 [21, 33]. The majority of these deaths are caused by CVD. Mortality because of CVD was more increased, ranging from 1.65 to 3.07. It is now generally accepted that the earlier the onset of preeclampsia occurs, the greater the resulting risk for death due to CVD. In a large Scandinavian study the risk of death due to CVD after early preeclampsia was estimated as 8.12 [33]. An American cohort study found an even higher hazard ratio for death due to CVD of 9.54 (95% CI 4.50–20.26) [34]. In another American cohort that was followed for 50 years after delivery, a difference in mortality risk was made between early- and late-onset preeclampsia. Hazard ratios for early- and late-onset disease were respectively 3.6 (95% CI 1.04–12.19) and 2.0 (95% CI 1.18–3.46) (Figure 22.7) [35].

Nevertheless, this increased mortality risk seems more or less confined to women that only had one pregnancy. More or less unexpected was the finding that women after a first pregnancy complicated by preeclampsia that had one or more children in uncomplicated pregnancies proved to have a lower risk on cardiovascular mortality than women that had no more pregnancies (Figure 22.8) [36].

The cumulative risk of cardiovascular mortality decreased from 9.2% to 1.1% after one or more uncomplicated pregnancies. The excessive risk of noncardiovascular death disappeared entirely in these women after one or more uneventful successive pregnancy. Women with two or more pregnancies complicated by preeclampsia had only slightly higher risk of cardiovascular death than after one preeclamptic pregnancy, with a hazard ratio of 1.5 (95% CI 1.2–1.9). Having preeclampsia not in the first pregnancy but in one of the following pregnancies gave a slightly higher hazard ratio of 2.0 (95% CI 1.2–3.3), which was irrespective of the occurrence of preeclampsia in the first pregnancy. An explanation for these findings of a so-called "healing effect" of a successive pregnancy may be found in the

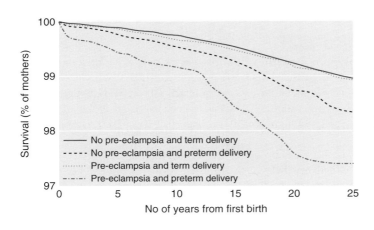

Figure 22.7 Long-term survival of primiparous mothers in relation to preeclampsia and/or preterm delivery.
(Source: Adapted from Irgens et al. [78])
(A black and white version of this figure will appear in some formats. For the color version, please refer to the plate section.)

Survival (% of mothers)

100
99
98
97

—— No pre-eclampsia and term delivery
- - - - No pre-eclampsia and preterm delivery
········· Pre-eclampsia and term delivery
—·—·— Pre-eclampsia and preterm delivery

0   5   10   15   20   25

No of years from first birth

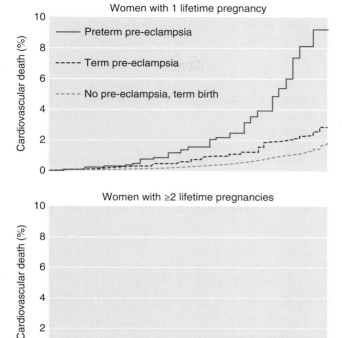

Figure 22.8 Cumulative risk of cardiovascular death for women according to preeclampsia status at first pregnancy and number of lifetime pregnancies. (Source: Adapted from Skjaerven et al. [79]) (A black and white version of this figure will appear in some formats. For the color version, please refer to the plate section.)

selection of women that decided and/or succeeded to have another pregnancy. Some women decided not to have another pregnancy; some were advised not to have a second pregnancy. No other studies have investigated this association so far. Also, no studies looked for CVD risks in this way. Only one small study investigated the increase of hypertension after more than one preeclamptic pregnancy. This study showed that more than one preeclamptic pregnancy may lead to increased incidence rates of hypertension [37].

Preterm Birth

Several studies show that following preterm birth, years after delivery blood pressure is significantly higher than after term births [38, 39, 40]. From these studies, it is not clear how many women really develop hypertension after preterm birth. The only study that tries to give odds ratios states that 10–25 years and >25 years after preterm delivery the odds ratios for developing hypertension were not significantly increased as compared to term delivery [40].

A large Scandinavian study describes how the risk of developing CVD increases with decreasing gestational age at delivery [41]. Using information on almost one million women having their first child, the hazard ratios for CVD in women were evaluated. CVD was defined as coronary heart disease, cerebrovascular events and heart failure. Compared to women who were delivered of a normally grown infant, the hazard ratios to develop CVD were 2.18 (95% CI 1.33–3.57) in extreme preterm (< 27 weeks) birth, 2.57 (95% CI 1.97–3.34) in very preterm birth (28–31 weeks) and 1.39 (95% CI 1. 22–1.58) in moderately preterm (32–36 weeks) birth. Reference was term delivery, and figures were adjusted for variables such as maternal age, birth year, pre-existing hypertension and diabetes mellitus, hypertensive disorders of pregnancy and smoking. The risk of coronary heart disease was higher than that of cerebrovascular disease. Delivering before 32 weeks of a nonSGA neonate gave a hazard ratio of 4.41 for coronary heart disease and 2.41 for cerebrovascular disease. A similar American study in almost 50,000 women showed that 10 years after a preterm birth cardiovascular hospitalizations were slightly increased (hazard ratio 1.4, 95% CI 1.2–1.6). This figure was adjusted for most important confounding factors. The risk increased if preterm birth occurred earlier or spontaneously [42].

Preterm delivery also predisposes to a higher CVD mortality risk, which was reported with a hazard ratio of 2.1 (95% CI 1.40–2.01) in an American study with a 50-year follow-up [35].

Fetal Growth Restriction

Many studies have shown that CVD risk is also increased after pregnancies complicated by fetal growth restriction [28]. Delivering a baby in the lowest birthweight quintile for gestational age places the mother at an increased risk of being admitted for ischemic heart disease or death (hazard ratio 1.9, 95% CI 1.5–2.4) [43]. The identical cardiovascular vascular changes in preeclampsia and fetal growth restriction link these complications strongly and suggest they are both surrogates of CVD during pregnancy [44].

In the earlier mentioned Scandinavian study, delivering of a very small neonate, defined as a fetal growth restriction more than 2 SD under the mean, irrespective of gestational age, gave a hazard ratio for CVD of 1.60 (95% CI 1.38–1.86) [41]. The combination of very small and very preterm gave a hazard ratio of 2.97 for CVD. Again, the hazard ratio for coronary heart disease (3.75, 95% CI 1.97–7.14) was higher than that for cerebrovascular disease (3.11, 95% CI 1.91–5.09).

Maternal CVD mortality is also increased after a pregnancy complicated by fetal growth restriction (hazard ratio 1.60, 95% CI 1.02–2.42) [35].

Gestational Diabetes Mellitus

It has been established that GDM increases the risk of developing type 2 diabetes mellitus in later life. Some studies have shown that GDM also increases the later risk of developing CVD [45, 46, 47]. However, this increase seems mainly related to the onset of type 2 diabetes mellitus. A large French study showed an association of GDM with overall CVD after adjusting for age and obesity (OR 1.25, 95% CI 1.09–1.43) within seven years after pregnancy. Angina pectoris (OR 1.68), myocardial infarction (OR 1.92) and hypertension (OR 2.72) were significantly correlated; cerebrovascular disease was not [48].

A meta-analysis showed that increased intima-media thickness, irrespective of other risk factors, remains increased in women years after pregnancies complicated by gestational diabetes mellitus (GDM) [49]. An increased intima-media thickness can be considered as a form of subclinical atherosclerosis. The increased intima-media thickness was in most cases of GDM already present during or shortly after pregnancy, and this correlation was stronger in obese women.

Practical problems in this respect are the diagnostic criteria for GDM, which vary, and the lag time between pregnancies and the development of CVD years later. Longitudinal and prospective studies are needed to elucidate and confirm the relationship between GDM and later CVD.

Placental Abruption

Being one of the least occurring pregnancy-related complications, not much data are available on the long-term effects of this disorder. In a large Scandinavian cohort, the hazard ratio for death due to CVD after placental abruption in any pregnancy was 1.8 (95% CI 1.5–2.2) [50]. (Mean follow-up was 23 years, and there was no difference in mortality hazard ratio for placental abruption in a first pregnancy or in any further pregnancy.) Another large study in Canada showed a hazard ratio of 1.7 (95% CI 1.3–2.2) after this complication [28]. Two smaller studies showed similar results but lacked a clear definition of CVD [51] or strict follow-up of all women [52].

Acute Fatty Liver of Pregnancy

Being primarily a disease of the liver and being a very rare disorder, long-term follow-up of patients with this disease is not described in the literature. In particular, risk of CVD is not described in this group of patients. On the basis of the pathophysiology of this disease, especially problems with liver function in later life could be expected.

Miscarriage

Although during pregnancies terminated by miscarriage the vascular system does not expand as much as during a pregnancy that lasts for a longer time, the risk to develop CVD in later life is probably also increased. In a Scottish cohort, two, three or more miscarriages, irrespective of whether this was consecutive, lead to arterial CVD with a hazard ratio of, respectively, 1.75 (95% CI 1.22–2.52) and 3.18 (95% CI 1.49–6.80) [53]. The risk for CVD in later life after only one miscarriage was not increased in this cohort. Earlier studies on this subject were summarized in a meta-analysis that showed that one miscarriage coincides with coronary heart disease (OR 1.45, 95% CI 1.19–1.78) but not with cerebrovascular disease [54]. A large American cohort study found a 10% increased risk for myocardial infarction, cerebrovascular infarction and hypertension after one miscarriage, with risks increasing by 10% to 20% with every new miscarriage [55].

Overall, the risk of developing CVD after a miscarriage is smaller than after other pregnancy complications; this risk, however, tends to increase after more miscarriages.

Other Pregnancy Complications

Excessive weight gain during pregnancy and weight retention postpartum are also considered as risk factors for developing CVD in later life. These risk factors are more related to the usual lifestyle risk factors such as obesity than to pregnancy complications. Women with excessive weight gain during their pregnancies are prone to be more obese years after their pregnancies [56]. In particular, maternal weight gain in the first trimester is correlated with maternal weight retention after pregnancy [57]. This may be explained by the deposition of an excess of fat during this period of pregnancy. More weight retention results in both higher maternal weight and higher systolic blood pressure years later.

Obesity during pregnancy creates a small increased risk of hospital admissions for CVD in later life (HR 1.26, 95% CI 1.01–1.57). This was irrespective of parity [58].

Mechanisms Leading to Future CVD After Pregnancy Complications

The underlying pathophysiological disorder in preeclampsia, endothelial dysfunction, remains present for a long time after these pregnancies. Endothelium lines the inner layer of the blood vessels and controls circulation and determines biochemical changes that determine cardiovascular homeostasis. Endothelial dysfunction causes hypertension, increased vascular permeability and activation of the coagulation cascade. The latter effects are called phase two of the disease. Phase one is defined by the release of angiogenic factors that are released by the dysfunctional placenta. Since preeclampsia is induced by factors that result from inadequate placentation or a dysfunctional placenta, it is likely that in cases of other placental syndromes endothelial dysfunction is also present.

During uncomplicated pregnancies certain features of metabolic syndrome, dyslipidemia and insulin resistance, arise temporarily, which possibly result in vascular dysfunction. Uncomplicated pregnancies show increases in plasma triglycerides and cholesterol concentrations. After pregnancy and after birth of the placenta these metabolic changes eventually disappear, but the metabolic effects of pathological pregnancies remain longer present. In pregnancies complicated by preeclampsia, these effects are already prominent before the clinical disease develops. Postpartum one to three years after delivery, women after preeclamptic pregnancies still have significant differences in lipid parameters and an increased susceptibility to lipoprotein oxidation in comparison with women with uncomplicated pregnancies [59].

Together with the changes in lipid metabolism, pregnancy is characterized by an increase in insulin resistance. In pregnancies complicated by preeclampsia, insulin resistance is already increased during the first trimester. This increased insulin resistance is also correlated with an increase in angiogenic factors [60]. Increased insulin resistance remains more prevalent in women until years after formerly preeclamptic pregnancies than after uncomplicated pregnancies [61].

Many studies demonstrate that endothelial dysfunction is still present for many years after complicated pregnancies. Eventually this feature seems not to disappear until more than ten years later when other cardiovascular risk factors still are present. This slow recovery may be indicative of the fact that pre-existing cardiovascular risk factors are already present before the index pregnancy [62, 63, 64]. Another possibility is that pre-existing cardiovascular risk factors are worsened by a preeclamptic pregnancy [19].

Follow-up Programs After Complicated Pregnancies

In some countries, follow-up programs have been developed for women after complicated pregnancies [65, 66, 67]. Most of these programs focus on women after pregnancies complicated by hypertensive disorders of pregnancy. According to the risks that exist also after other pregnancy complications, a wider range of women would be eligible for follow-up. More than 20% of all pregnancies are complicated by pregnancy-related complications [15]. The goals of this follow-up should be focused on the identification and possible (early) therapy of cardiovascular risk factors. It may be worthwhile to treat cardiovascular risk factors at lower thresholds than in women after uncomplicated pregnancies.

Preventive Programs After Complicated Pregnancies

With the knowledge of an increased risk to develop CVD after complicated pregnancies, it seems feasible to introduce prevention programs in this group of women. It is still questionable whether these programs will lead to positive results. Many of these programs depend on motivation of those women [65]. Since most of these women suffered severe pregnancy complications, it is suggested that they would be more motivated to be part of and to continue prevention programs. The period immediately after a complicated pregnancy is therefore called in literature "The window of opportunity." It can be assumed that early intervention is more effective than later intervention. The more emotional or physical this complication was, the more motivated women are. Obviously this is especially true for women after preeclamptic pregnancies. Preliminary studies show that, at least in the first year after delivery, a prevention program may improve maternal health [67, 68, 69]. Since women have to continue these intervention programs for many years, these programs have to be tailored very accurately to make them successful. This means that specific prevention programs are needed for this group of women.

Conclusions

More than 20% of pregnancies will be complicated by pregnancy-related complications such as hypertensive disorders, fetal growth restriction, gestation diabetes mellitus and preterm delivery. Most of these complications result in an increased risk of developing CVD in later life. The overall chance of developing these complications is more or less doubled. The chance to develop cerebrovascular events is, with the exception of the period during and some time after pregnancy, less prominent. A combination of pregnancy-related complications and increasing severity may increase these risks more than sevenfold. Specific follow-up programs may be instituted to detect cardiovascular risk factors at an early stage. Specific prevention programs may help to decrease these risks.

Key Points

- Twenty percent of all pregnancies are complicated by pregnancy-related complications.
- Pregnancy-related complications predispose to development of cardiovascular complications in later life.
- After complicated pregnancies, the risk of developing cardiovascular complications is increased almost twofold.
- A combination of pregnancy-related complications and/or an increased severity increases the risk of developing cardiovascular complications more than sevenfold.
- Early intervention programs influencing cardiovascular risk factors might reduce the risk of developing cardiovascular complications after complicated pregnancies.

References

1. Magnussen EB, Vatten LJ, Lund-Nilsen TI, Salvesen KA, Davey Smith G, Romundstad PR. Prepregnancy cardiovascular risk factors as predictors of pre-eclampsia: population based cohort study. *BMJ* 2007;**335**:978.

2. Spiegelberg O. The pathology and treatment of puerperal eclampsia. *Trans Am Gynecol Soc* 1878;**2**:161–74.

3. Chesley LC. History and epidemiology of preeclampsia-eclampsia. *Clin Obstet Gynecol* 1984;**27**:801–20.

4. Chesley LC, Annitto JE, Cosgrove RA. The remote prognosis of eclamptic women. Sixth periodic report. *Am J Obstet Gynecol* 1976;**124**:446–59.

5. Williams GC. Pleiotropy, natural selection, and the evolution of senescence. *Evolution* 1957;**11**:635–32.

6. Kirkwood TBL. Evolution of aging. *Nature* 1977;**270**:301–4.

7. Ness RB, Harris T, Cobb J. et al. Number of pregnancies and the subsequent risk of cardiovascular disease. *N Engl J Med* 1993;**328**:1528–33.

8. Parikh NI, Cnattingius S, Dickman PW, Mittleman MA, Ludvigsson JF, Ingelsson E. Parity and risk of later-life maternal cardiovascular disease. *Am Heart J* 2010;**159**:215–221.

9. Kuningas M, Altmäe S, Uitterlinden AG, Hofman A, van Duijn CM, Tiemeier H. The relationship between fertility and lifespan in humans. *Age (Dordr)* 2011;**33**: 615–22.

10. Grundy EM, Tomassini C. Marital history, health and mortality among older men and women in England and Wales. *BMC Public Health* 2010;**10**:554.

11. Grundy E, Tomassini C. Fertility history and health in later life: a record linkage study in England and Wales. *Soc Sci Med* 2005;**61**:217–28.

12. Grundy E, Kravdal Ø. Do short birth intervals have long-term implications for parental health? Results from analyses of complete cohort Norwegian register data. *J Epidemiol Community Health* 2014;**68**: 958–64.

13. Ngo AD, Roberts CL, Figtree G. Association between interpregnancy interval and future risk of maternal cardiovascular disease—a population-based record linkage study. *BJOG* 2016;**123**(8):1311–8.

14. Conde-Agudelo A, Belizán JM. Maternal morbidity and mortality associated with interpregnancy interval: cross sectional study. *BMJ* 2000;**321**:1255–9.

15. Smith GN, Pudwell J, Roddy M. The Maternal Health Clinic: a new window of opportunity for early heart disease risk screening and intervention for women with pregnancy complications. *J Obstet Gynaecol Can* 2013;**35**:831–9.

16. Sattar N, Greer IA. Pregnancy complications and maternal cardiovascular risk: opportunities for intervention and screening? *BMJ* 2002;**20**;325(7356): 157–60.

17. Mosca L, Benjamin EJ, Berra K, et al. American Heart Association. Effectiveness-based guidelines for the prevention of cardiovascular disease in women – 2011 update: a guideline from the American Heart Association. *J Am Coll Cardiol* 2011; **57**:1404–23.

18. Cirillo PM, Cohn BA. Pregnancy complications and cardiovascular disease death: 50-year follow-up of the Child Health and Development Studies pregnancy cohort. *Circulation* 2015;**132**: 1234–42.

19. Berks D, Hoedjes M, Raat H, Duvekot JJ, Steegers EA, Habbema JD. Risk of cardiovascular disease after pre-eclampsia and the effect of lifestyle interventions: a literature-based study. *BJOG* 2013;**120**: 924–31.

20. Burgess A, Founds S. Cardiovascular implications of preeclampsia. *MCN Am J Matern Child Nurs* 2016;**41**:8–15.

21. Charlton F, Tooher J, Rye KA, Hennessy A. Cardiovascular risk, lipids and pregnancy: preeclampsia and the risk of later life cardiovascular disease. *Heart Lung Circ* 2014;**623**:203–12.

22. Bellamy L, Casas JP, Hingorani AD, Williams DJ. Pre-eclampsia and risk of cardiovascular disease and cancer in later life: systematic review and meta-analysis. *BMJ* 2007;**335**(7627):974.

23. Berks D, Steegers EA, Molas M, Visser W. Resolution of hypertension and proteinuria after preeclampsia. *Obstet Gynecol* 2009;**114**:1307–14.

24. Ferrazzani S, De Carolis S, Pomini F, Testa AC, Mastromarino C, Caruso A. The duration of hypertension in the puerperium of preeclamptic women: relationship with renal impairment and week of delivery. *Am J Obstet Gynecol* 1994 **171**:506–12.

25. Scantlebury DC, Kane GC, Wiste HJ, et al. Left ventricular hypertrophy after hypertensive pregnancy disorders. *Heart* 2015;**101**:1584–90.

26. Ghossein-Doha C, Peeters L, van Heijster S, van Kuijk S, Spaan J, Delhaas T, Spaanderman M. Hypertension after preeclampsia is preceded by changes in cardiac structure and function. *Hypertension* 2013;**62**:382–90.

27. Melchiorre K, Sutherland GR, Liberati M, Thilaganathan B. Preeclampsia is associated with persistent postpartum cardiovascular impairment. *Hypertension* 2011;**58**:709–15.

28. Ray JG, Vermeulen MJ, Schull MJ, Redelmeier DA. Cardiovascular health after maternal placental syndromes (CHAMPS): population-based retrospective cohort study. *Lancet* 2005;**366**(9499):1797–803.

29. Wilson BJ, Watson MS, Prescott GJ, et al. Hypertensive diseases of pregnancy and risk of hypertension and stroke in later life: results from cohort study. *BMJ* 2003;**326** (7394):845.

30. Wikström AK, Haglund B, Olovsson M, Lindeberg SN. The risk of maternal ischaemic heart disease after gestational hypertensive disease. *BJOG* 2005;**112**:1486–91.

31. Lykke JA, Langhoff-Roos J, Sibai BM, Funai EF, Triche EW, Paidas MJ. Hypertensive pregnancy disorders and subsequent cardiovascular morbidity and type 2 diabetes mellitus in the mother. *Hypertension* 2009;**53**:944–51.

32. Lin YS, Tang CH, Yang CY, et al. Effect of pre-eclampsia-eclampsia on major cardiovascular events among peripartum women in Taiwan. *Am J Cardiol* 2011;**107**: 325–30.

33. Irgens HU, Reisaeter L, Irgens LM, Lie RT. Long term mortality of mothers and fathers after pre-eclampsia: population based cohort study. *BMJ* 2001;**24**;323(7323): 1213–7.

34. Mongraw-Chaffin ML, Cirillo PM, Cohn BA. Preeclampsia and cardiovascular disease death: prospective evidence from the child health and development studies cohort. *Hypertension* 2010;**56**:166–71.

35. Cirillo PM, Cohn BA. Pregnancy complications and cardiovascular disease death: 50-year follow-up of the Child Health and Development Studies pregnancy cohort. *Circulation* 2015;**132**: 1234–42.

36. Skjaerven R, Wilcox AJ, Klungsøyr K, et al. Cardiovascular mortality after pre-eclampsia in one child mothers: prospective, population based cohort study. *BMJ* 2012;**345**:e7677.

37. Sibai BM, el-Nazer A, Gonzalez-Ruiz A. Severe preeclampsia-eclampsia in young primigravid women: subsequent pregnancy outcome and remote prognosis. *Am J Obstet Gynecol* 1986;**155**:1011–16.

38. Catov JM, Lewis CE, Lee M, Wellons MF, Gunderson EP. Preterm birth and future maternal blood pressure, inflammation, and intimal-medial thickness: the CARDIA study. *Hypertension* 2013;**61**:641–6.

39. Perng W, Stuart J, Rifas-Shiman SL, Rich-Edwards JW, Stuebe A, Oken E. Preterm birth and long-term maternal cardiovascular health. *Ann Epidemiol* 2015;**25**:40–5.

40. Xu J, Barinas-Mitchell E, Kuller LH, Youk AO, Catov JM. Maternal hypertension after a low-birth-weight delivery differs by race/ethnicity: evidence from the National Health and Nutrition Examination Survey (NHANES) 1999–2006. *PLoS One* 2014;**9**:e104149.

41. Bonamy AK, Parikh NI, Cnattingius S, Ludvigsson JF, Ingelsson E. Birth characteristics and subsequent risks of maternal cardiovascular disease: effects of gestational age and fetal growth. *Circulation* 2011;**124**:2839–46.

42. Kessous R, Shoham-Vardi I, Pariente G, Holcberg G, Sheiner E. An association between preterm delivery and long-term maternal cardiovascular morbidity. *Am J Obstet Gynecol* 2013;**209**:368.e1–8.

43. Smith GC, Pell JP, Walsh D. Pregnancy complications and maternal risk of ischaemic heart disease: a retrospective cohort study of 129,290 births. *Lancet* 2001;**357**(9273):2002–6.

44. Stergiotou I, Bijnens B, Cruz-Lemini M, Figueras F, Gratacós E, Crispi F. Maternal subclinical vascular changes in fetal growth restriction with and without pre-eclampsia. *Ultrasound Obstet Gynecol* 2015;**46**:706–12.

45. Lind JM, Hennessy A, McLean M. Cardiovascular disease in women: the significance of hypertension and gestational diabetes during pregnancy. *Curr Opin Cardiol* 2014;**29**:447–53.

46. Retnakaran R, Shah BR. Mild glucose intolerance in pregnancy and risk of cardiovascular disease: a population-based cohort study. *CMAJ* 2009;**181**:371–6.

47. Shah BR, Retnakaran R, Booth GL. Increased risk of cardiovascular disease in young women following gestational diabetes mellitus. *Diabetes Care* 2008;**31**:1668–9.

48. Goueslard K, Cottenet J, Mariet AS, et al. Early cardiovascular events in women with a history of gestational diabetes mellitus. *Cardiovasc Diabetol* 2016;**15**:15.

49. Li JW, He SY, Liu P, Luo L, Zhao L, Xiao YB. Association of gestational diabetes mellitus (GDM) with subclinical atherosclerosis: a systemic review and meta-analysis. *BMC Cardiovasc Disord* 2014;**14**:132.

50. DeRoo L, Skjærven R, Wilcox A, Klungsøyr K, Wikström AK, Morken NH, Cnattingius S. Placental abruption and long-term maternal cardiovascular disease mortality: a population-based registry study in Norway and Sweden. *Eur J Epidemiol* 2015 Jul 16.**31**(5):501–11.

51. Lykke JA, Langhoff-Roos J, Lockwood CJ, Triche EW, Paidas MJ. Mortality of mothers from cardiovascular and non-cardiovascular causes following pregnancy complications in first delivery. *Paediatr Perinat Epidemiol* 2010;**24**:323–30.

52. Pariente G, Shoham-Vardi I, Kessous R, Sherf M, Sheiner E. Placental abruption as a significant risk factor for long-term cardiovascular mortality in a follow-up period of more than a decade. *Paediatr Perinat Epidemiol* 2014;**28**:32–8.

53. Wagner MM, Bhattacharya S, Visser J, Hannaford PC, Bloemenkamp KW. Association between miscarriage and cardiovascular disease in a Scottish cohort. *Heart* 2015;**101**:1954–60.

54. Oliver-Williams CT, Heydon EE, Smith GC, Wood AM. Miscarriage and future maternal cardiovascular disease: a systematic review and meta-analysis. *Heart* 2013;**99**:1636–44.

55. Ranthe MF, Andersen EA, Wohlfahrt J, Bundgaard H, Melbye M, Boyd HA. Pregnancy loss and later risk of atherosclerotic disease. *Circulation* 2013;**127**:1775–82.

56. McClure CK, Catov JM, Ness R, Bodnar LM. Associations between gestational weight gain and BMI, abdominal adiposity, and traditional measures of cardiometabolic risk in mothers 8 y postpartum. *Am J Clin Nutr* 2013;**98**:1218–25.

57. Walter JR, Perng W, Kleinman KP, Rifas-Shiman SL, Rich-Edwards JW, Oken E. Associations of trimester-specific gestational weight gain with maternal adiposity and systolic blood pressure at 3 and 7 years postpartum. *Am J Obstet Gynecol* 2015;**212**(499):e1–12.

58. Lee KK, Raja EA, Lee AJ, et al. Maternal obesity during pregnancy associates with premature mortality and major cardiovascular events in later life. *Hypertension* 2015;**66**:938–44.

59. Gratacós E, Casals E, Gómez O, et al. Increased susceptibility to low density lipoprotein oxidation in women with a history of pre-eclampsia. *BJOG* 2003;**110**: 400–4.

60. Thadhani R, Ecker JL, Mutter WP, et al. Insulin resistance and alterations in angiogenesis: additive insults that may lead to preeclampsia. *Hypertension* 2004; **43**: 988–92.

61. Al-Nasiry S, Ghossein-Doha C, Polman SE, et al. Metabolic syndrome after pregnancies complicated by pre-eclampsia or small-for-gestational-age: a retrospective cohort. *BJOG* 2015; **122**: 1818–23.

62. Östlund E, Al-Nashi M, Hamad RR, et al. Normalized endothelial function but sustained cardiovascular risk profile 11 years following a pregnancy complicated by preeclampsia. *Hypertens Res* 2013; **36**: 1081–7.

63. Yinon Y, Kingdom JC, Odutayo A, et al. Vascular dysfunction in women with a history of preeclampsia and intrauterine growth restriction: insights into future vascular risk. *Circulation* 2010;**122**: 1846–53.

64. Sandvik MK, Leirgul E, Nygård O, et al. Preeclampsia in healthy women and endothelial dysfunction 10 years later. *Am J Obstet Gynecol* 2013;**209**:569.e1–569.e10.

65. Hoedjes M, Berks D, Vogel I, et al. Motivators and barriers to a healthy postpartum lifestyle in women at increased cardiovascular and metabolic risk: a focus-group study. *Hypertens Pregnancy* 2012;**31**:147–55.

66. Smith GN. The Maternal Health Clinic: Improving women's cardiovascular health. *Semin Perinatol* 2015;**39**:316–9.

67. Janmohamed R, Montgomery-Fajic E, Sia W, et al. Cardiovascular risk reduction and weight management at a hospital-based postpartum preeclampsia clinic. *J Obstet Gynaecol Can* 2015;**37**: 330–7.

68. Scholten RR, Thijssen DJ, Lotgering FK, Hopman MT, Spaanderman ME. Cardiovascular effects of aerobic exercise

69. Rich-Edwards JW, Fraser A, Lawlor DA, Catov JM. Pregnancy characteristics and women's future cardiovascular health: an underused opportunity to improve women's health? *Epidemiol Rev* 2014; **36**:57–70.

70. Yusuf S, Hawken S, Ounpuu S, et al. INTERHEART Study Investigators. Effect of potentially modifiable risk factors associated with myocardial infarction in 52 countries (the INTERHEART study): case-control study. *Lancet* 2004;**364**(9438): 937–52.

71. Umans-Eckenhausen MA, Sijbrands EJ, Kastelein JJ, Defesche JC. Low-density lipoprotein receptor gene mutations and cardiovascular risk in a large genetic cascade screening population. *Circulation* 2002;**106**:3031–6.

72. Parikh NI, Cnattingius S, Dickman PW, Mittleman MA, Ludvigsson JF, Ingelsson E. Parity and risk of later-life maternal cardiovascular disease. *Am Heart J* 2010; **159**:215–221.e6).

73. Kuningas M, Altmäe S, Uitterlinden AG, Hofman A, van Duijn CM, Tiemeier H. The relationship between fertility and lifespan in humans. *Age (Dordr)* 2011; **33**:615–22.

74. Ngo AD, Roberts CL, Figtree G. Association between interpregnancy interval and future risk of maternal cardiovascular disease – a population-based record linkage study. *BJOG* 2015 Oct 20.

75. Sattar N, Greer IA. Pregnancy complications and maternal cardiovascular risk: opportunities for intervention and screening? *BMJ* 2002; 20;**325** (7356):157–60.

76. Bellamy L, Casas JP, Hingorani AD, Williams DJ. Pre-eclampsia and risk of cardiovascular disease and cancer in later life: systematic review and meta-analysis. *BMJ* 2007; **335**(7627):974.

77. Bellamy L, Casas JP, Hingorani AD, Williams DJ. Pre-eclampsia and risk of cardiovascular disease and cancer in later

life: systematic review and meta-analysis. *BMJ* 2007; **335**(7627):974.

78. Irgens HU, Reisaeter L, Irgens LM, Lie RT. Long term mortality of mothers and fathers after pre-eclampsia: population based cohort study. *BMJ* 2001 24;**323** (7323):1213–17.

79. Skjaerven R, Wilcox AJ, Klungsøyr K, Irgens LM, Vikse BE, Vatten LJ, Lie RT. Cardiovascular mortality after pre-eclampsia in one child mothers: prospective, population based cohort study. *BMJ* 2012; **345**: e7677.

Index